THE MOUNT SINAI MEDICAL CENTER

FAMILY GUIDE
to
DENTAL
HEALTH

THE MOUNT SINAI MEDICAL CENTER

FAMILY GUIDE
to
DENTAL HEALTH

JACK KLATELL, D.D.S.
ANDREW KAPLAN, D.M.D.
GRAY WILLIAMS, JR.

Illustrations by Caroline Meinstein

MACMILLAN PUBLISHING COMPANY / NEW YORK

Maxwell Macmillan Canada / Toronto

Maxwell Macmillan International
New York / Oxford / Singapore / Sydney

DISCLAIMER

This book is not intended as a substitute for the professional advice of dentists. The reader should regularly consult a dentist in matters relating to his or her dental health, particularly any symptoms that may require diagnosis or treatment.

Macmillan Publishing Company
866 Third Avenue
New York, NY 10022

Maxwell Macmillan Canada, Inc.
1200 Eglinton Avenue East
Suite 200
Don Mills, Ontario M3C 3N1

Macmillan Publishing Company is part of the Maxwell Communication Group of Companies.

Library of Congress Cataloging-in-Publication Data
Klatell, Jack.
    The Mount Sinai Medical Center family guide to dental health/
Jack Klatell, Andrew Kaplan, Gray Williams, Jr.
        p.   cm.
    Includes index.
    ISBN 0-02-563675-8
    1. Teeth—Care and hygiene. 2. Dentistry—Popular works.
I. Kaplan, Andrew S., date.   II. Williams, Gray, date.
III. Mount Sinai Medical Center (New York, N.Y.) IV. Title.
RK61.K548 1991   90-23865 CIP
617.6—dc20

Macmillan books are available at special discounts for bulk purchases for sales promotions, premiums, fund-raising, or educational use. For details, contact:
                Special Sales Director
                Macmillan Publishing Company
                866 Third Avenue
                New York, NY 10022

Design by Robert Bull Design

10 9 8 7 6 5 4 3 2 1

Printed in the United States of America

To my parents, who encouraged my love for dentistry; to my wife, Arla, and my sons, Robert and David, who have understood and supported it; and to my colleagues and patients, who invigorate it every day.

J.K.

To my wife, Sandra, and my children, Daniel and Laura Emily, who give my work purpose; and to my patients, from whom I constantly learn.

A.K.

To Marian, who makes everything possible.

G.W.

CONTRIBUTORS

Jack Klatell, D.D.S.
Chairman of Dentistry and Professor,
    Mount Sinai School of Medicine
Director and Chief, Department of
    Dentistry, The Mount Sinai Hospital

Andrew S. Kaplan, D.M.D.
Assistant Clinical Professor, Mount Sinai
    School of Medicine
Assistant Attending, Department of
    Dentistry (Temporomandibular
    Disorders), The Mount Sinai Hospital

Kenneth W. Aschheim, D.D.S.
Assistant Clinical Professor, Mount Sinai
    School of Medicine
Assistant Attending, Department of
    Dentistry (General Dentistry), The Mount
    Sinai Hospital

Melvin Blake, D.D.S.
Associate Clinical Professor, Mount Sinai
    School of Medicine
Associate Attending, Department of
    Dentistry (Oral Pathology, Oral and
    Maxillofacial Surgery), The Mount Sinai
    Hospital

Morton R. Brenner, D.D.S.
Assistant Clinical Professor, Mount Sinai
    School of Medicine
Associate Attending, Department of
    Dentistry (Endodontics), The Mount
    Sinai Hospital

Daniel Buchbinder, D.M.D.
Assistant Professor, Mount Sinai School of
    Medicine
Assistant Attending, Department of
    Dentistry (Oral and Maxillofacial
    Surgery), The Mount Sinai Hospital

Alfred Carin, D.D.S.
Assistant Clinical Professor, Mount Sinai
    School of Medicine
Associate Attending, Department of
    Dentistry (General Dentistry), The Mount
    Sinai Hospital

Charles I. Cohen, D.D.S.
Associate Clinical Professor, Mount Sinai
    School of Medicine
Associate Attending, Department of
    Dentistry (Periodontics), The Mount Sinai
    Hospital

Barry G. Dale, D.M.D.
Assistant Clinical Professor, Mount Sinai
    School of Medicine
Assistant Attending, Department of
    Dentistry (General Dentistry), The Mount
    Sinai Hospital

Alexander E. Eitches, D.D.S.
Assistant Clinical Professor, Mount Sinai
    School of Medicine
Assistant Attending, Department of
    Dentistry (Prosthodontics), The Mount
    Sinai Hospital

Arthur C. Elias, D.M.D.
Assistant Clinical Professor, Mount Sinai
    School of Medicine
Associate Attending, Department of
    Dentistry (Oral and Maxillofacial
    Surgery), The Mount Sinai Hospital

Bruce E. Evans, D.M.D. (deceased)
Assistant Clinical Professor, Mount Sinai
    School of Medicine
Assistant Attending, Department of
    Dentistry (Oral and Maxillofacial
    Surgery), The Mount Sinai Hospital

Gordon C. Gaynor, D.D.S.
Assistant Clinical Professor, Mount Sinai
    School of Medicine
Assistant Attending, Department of
    Dentistry (Orthodontics), The Mount
    Sinai Hospital

Stanley Gibbs, D.D.S.
Assistant Clinical Professor, Mount Sinai
    School of Medicine
Adjunct Assistant Attending, Department
    of Dentistry (Orthodontics), The Mount
    Sinai Hospital

Jerome Goldhuber, D.D.S.
Clinical Instructor, Mount Sinai School of
    Medicine
Clinical Assistant, Department of Dentistry
    (General Dentistry), The Mount Sinai
    Hospital

Jack Hirsch, D.D.S.
Assistant Clinical Professor, Mount Sinai
    School of Medicine
Associate Attending, Department of
    Dentistry (General Dentistry), The Mount
    Sinai Hospital

H. Jinder Khurana, D.D.S.
Clinical Instructor, Mount Sinai School of
    Medicine
Assistant Attending, Department of
    Dentistry (Periodontics), The Mount Sinai
    Hospital

Jeffrey G. Leeds, D.D.S.
Clinical Instructor, Mount Sinai School of
    Medicine
Clinical Assistant, Department of Dentistry
    (Pediatric Dentistry), The Mount Sinai
    Hospital

Marc Lorinsky, D.M.D.
Assistant Clinical Professor, Mount Sinai
    School of Medicine
Assistant Attending, Department of
    Dentistry (Prosthodontics), The Mount
    Sinai Hospital

Brian B. Pollack, D.D.S.
Associate Professor, Mount Sinai School of
    Medicine
Associate Attending, Department of
    Dentistry (General Dentistry), The Mount
    Sinai Hospital

Marie Ramer, D.D.S.
Lecturer, Mount Sinai School of Medicine
Clinical Assistant, Department of Dentistry
    (Oral Pathology), The Mount Sinai
    Hospital

J. Gordon Rubin, D.D.S.
Associate Clinical Professor, Mount Sinai
    School of Medicine
Associate Attending, Department of
    Dentistry (Dental Phobia), The Mount
    Sinai Hospital

Sheryl L. Silverstein, D.M.D.
Assistant Clinical Professor, Department of
  Geriatrics and Adult Development,
  Mount Sinai School of Medicine
Attending Staff, Long Island
  Jewish–Hillside Medical Center
Coordinator of Outpatient Dental Clinic,
  Parker Jewish General Institute for
  Geriatric Care

Berry Stahl, D.M.D.
Clinical Instructor, Mount Sinai School of
  Medicine
Clinical Assistant, Department of Dentistry
  (Anesthesiology), The Mount Sinai
  Hospital

David V. Valauri, D.D.S.
Assistant Clinical Professor, Mount Sinai
  School of Medicine
Assistant Attending, Department of
  Dentistry (Oral and Maxillofacial
  Surgery), The Mount Sinai Hospital

Samuel Weber, D.D.S.
Clinical Assistant, Mount Sinai School of
  Medicine
Assistant Attending, Department of
  Dentistry (Implantology), The Mount
  Sinai Hospital

CONTENTS

PART IV   ORAL PATHOLOGY

INTRODUCTION

Today, our society is in the midst of what might be called a dental revolution. More and more children are reaching adulthood with teeth that require few fillings or none at all. More and more adults go through life with all or most of their natural teeth in good working order. More and more people are undergoing new and innovative forms of treatment, such as aesthetic dentistry, bone-integrated implantation, and adult orthodontics—treatments that not only contribute to the health of their teeth but also to their self-image and their quality of life.

This revolution has come about partly through advances in dental science, which in recent decades have been enormous. But just as important has been a fundamental change in public attitude. People today simply care more about their teeth and about keeping them healthy.

Perhaps the main reason people care more about their teeth is that they have much more reason for long-term optimism about them. Not so many years ago, it was common wisdom that the inevitable fate of teeth was to be lost. It was widely believed that women would lose "a tooth for every child" through the rigors of childbearing. Dental care promised, not to make teeth last a lifetime, but merely to postpone their removal. Almost no one expected, or could expect, to reach old age with any significant number of sound teeth. In fact, it was all too customary, once most of the teeth were gone, for the rest to be extracted "before they started giving trouble," and replaced with dentures.

Moreover, dentistry carried a heavy burden of unpleasant associations. "Going to the dentist" used to be a familiar synonym for pain. The prospect of drilling or extraction filled patients with terror. The ordeal of treatment was tolerable only in the relief it offered from the greater agonies of toothache.

Modern dentistry has taken away much of the justification for this fear. Tooth decay is still an epidemic, but it is a needless epidemic. We now know that advanced tooth decay can be prevented, with collaborative care by dentist and patient, and that such care need not be difficult, burdensome, or costly. If you take proper care of your teeth, they can indeed last a lifetime.

The emphasis of dental treatment has changed as well. Today, dentists try not to extract teeth except when it is absolutely necessary; they try to save every tooth, or salvageable portion of tooth, they can. Within the last few decades, modern materials and techniques have enormously expanded our abilities to make teeth look better and work better. Almost any tooth, no matter how damaged, can now be restored. And if teeth must be replaced, we can make the substitutes nearly identical to natural teeth, and can fit them to be both comfortable and efficient.

Even full dentures have come a long way from the obviously artificial, ill-fitting "choppers" of the past. Modern materials can make them nearly indistinguishable from natural teeth—we can even position and color them so they won't look "too good to be true." And modern implantation techniques allow us to attach them more firmly and permanently.

There have been advances in virtually every field of dentistry. For example, orthodontics used to be limited almost entirely to the flexible jaws of children. For adults, the process was thought to be too painful, too unsightly, and too uncertain of outcome. But with techniques now available, the orthodontist can achieve results with adults that are just as extensive and just as long-lasting as those with children. Also, dentists are combining traditional and new techniques to create comprehensive programs of aesthetic dentistry, which improve the appearance not only of the teeth but also of the patient's whole face—often quite dramatically.

Perhaps the most important revolution, from the patient's point of view, has been the reduction of pain. "Painless dentistry" used to be at best an empty promise, at worst a bad joke. Now the promise comes close to fulfillment. Not only has anesthesia become safer and more widely used, but equipment such as high-speed "cool" drills eliminate pain at the source. There are also many promising new developments in pain relief, such as the use of electrical stimulation of the nerves. Going to the dentist may still not be a pleasure, but it should cause you little more trepidation than visiting the office of any other health professional.

You now have very good reasons to place your confidence in proper dental care, as a long-term investment in good looks, good health, and comfort. This book is designed to help you get the most professional treatment, and to contribute effectively to your own dental health. It is organized into four parts:

Part One is an introduction and reference section containing two chapters. The first describes and illustrates the anatomy of the mouth. The second explains the dental profession and its various specialties, and gives advice on how to find good dental treatment.

Part Two is a guide to basic dental care, with an emphasis on the prevention of dental problems. It explains routine professional care, describes an effective program of home care, and outlines first aid procedures you can use in dental emergencies. It provides guidance on overcoming dental fear, and describes the anesthetics and medications used to control pain. It explains basic procedures such as filling cavities and treating periodontal tissues, and it offers detailed information on the special care needed for children and older people.

Part Three is an overview of advanced professional treatment, from endodontics to oral surgery. It covers such recent developments as aesthetic dentistry, and the treatment of temporomandibular disorders. It also discusses the special needs of "medically compromised" patients, whose medical problems require special dental procedures.

The final chapter in this part gives you advice as a dental consumer. It analyzes the costs of dental care, outlines the various kinds of dental insurance, and shows you how to avoid dental fraud and quackery.

Part Four is devoted to dental pathology: medical disorders that are often diagnosed or treated by dentists. It contains three sections, covering disorders of the teeth, the soft tissues of the mouth, and the bones of the jaws.

This guide represents the accumulated knowledge and experience of professionals in every field of dentistry. Here at the dental department of the Mount Sinai Medical Center, we treat more than 7,000 patients each year, and we are active in research and teaching as well. It is our aim to provide you with a comprehensive overview of all major aspects of dental science and dental care, to help you understand any treatment you may be receiving or contemplating, to give you information about your mouth and teeth and what can go wrong with them, and to offer you practical guidance in looking after your own dental health.

We cannot emphasize too much that

achieving dental health must be a collaborative effort by both dentist and patient. You can't achieve it by simply sitting in a dentist's chair every six months and opening your mouth. You certainly can't achieve it by avoiding dental treatment except when something goes wrong. If this guide helps you establish a more effective working relationship with your dentist, and encourages you to participate actively and faithfully in a program of dental self-care, then we will have achieved our purpose.

PART I

INTRODUCTION TO DENTAL HEALTH

O N E

The Teeth, the Jaws, and the Mouth

Your dental health depends not only upon the soundness of your teeth but also upon the condition of the other parts of your mouth. These include both *hard* and *soft* tissues. The hard tissues include the bones of your upper and lower jaws, as well as your teeth. The soft tissues include the gums, the tongue, the lips and cheeks, and the salivary glands. Moreover, it is essential that all these components work together harmoniously to form an effective *occlusion*, or bite.

KINDS OF TEETH

In the adult mouth, there are up to 32 *permanent* teeth, 16 in each jaw. Young children have only 20 *primary* teeth, which are replaced by the permanent teeth (see chart, page 4).

The main function of your teeth is to break up food into fragments small enough for you to swallow and digest. Human beings are *omnivores*—that is, they eat both animal and vegetable food. Human teeth have two basic shapes, to chew both.

The six front teeth in each jaw have single, sharp edges—like knives. The edges of the four *incisors* are straight, for cutting off pieces of food. The edges of the two *canines* (also called *cuspids* or *eye teeth*) come to a point, for tearing food as well. Each of these teeth has a single root.

The ten back teeth in each jaw—five on each side—have wide chewing surfaces, to grind food. Each chewing surface contains two or more low mounds, called *cusps*, separated by hollows and grooves. On each side of the jaw are two *premolars* (sometimes called *bicuspids*) and up to three *molars*. The premolars are smaller than the molars, and have one or two roots. The upper molars usually have three roots; the lower molars have two or three. The additional roots brace these teeth against the heaviest pressures of chewing.

The parts of your teeth most susceptible to decay are the chewing surfaces of the back teeth, surfaces where adjacent teeth meet, and surfaces nearest the gumline. The decay process is discussed in Chapter 8.

PERMANENT TEETH

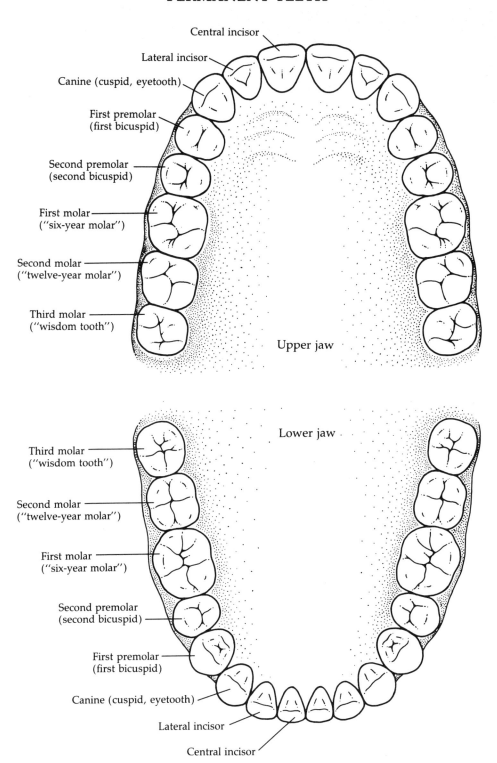

Central incisor

Lateral incisor

Canine (cuspid, eyetooth)

First premolar
(first bicuspid)

Second premolar
(second bicuspid)

First molar
("six-year molar")

Second molar
("twelve-year molar")

Third molar
("wisdom tooth")

Upper jaw

Lower jaw

Third molar
("wisdom tooth")

Second molar
("twelve-year molar")

First molar
("six-year molar")

Second premolar
(second bicuspid)

First premolar
(first bicuspid)

Canine (cuspid, eyetooth)

Lateral incisor

Central incisor

4

ANATOMY OF THE TOOTH

A tooth has two principal parts. The *crown* is the part visible above the gum, and contains the hard biting surfaces. The *root* is the part normally located below the gum; it rests in a socket in the bone of the jaw.

The crown has an outer layer of *enamel,* which protects it from wear and decay. Enamel is made up almost entirely of the minerals calcium and phosphorus, and is the hardest substance in your body. The less-exposed root is covered with a bonelike material called *cementum,* which is thinner than enamel and not as hard.

Within these outer layers is the main structure of the tooth, the *dentin.* Dentin is less dense than enamel but somewhat denser than cementum. It contains numerous fine channels, called *tubules,* inside which are threadlike extensions of living cells called *odontoblasts.*

At the core of the tooth is a channel that extends from mid-crown to root. It contains soft tissue called *pulp.* The outer layer of the pulp is made up of the odontoblasts that protrude into the dentin tubules. The rest is composed largely of nerves and blood vessels. The blood vessels carry nourishment to the tooth, and the nerves are sensitive to pressure, heat, cold, electricity, and certain chemicals.

The inner structure of the tooth is discussed in more detail in Chapter 12.

SUPPORTING TISSUES OF THE TEETH

The root of each tooth fits into a socket in your upper or lower jawbone. The arch-shaped line of sockets in each jaw is known as the *alveolar ridge,* and is composed of *alveolar bone (alveolar* comes from a word meaning "socket"). Each tooth is anchored in place and cushioned against chewing pressures by

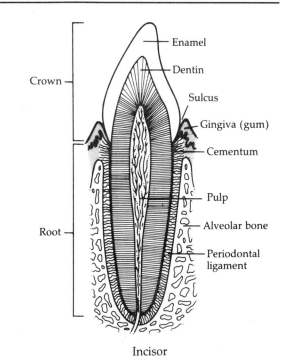

Incisor

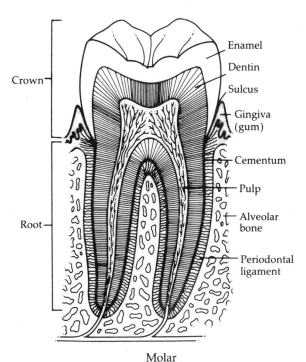

Molar

a network of *periodontal ligament* that extends between the bone and the cementum of the root.

Some of the root extends out of the socket in the alveolar ridge. This exposed root and the surface of the bone are covered and protected by soft tissue called *gingiva,* the gum. Where the gum meets the tooth, at the base of the enamel, it forms a small cuff, which encloses a shallow, V-shaped hollow called a *sulcus.*

When *plaque* and *calculus* are allowed to collect in the sulcus, *periodontal disease* is likely to result. This process is discussed more fully in Chapter 9.

OTHER SOFT TISSUES OF THE MOUTH

THE TONGUE

Your tongue is a complex organ with several functions. Its muscles move food into contact with your teeth and initiate the process of swallowing. It may also be used to dislodge food particles left in your mouth after eating, but its action cannot replace regular brushing and flossing.

The tongue muscles are essential for speech. People can (and do) speak intelligibly without teeth—but not without a tongue. The tongue also exerts a slight but significant pressure against the teeth. It helps guide erupting teeth into their proper positions, and then helps hold them there.

Finally, your tongue (supplemented by your nose) registers sensations of taste. On the upper surface of the tongue, especially near its edges and across its back, are the *taste buds.* Taste buds identify just four flavors: sweet, sour, salty, and bitter—all other flavors are mixtures of these.

Disorders of the tongue are described in Chapter 19.

THE LIPS AND CHEEKS

The principal functions of the lips and cheeks are to shape your mouth into a muscular container for food and to keep its interior moist. Like your tongue, your lips are essential to speech. And just as your tongue exerts pressure upon the teeth from within, the muscles of your lips and cheeks exert pressure from without, helping to hold your teeth in proper position.

Disorders of the lips and cheeks are described in Chapter 19.

THE SALIVARY GLANDS

The interior of your mouth is kept constantly moist, partly by mucus secreted by the cheeks, lips, and palate. But most of the moisture is saliva, a slippery liquid secreted by the salivary glands.

There are three pairs of *major* salivary glands. In addition, there are many *minor* glands inside your lips and cheeks.

Normally, the salivary glands generate and release small but steady flows of saliva into your mouth. But food, or even the prospect of food, stimulates the glands to produce extra quantities of saliva, causing your mouth to "water."

Saliva is a complex mixture of water, mucus, and other substances, which serves several functions. The most important of these is to moisten and bind together chewed particles of food, which your tongue shapes into a ball, or *bolus,* for swallowing. Saliva also contributes to sensations of taste. The taste buds of your tongue react only to moist food; saliva, mixing with dry food, enables you to taste it.

Saliva helps in resisting tooth decay. Assisted by your tongue, it washes food particles from your teeth and gums. Since it is slightly alkaline, it neutralizes, or *buffers,* some of the acids produced by bacteria in your mouth. It also acts upon bacteria di-

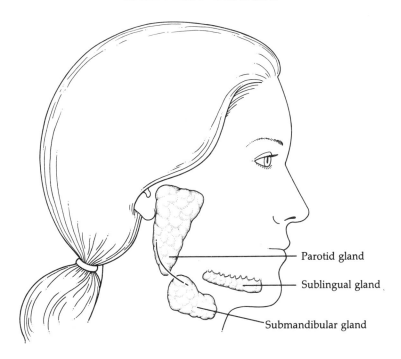

Parotid gland

Sublingual gland

Submandibular gland

rectly, somewhat limiting their growth. Finally, it contains the minerals calcium and phosphorus, which your teeth can draw upon to strengthen their enamel.

But saliva also contributes, at least slightly, to the formation of acids in your mouth. It contains an enzyme, *amylase*, that breaks down starches into sugars—an essential step in digestion. But these sugars also provide food for mouth bacteria, which create acids as an inevitable by-product of digestion (see page 59).

The most familiar disorder of the salivary glands is mumps—an infectious viral disease of the largest glands, the parotids. This and other salivary gland disorders are described in Chapter 19.

BONES OF THE MOUTH

There are five principal bones in your mouth. They are the single lower jawbone (*mandible*),

the two bones of the upper jaw (*maxilla*), and the two bones that form the roof of the mouth (*palate*).

THE MANDIBLE

The shape of your lower jawbone is basically an arch. At each end of the arch is an upward extension, or *ramus* (from a word meaning "branch"), which is topped by a rounded knob called a *condyle*.

The mandible is the densest and strongest bone in your skull. Like other bones, it is fairly flexible in childhood and becomes more rigid during adolescence. One portion of it—the *alveolar ridge*, which contains the tooth sockets—remains relatively flexible even into adulthood.

When your mouth opens and closes, only the mandible moves. The condyles pivot and slide at the *temporomandibular joints,* or *TMJs* (see page 199).

BONES OF THE JAWS

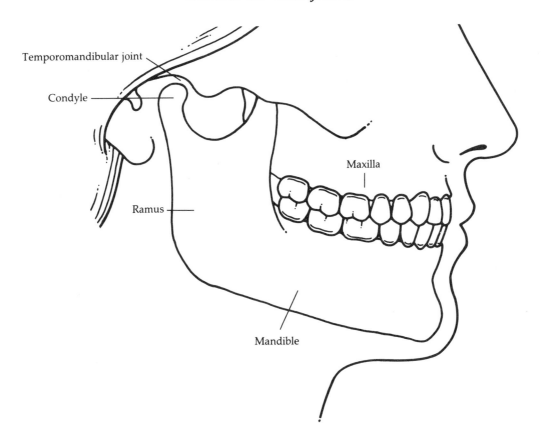

Temporomandibular joint

Condyle

Ramus

Maxilla

Mandible

THE MAXILLA

The two bones of your upper jaw extend upward from the teeth to the bases of the cheek and nose bones. The structure of the maxilla is generally less dense than that of the mandible.

Ideally, the arches of the maxilla and mandible should match closely in size and shape. For hereditary and other reasons, they often don't, resulting in faulty *occlusion* (see below).

THE PALATAL BONES

Like other bones of the cranium, the two bones of the palate are joined together by a thin line of connective tissue called a *suture.* During infancy and childhood, the suture is flexible and easily stretched, but it becomes stronger and more rigid in adolescence. This change has important implications for orthodontic treatment (see page 175).

Disorders of the bones of the mouth are described in Chapter 19.

OCCLUSION, OR BITE

When your jaws close, the teeth meet in *occlusion,* or bite. A proper occlusion is essential to effective chewing. Your upper front teeth should overlap the lowers, and the biting edges of the lower teeth should lightly touch

OCCLUSION (BITE)

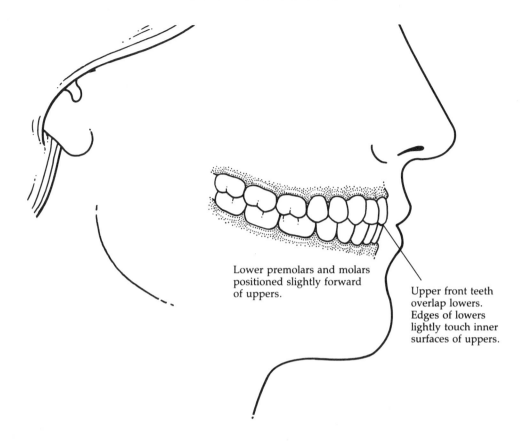

Lower premolars and molars positioned slightly forward of uppers.

Upper front teeth overlap lowers. Edges of lowers lightly touch inner surfaces of uppers.

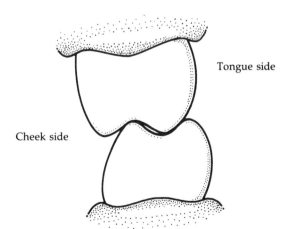

Tongue side

Cheek side

Occlusion, upper and lower molars (Lower molar slightly inside upper. Outside ridge meshes with central groove.)

the inner surfaces of the uppers. Your back teeth, the premolars and molars, should meet evenly. The chewing surfaces of the lower teeth should be slightly *inside* the uppers, so that their outer cusps mesh with the central grooves of the uppers. Ideally, the lower molars and premolars should also be positioned slightly *forward* of the corresponding upper teeth.

The many forms of faulty occlusion, or *malocclusion,* are described in detail in Chapter 16.

T W O

The Dental Profession

Since the dawn of history, human beings have had trouble with their teeth—from decay, from wear, from injury, and from gum disease. And so, dating from the earliest human civilizations, there have been dentists attempting to remedy these ills. The earliest reference to "physicians who treat the teeth" appears in an Egyptian hieroglyphic relief of about 2600 B.C.

But up to fairly recent times, dental treatment was almost entirely limited to the extraction of diseased teeth, and their replacement with artificial substitutes. Cleaning the teeth was also practiced, but more for cosmetic than for health reasons. The causes of decay were not understood.

Modern dentistry had its origins in the nineteenth century, with such developments as the dental drill, silver amalgam fillings, and anesthesia. The first American dental school opened in 1840, in Baltimore, Maryland, and dentistry has since evolved into a recognized profession, requiring formal training, subject to professional standards, and backed up by reliable scientific research.

GENERAL DENTAL EDUCATION

The dental profession today is organized somewhat like the medical profession, and the training is similar. Just as prospective physicians go to medical school after graduating from college, those training to become dentists attend dental school. Both medical and dental schools customarily require four years of study.

Dental students must pass two nationwide examinations, known as National Boards. The first, given after the first two years of study, concentrates upon academic subjects, such as biology, chemistry, and anatomy. The second is given during the senior year, and stresses knowledge of actual clinical practice. In addition, dental school graduates must pass state or regional licensing examinations. Like the National Boards, State or Regional Boards test both academic and clinical mastery.

When they graduate from dental school, dentists receive a degree that corresponds to M.D. (Doctor of Medicine). Some institutions use the term *D.D.S.* (Doctor of Dental Surgery), and others, the term *D.M.D.* (Doctor of Dental Medicine). There is no difference between the two.

After passing their Boards, dental school graduates are entitled to get a license to practice as general dentists. Some graduates go directly into practice, but many others seek further training. They may enter a one- or two-year residency program in general dentistry, or they may train for one of the dental specialties.

DENTAL SPECIALTIES

There are eight recognized professional specialties, each supervised by its own association, or *board*. Each specialty requires from two to four years (or more) of postgraduate training. Once that training is completed, specialist dentists are described as *board eligible*. Then, if they pass the board examinations in their specialty, they become *board certified*.

Most of the eight specialties concentrate upon some specific type of dental treatment or kind of patient:

- *Pediatric dentistry:* Pediatric dentists, like pediatricians in medicine, specialize in the treatment of children. Their work is described in detail in Chapter 10.
- *Periodontics. Peri-* means "around"; *odont* means "tooth." Periodontists treat the tissues "around the teeth"—the gums and supporting bone. Their work is described in Chapter 9.
- *Endodontics. Endo-* means "inside." Endodontists treat the inner parts of the teeth, particularly the soft pulp. The most common treatment they provide is cleansing, sterilizing, and filling root canals. Their work is described in Chapter 12.
- *Prosthodontics. Prostho-* comes from a word meaning "replacement." Prosth-

odontists replace all or parts of damaged or missing teeth, using inlays, crowns, bridges, or dentures. Their work is described in Chapter 13.
- *Orthodontics. Ortho-* means "straight" or "correct." Orthodontists use appliances to make teeth move into healthier, more efficient, better-looking positions. Their work is described in Chapter 16.
- *Oral and maxillofacial surgery.* Oral surgeons perform operations upon the mouth, the jaws, and adjoining parts of the face. They also perform complex or difficult extractions, such as the removal of impacted third molars, or "wisdom teeth." Their work is described in Chapter 15.
- *Oral pathology.* Oral pathologists, like medical pathologists, study tissue from the mouth and teeth to diagnose disorders and to make recommendations concerning treatment. Some pathologists have private practices, but many work in laboratories, universities, hospitals, or other research institutions.
- *Public health dentistry.* In this specialty, the patient is the community. Public health dentists customarily work in either education or government. They study trends in dental disease and related disorders. They set up and supervise programs of prevention and treatment in communities and institutions. They train other dentists in public-health concerns, and disseminate information to both their colleagues and the general public.

General dentists often supplement their education with additional courses, lectures, and seminars in various aspects of dentistry. Many belong to the Academy of General Dentistry, which requires and monitors such postgraduate study. As a result, many general dentists provide at least some kinds of specialized treatment—especially periodontics, endodontics, and prosthodontics. Dentists who complete a specialist training program are more likely to limit their practice to that specialty. And it is very unusual for a dentist to be board eligible or board certified in more than one specialty.

HOW TO FIND A GENERAL DENTIST

Let's suppose you've just moved to a new community. How do you go about finding a good general dentist—not only a dentist who is professionally well qualified, but also one who will meet your individual needs?

One very good way is obvious: personal recommendation. Ask the advice of your neighbors, or others in the community. If a dentist is warmly recommended by satisfied patients, there is a reasonable chance that you will be satisfied, too.

Another good source of information is your own former dentist. Like professionals in other fields, dentists have networks of associates, friends, and fellow dental school alumni. Your former dentist may not personally know a good dentist in your new community but may know somebody who does.

You can also seek help from local professionals. You can call the local hospital or medical center and get the names of the *attending* dentists—those whose credentials are periodically reviewed by the institution and who are granted the privilege of treating patients there.

Similarly, you can call the nearest dental school, or other dental training facility (such as a hospital with a dental residency program), for the names of faculty. Dentists who teach others are often well qualified to provide treatment themselves.

Another useful source of information is the American Dental Association (ADA), to which a very large majority of dentists belong. The ADA serves as the principal voice and representative of the dental profession, and is especially active in education. It sponsors school programs and publications for the general public, and postgraduate courses and workshops for professionals. It reviews dental materials and equipment for effectiveness and safety (you are probably familiar with the ADA seal of approval that appears on some brands of toothpaste). And ADA peer-review boards help resolve complaints and disputes between dentists and patients.

The ADA has branch societies in every state and in some metropolitan areas as well. You can find the number of the closest local society in the telephone directory white pages, usually under *Dental Society*. The society will supply you with a list of members in the area. The list won't be complete, since not all dentists belong to the ADA.

HOW TO FIND A SPECIALIST

If you need to see a dental specialist, usually your general dentist or another specialist will refer you to one. But sometimes you may have to—or may prefer to—conduct the search yourself.

The methods you will use are mostly the same as those for finding a general dentist. In addition, specialists often belong to special organizations in their field, and these organizations will provide you with the names of members. Many of them are listed in the Appendix. Since the main function of such organizations is the exchange of information, dentists who belong to them are likely to be not only professionally qualified but also familiar with up-to-date treatment and research.

HOW TO EVALUATE A DENTIST

Determining whether you have found a good dentist is not easy, if only because personal reactions and personal needs vary so much. Nonetheless, there are some general guidelines that may help you reach a decision.

THE OFFICE

The waiting room and the treatment rooms should be clean, neat, and well-kept. Clutter suggests carelessness or inattention to detail—not good qualities in a dentist. The equipment should look new, or at least not seriously worn.

CREDENTIALS

The dentist's dental-school diploma, license, and other educational records should be in plain sight. For a specialist, these should include a certificate of advanced education in that field, and possibly a document of board certification as well. However, there is no harm in asking what training and experience the dentist has had. Ask what courses or training programs he or she has taken. Recent postgraduate work, in particular, indicates an effort to stay up-to-date.

THE CHAIRSIDE MANNER

No professional should be judged solely on the basis of personal charm. At the same time, you have a right to expect a reasonable degree of courtesy, patience, and above all, concern for you as an individual patient. The following guidelines may be helpful:

- The dentist should be reasonably prompt in keeping appointments. If he or she chronically overschedules, or otherwise fails to see patients on time, it may signify a less than satisfactory commitment to patient welfare.

- You should be given a thorough examination. Unless your first visit is purely introductory, the dentist should take a complete history and provide the kind of dental examination described in Chapter 3. If the dentist is a specialist, you should be given the type of examination described in the chapter on that specialty.

- The dentist should listen to you. There's an old saying among physicians and dentists: "If you listen, the patient will tell you the diagnosis." If the dentist doesn't allow you to complete your history and describe any symptoms you may have, or frequently interrupts or contradicts you or generally fails to hear you out, you have reason to be cautious.

- The dentist should give you undivided attention. If, during your visit, the dentist is frequently distracted by phone calls or divides your time with other patients or delegates virtually the whole interview and examination to assistants, you may not be receiving the professional commitment you deserve.

- The dentist should inform you fully of any diagnosis and should explain to you any intended treatment. You have a right to know what to expect, and what treatment options are available. You should also be told the likely results of *not* undergoing treatment. If treatment of your condition doesn't always produce successful results, or if it involves possible risks or side effects, you must be given enough information to give what is known as *informed consent*.

PROFESSIONAL SUPPORT

Very few dentists work entirely alone. They are usually assisted by a professional staff and backed up by a network (formal or informal) of their colleagues. The quality of this support is an important factor in the overall quality of care.

The staff may include dental assistants, hygienists, and receptionists, who should meet many of the same standards as dentists. They, too, should be courteous, painstaking, attentive, and concerned with you as an individual. One important staff service is often undervalued: an efficient system for making appointments, changing them if necessary, and reminding you of them as they approach.

The backup network, too, is important. No professional can always be available in person. You should be able to reach the office outside regular office hours, and you should be told whom to call in an emergency if your own dentist is not available. As every dentist knows, a toothache is most likely to occur in the middle of the night or on a weekend.

BUSINESS ARRANGEMENTS

Dentistry is a profession, but it is also a business, and you and your dentist must come to an agreement about your business relationship. You should know what the dentist's fees are, and you shouldn't hesitate to ask. This is a particularly important issue when extensive treatment is involved.

You should also know when and under what circumstances payments are to be made: upon receipt of a monthly bill, say, or at the time of your visit. If you wish to spread payments over time, you will have to make such an arrangement with the dentist in advance.

Finally you should be familiar with the dentist's policies regarding insurance (see Chapter 2).

THE HUMAN FACTOR

All these guidelines must be tempered by the "human factor." That is, regardless of the dentist's qualifications, *you* should be comfortable with your choice. You must have enough confidence in the dentist to place yourself in his or her care, and to be open and frank. This is especially true if you have any feelings of anxiety concerning dental treatment.

This "human factor" is the very personal reaction of an individual patient to a particular practitioner. But it is just as important as any other criterion.

COMPARATIVE SHOPPING, SECOND OPINIONS, AND SWITCHING

There is no reason why you should have to choose a dentist with whom you don't feel comfortable, or to continue being treated by one with whom you are not satisfied. The old advertising slogan, "Select, don't settle," applies to dental treatment just as it does to any other product or service.

There is nothing wrong (and much that is right) in interviewing more than one general dentist, using the guidelines listed above, before making your choice. You should not hesitate to inform each dentist that you are doing so. If any dentist responds negatively, or seems affronted, that alone can be a reason for choosing someone else.

Similarly, whenever you are advised to undertake an extensive—and expensive—course of dental treatment, you should seek at least one additional expert opinion. If the treatment is to be paid for by insurance, the insurance company is likely to insist on a second opinion, and possibly a third as well. If you need an additional opinion, you can use the approaches outlined above to find other practitioners.

Finally, for any of a number of reasons, you may decide later that you are dissatisfied with your dentist. If so, you are not obliged to continue treatment and are free to find someone else. You should certainly not worry about hurting the dentist's feelings.

If you do decide to switch dentists, you are entitled, under the laws of most states, to obtain copies of your dental X-rays at a reasonable charge for their duplication. The same rule applies to your dental records (your *chart*) and any casts that the dentist may have made of your jaws.

WHAT YOUR DENTIST EXPECTS OF YOU

Just as there are professional standards that you have a right to expect your dentist to meet, there are certain standards that your dentist expects you to meet. To a considerable extent, your own attitudes and behavior will affect the level of care you receive.

The dentist's main resource is time, and it shouldn't be wasted. You should be on time for your appointments, and if you are delayed, you should make an effort to get word to the office. If you cannot keep an appointment, you should provide as much warning as possible—at least a day, except in an unexpected emergency.

For some patients, the underlying reason for being late for appointments, or missing them entirely, is fear of treatment. The only remedy is to face the problem honestly, and to accept the dentist's help in treating it (see Chapter 6).

You should pay your dental bills on time. If special arrangements for payment are needed, you and the dentist should agree on them before treatment. If unexpected financial problems arise during treatment, making it difficult or impossible for you to pay promptly, discuss the matter openly and fully with the dentist. Often, an agreement to defer payment can be reached.

You should cooperate with the dentist in your treatment. You cannot hope to be treated successfully otherwise. In particular, you should conscientiously follow a program of oral home care (see Chapter 4). You should also be prepared to follow instructions. If your dentist prescribes a certain medication, it must be taken as prescribed. If your dentist tells you to wear an appliance at certain times for certain periods, wear it. And if you are told to return for another visit at a certain time, return on schedule.

Finally, you should be forthright in expressing your concerns—especially negative concerns. Your dentist expects patients to be nervous and apprehensive about treatment, and is prepared to deal with these feelings effectively. Similarly, if a treatment causes you significant discomfort, or if you are not satisfied with its pace or its results, you should not hesitate to discuss the matter with the dentist.

PART II

BASIC DENTAL CARE

T H R E E

BASIC PROFESSIONAL CARE

The main purpose of modern dental treatment is *prevention*—prevention of decay, gum disease, and other disorders that endanger the health of the teeth and mouth. It can be accomplished only with regular professional attention—a visit to the dentist at least once every six months.

Tooth decay, for example, seldom stops or goes away by itself. Instead, it spreads and penetrates, often without you being aware of it. Similarly, gum disease is likely to worsen slowly, without your knowledge, until it threatens the stability of your teeth. These are just two of the many conditions that can often be halted or corrected if they are caught early.

Your initial consultation with a general dentist will consist of three main elements: a history, a dental examination, and (time permitting) a professional cleaning. If you suffer from anxiety about dental treatment, the dentist may suggest a variety of measures to re-duce or overcome it (see Chapter 6) and may limit the first consultation to an interview.

DENTAL AND MEDICAL HISTORY

Before you are examined, the dentist or an assistant will ask you to provide both a dental and a medical history. You may be asked to give this information orally or to fill out a questionnaire or both. Your dental history will include a record of past dental problems and treatment, and any current complaints. Your medical history will include information concerning not only your general state of health, but also past and present disorders, medications and other medical treatment, and special conditions such as allergies and chemical sensitivities.

Although the details of your medical history may not seem obviously relevant, they deeply affect your dental health and your

THE DENTAL OFFICE AND ITS EQUIPMENT

The offices of general dentists are generally similar in layout, and contain a nucleus of standard equipment. An office is likely to be divided into at least five functional areas:

- A waiting room for patients.
- One or more *operatories*, or patient treatment rooms.
- A room or an area for the storage of patient records, sometimes combined with an office for clerical record-keeping and appointment-making.
- A laboratory for the fabrication and adjustment of dental appliances, and the sterilization of instruments.
- A darkroom or an area in which X-ray films are developed.

An operatory is likely to contain the following equipment:

- Cabinets for the storage of dental instruments and materials.
- An electrically controlled reclining chair, providing support from head to foot when the patient is recumbent upon it.
- A *dental unit*, which is usually attached to the chair or free standing.

The dental unit contains several pieces of equipment: an adjustable overhead light, a small sink, a *saliva ejector*, air hoses for *handpieces*, and a tray for instruments.

- The overhead spotlight focuses a high-intensity beam on the mouth. When properly set, it should not glare in the patient's eyes.
- A small sink is used by the patient to periodically rinse the mouth during treatment.
- The saliva ejector is a small suction pump, attached to a hose with a disposable plastic tip. It is placed in the mouth to keep the working area relatively dry during treatment.

- The hoses convey air from an electric compressor to power either a low-speed or a high-speed rotary *handpiece*. Drilling and grinding burs, cleaning heads, and other devices can be attached to the handpiece.

The instrument tray is likely to hold the following:

- A ¾-inch round mirror, with an angled handle, for examining the inside of the mouth.
- One or more *explorers*, pointed probes that function as an extension of the dentist's fingers, to explore crevices, cavities, etc.
- A *periodontal probe*, to measure the depth of the "pockets" between teeth and their adjacent gums.
- Narrow-bladed *scalers, curettes*, and *root-planers*, which are used to scrape plaque and its products from the crowns and roots of the teeth.
- Tweezers (often called *cotton forceps*) for picking up small objects.
- A second handpiece, high or low speed, and the heads that can be attached.
- Other instruments or materials, depending on the nature of the treatment, such as cleaning compound, filling materials, and a hypodermic syringe for anesthetic.

The operatory is also likely to contain an X-ray machine, which often extends from the wall; it is used to take diagnostic films of the mouth and teeth. Some operatories are also equipped with an *ultrasonic cleaning machine* for the removal of plaque and tartar.

Basic dental equipment also includes machines and materials to prevent and control infection. Many dental supplies are used once and then discarded. Others are sterilized in an *autoclave*, or submerged in an antiseptic solution. Dentists now customarily wear disposable latex gloves. Many cover their mouths and noses with surgical masks, and protect their eyes as well.

dental treatment. For instance, certain medical disorders and medications can damage the teeth and gums, and certain diseases and allergies may limit or alter the kind of treatment you can be offered (see Chapters 19 and 20). Before starting treatment, the dentist may wish to consult with your physician concerning your medical history and state of health.

DENTAL EXAMINATION

Once your history is recorded, the dentist will perform a dental examination. It will explore three main areas: your teeth, your gums, and other tissues of your mouth. In addition, the dentist may examine the temporomandibular joints (TMJs)of your jaws.

The dentist will either enter the examination results directly on your chart, or permanent record, or will dictate the findings to an assistant. To identify specific teeth, the dentist will use a system that assigns a number (for permanent teeth) or letter (for primary teeth) to each one.

TEETH

Using a mirror and a probe, the dentist will examine the visible crown of each tooth, looking in particular for the buildup of plaque and evidence of looseness and decay. *Pulp tests* may also be performed, to assess conditions inside the tooth (see page 118).

The dentist will also check the way your teeth mesh together in *occlusion*, or bite. If further study is required, *impressions* of the upper and lower jaws may be taken (see page 24).

GUMS

The dentist will examine the general condition of your gums, which should be firm and

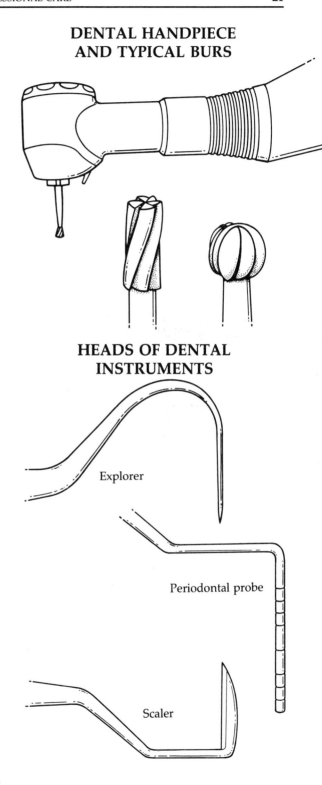

DENTAL HANDPIECE AND TYPICAL BURS

HEADS OF DENTAL INSTRUMENTS

Explorer

Periodontal probe

Scaler

pink, and not soft, swollen, or inflamed. A periodontal probe will be used to check the depth of the *sulcus*, the slight depression where each tooth meets the gum. Overly deep depressions, called *pockets*, are evidence of gum disease.

OTHER TISSUES OF THE MOUTH

The dentist will examine your lips, cheeks, tongue, and other areas of your mouth for irregularities and disorders that might require not only dental but also medical attention. Your dentist may be the first to spot and diagnose conditions, such as cancer, which can profoundly affect your general health.

THE TEMPOROMANDIBULAR JOINTS

The dentist may perform a special examination of the temporomandibular joints that connect your lower jawbone (the *mandible*) to your skull. The dentist is especially likely to conduct such an examination if you have difficulty in opening or closing your mouth or if you have reported such symptoms as recurrent headaches or facial pain (see Chapter 18).

X-RAYS

The dentist will supplement the direct examination of the visible parts of your teeth and mouth by taking X-rays that show the parts that cannot be seen by eye.

Some patients are concerned about exposure to radiation. When properly used, dental X-rays are not dangerous. First of all, modern X-ray film requires relatively little radiation. Moreoever, the radiation is carefully filtered, and focused upon the area to be examined. Protective devices such as lead aprons further protect the rest of the body from exposure.

An X-ray can be thought of as a powerful, penetrating beam of light, and the image on the film as a shadow cast by this beam as it passes through various substances. A more pronounced shadow will be cast by a dense substance, such as a tooth or bone, than by softer tissue. The hard, outer enamel of a tooth, for example, will cast more of a shadow than the softer dentin, and tissues such as pulp and gum will cast almost none. Since the film image is a *negative*, the densest substances will appear lightest.

There is no substitute for X-ray studies to reveal conditions within the teeth and bones. Tooth decay, which is relatively soft, shows up as slightly darker than the surrounding healthy tooth tissue. Abscesses and other lesions in bone also show up darker than normal, and fractures and bone loss are readily apparent. So are teeth, such as "wisdom" teeth, that have failed to erupt, and remain buried under the gum. Metal restorations, such as fillings, are *radiopaque* and show up as near-white patches on the film.

During the first visit, the general dentist is likely to take at least two types of X-ray views—*periapical* and *bitewing*—and may take *occlusal* or *panoramic* views as well.

Periapical X-ray films for adults are about 1¼ by 1¾ inches (films for children are smaller). They provide complete side views of about four teeth, from the roots to the tops of the crowns. A complete series will consist of 16 to 24 views, showing each tooth at least twice, from somewhat different angles.

Bitewing films are the same size, but show only the crowns and parts of the roots of two or three pairs of opposing teeth. These provide a sharp view of decay, especially between adjacent teeth.

Bitewing films are customarily used for periodic checkups, and are routinely taken at intervals of about 18 months. A full-mouth set of periapical X-rays is usually taken when it is needed for a specific diagnosis, or at intervals of no less than three to five years.

Occlusal films are larger than periapical or bitewing types—about 2¼ by 3 inches. They are held between the teeth, and the X-ray machine is focused on them from either above or below. They show the full arch of the bite, and are especially useful in locating abscesses and other disorders in the jawbones. Most patients do not need them.

Panoramic films (sometimes called *Panorex*, from the name of a common brand) provide a two-dimensional view of the complete extent of both jaws, from ear to ear. They require a special setup: the X-ray generator and the film holder are mounted on tracks, and circle halfway around the head as a series of exposures is made. They, too, are especially useful in determining conditions in the bones of the jaw, and are becoming more commonly used in general dental practice.

X-ray films, or *radiographs*, can be developed in a few minutes at most. They are then mounted on a back-lit board or table for viewing, either during your visit or later on.

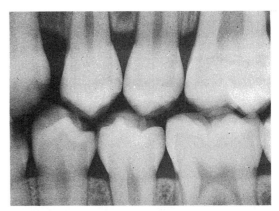

Bite-wing X-ray

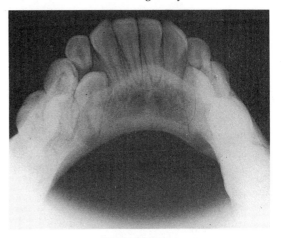

Occlusal X-ray

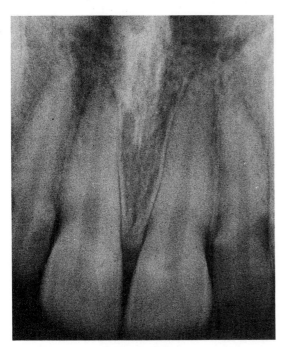

Periapical X-ray

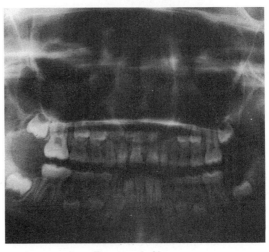

Panoramic X-ray

IMPRESSIONS AND MODELS

The dentist may wish to have a record of the precise position of your teeth and of the relationship between your jaws. Such a record is useful in general treatment, and it is essential if extensive restorative treatment or orthodontics is contemplated. The record customarily takes the form of plaster *models*, cast from *impressions* of your teeth and jaws.

Impressions are customarily taken of both jaws. A bow-shaped *impression tray* is filled with a special paste, and pressed over the teeth of one jaw.

Within a few minutes, the paste sets to a firm but rubbery consistency, and the tray is removed. This procedure is repeated for the other jaw. Later, in the laboratory, plaster models are cast from the impressions of each jaw, and mounted on an armature, or *articulator*, to show the relationship between the jaws.

PLAN OF TREATMENT

The dentist will use the results of your examination to formulate an overall *plan of treatment*, and will present it to you at either your first visit or a subsequent one. This plan can vary widely. The dentist may recommend only periodic checkups and cleaning, or the filling of cavities. At the other extreme, the dentist may recommend extensive treatment by one or more dental specialists. In any event, you should receive the following:

- A diagnosis of your dental health, in general, and of any specific problems that may exist.
- An explanation of treatment options—including the option of foregoing treatment entirely.
- An assessment of the likely outcome of treatment.

- An estimate of the likely cost, especially when extensive treatment is being considered.

In addition, the dentist will discuss a program of self-care you should undertake at home, to prevent dental problems from arising or to help correct problems that already exist (see Chapter 4). Such home care is just as important as professional care, if not even more so.

PROFESSIONAL CLEANING

Even if you faithfully brush and floss your teeth, they will need professional cleaning every six months. Home care cannot reach all tooth surfaces efficiently. Plaque inevitably builds up and forms hard compounds called *tartar* or *calculus*, especially in hard-to-reach areas near the gumline.

Professional cleaning is performed either by the dentist, or by a dental hygienist—a specially trained and licensed dental nurse. Cleaning consists mainly of scraping off hard deposits using manual scalers (see illustration 3.2) or an *ultrasonic* machine. An ultrasonic machine generates high-frequency sound waves, which are transmitted through a probe-like tip, and vibrate plaque deposits loose. The plaque particles are then flushed off with a stream of cool water.

To head off periodontal disease, the sides of the roots, as well as the crowns, must often be cleaned. To avoid discomfort, a *topical* anesthetic may be applied to the gums; it is occasionally supplemented with an injected *local* anesthetic (see pages 51 and 52).

Once the teeth are cleaned, they are polished. The dentist may apply a mildly abrasive compound from a special cup-shaped head attached to the handpiece, or may spray on a mixture of abrasive, air, and water. This process helps clean the crowns of stains, but

TAKING AN IMPRESSION

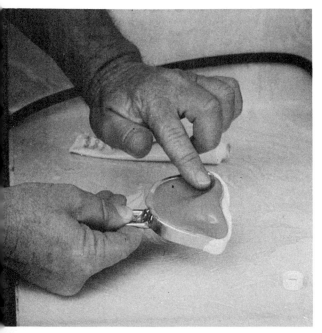

Impression tray containing impression material

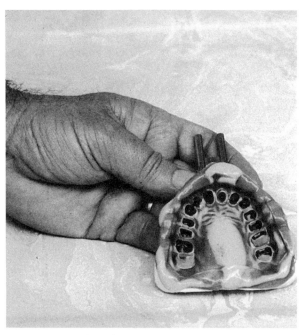

Hardened material, containing impression

Photographs by Alfred Carin

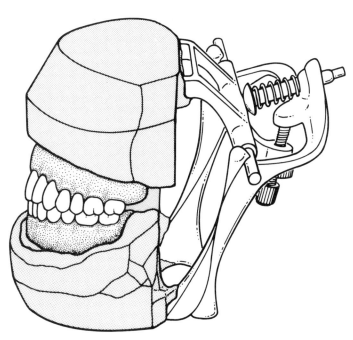

Models of jaws, mounted on articulator

it also smooths their surfaces, making it harder for plaque to stick to them.

Finally, the dentist or hygienist may treat your teeth with a fluoride compound or a sealant to help prevent decay. However, these treatments are recommended more commonly for children and adolescents than they are for adults (see page 101).

FOLLOW-UP

At the conclusion of your visit, the dentist or an assistant will arrange future visits. To be effective, professional treatment must continue—at least every six months—virtually for the rest of your life.

F O U R

HOME CARE: YOUR ROLE IN MAINTAINING DENTAL HEALTH

The two main enemies of dental health are tooth decay and periodontal disease. Both have the same basic cause: the buildup of plaque on exposed surfaces of the teeth (page 61). Hence, the main purpose of dental care is the control of plaque. In particular, it must be kept from adhering to your teeth for more than 24 hours. To accomplish this goal, you should remove plaque from your teeth at least once a day, every day. Semiannual cleaning by your dentist won't suffice—you'll have to do the job yourself, regularly and thoroughly.

For the removal of plaque, we recommend a three-step program, performed twice a day—at bedtime and after breakfast. The three steps are *brushing, flossing,* and cleaning the gumlines with an *interdental stimulator*.

BRUSHING

Brushing has long been established as an effective method of cleaning the teeth. But it must be done correctly, and its limits must be recognized.

For example, many people think that the toothpaste is what cleans the teeth and that the main function of the toothbrush is to apply the paste. Wrong. Plaque sticks to the teeth, and toothpaste won't dislodge it. Thorough, frequent brushing is needed to scrape plaque loose so it can be rinsed away.

The first step in effective brushing is the choice of a toothbrush. There are many shapes and styles on the market, and most of them will do a satisfactory job. The bristles are usually nylon, which doesn't go limp when it gets wet. But the bristles should be relatively soft, with rounded tips. Not much pressure is needed to loosen plaque; bristles that are stiff and sharp can injure your gums and wear away your teeth. They should be stiff enough, though, to stand up straight. You should replace the brush when the bristles begin to bend out of line.

You can use an electric toothbrush if you prefer—though an ordinary manual brush will work just as well for most people. There

HOW TO BRUSH YOUR TEETH

1. Imagine that your mouth is divided into four equal sections. Each section has an inside and an outside surface, making eight surfaces in all.
2. Brush one of these eight surfaces at a time. The exact order doesn't matter, but there should *be* an order, which becomes a habit through repetition.
3. You can brush with toothpaste or without. The brush can be wet or dry, so long as the bristles are upright.
4. The back teeth are the hardest to reach and the most often neglected. So, when brushing each surface, start in back, and work forward. You will find it easier to reach the outside surfaces, especially of the back teeth, if you open your mouth only slightly. Opening wide stretches the cheek muscles taut against the teeth.
5. Hold the brush horizontally, and place the bristles on one side of the teeth, close to the gumline. They will cover about three teeth at a time. Tilt the brush so that the bristles form an angle of about 45 degrees (one half a right angle) with the teeth. Exert enough pressure so that the bristles splay out slightly, and penetrate the groove, or *sulcus*, at the gumline.
6. Brush back and forth horizontally with *very* short strokes—no wider than a quarter of an inch or so. Continue for ten seconds.
7. Move the brush to the next group of teeth, and repeat the process. Continue until all surfaces of all four sections have been brushed.
8. If the chewing surfaces of the back teeth haven't been thoroughly brushed along with the inside and outside surfaces, brush them, too.
9. Brushing the top surface of the tongue refreshes the mouth and can reduce bad breath. It has no known effect on dental plaque.
10. After brushing, rinse the mouth thoroughly with water. A small amount of salt in warm water (¼ teaspoon in 8 ounces) will serve as a refreshing mouthwash, if you want one. If you enjoy the taste of a commercial mouthwash, use it, but be aware that such mouthwashes have no proven value in preventing tooth decay or gum inflammation.

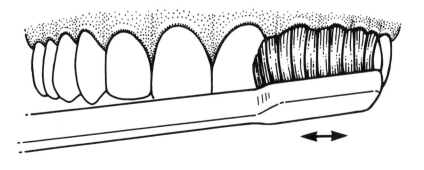

are three basic types of electric toothbrushes: One has bristles that make short back-and-forth strokes. The second has bristles that rotate from side to side. The third has individual tufts of bristles that rotate in their sockets. All three types are effective.

An electric toothbrush is especially useful to people who have limited manual dexterity, or who suffer from ailments such as arthritis, Parkinson's disease, or the aftereffects of a stroke (see page 110).

Toothpaste does have its uses, however. It contains agents that help carry away loosened plaque and food debris, and it refreshes the mouth. You should choose one of the fluoride-containing brands approved by the American Dental Association. The topical application of fluoride strengthens tooth enamel against decay. It is most effective on the teeth of children and adolescents (see page 86), but it can also be beneficial for adults, especially in later life (see page 110).

Many systems of brushing have been used. One that we have found effective is outlined on page 28. Whatever procedure you use should conform with the following principles.

- Every reachable surface of every tooth must be brushed. In order not to miss any surface, it is wise to brush your teeth in a fixed order, which will become habitual. You should also take care not to pass over relatively hard-to-reach teeth such as the back molars.
- Light brushing pressure is enough to loosen plaque. Heavy pressure, especially with a stiff-bristled brush, can damage your teeth—particularly in the areas near the gums.
- The gums near the teeth should be brushed as well, to make sure that plaque is cleaned out of the groove, or *sulcus*, where each tooth emerges from the gum. Brushing also stimulates and strengthens the gums. Unless you are suffering from periodontal disease, brushing shouldn't ordinarily make your gums bleed.

Brushing takes time, but it's worth the effort. Regular, thorough brushing is essential to your dental health.

FLOSSING

Many people don't floss their teeth at all, or floss infrequently and for the wrong reason. Many of those who do floss are simply trying to dislodge food particles caught between particular teeth. Yet there is a far more important reason to floss between all the teeth, every day.

Brushing doesn't reach all tooth surfaces.

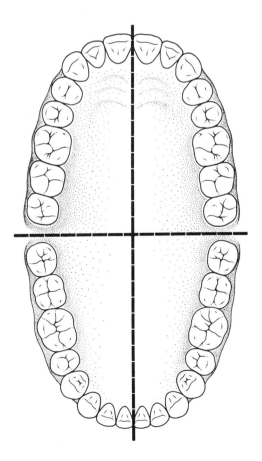

It inevitably misses the *proximal* surfaces—between the teeth. It also tends to miss the V-shaped sulcus between the gum and each tooth. Plaque tends to build up in these areas, leading to decay and periodontal disease. That's why flossing is important. It loosens plaque from each proximal surface and from at least part of the area enclosed by the sulcus. Flossing, before or after brushing, should be a regular part of your program of plaque control. If your gums are healthy, you should floss when you brush, after breakfast and at bedtime. If you have periodontal disease, you should brush and floss after lunch as well.

Types of floss available include waxed and unwaxed floss, flossing tape, and fuzzy "superfloss." They are all effective. Use the one your dentist recommends, or the one that is easiest for you to use.

If your teeth are so tightly spaced that you cannot readily force the floss between them, you can use a *floss threader*, a device that enables you to insert one end of the floss through the interproximal spaces below the contact points. A floss threader is especially useful for inserting floss under a fixed bridge. And if you have difficulty holding the ends of the floss with your fingers, you can place it in a more easily held *floss holder*.

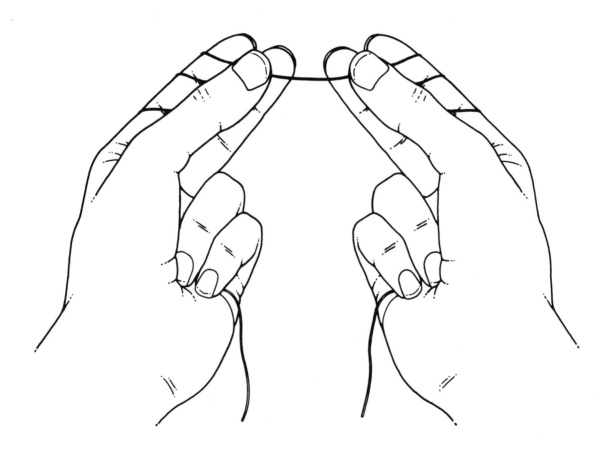

HOW TO FLOSS YOUR TEETH

1. Take a length of floss about 18 inches long from the floss dispenser. Wrap the ends three or four times around your index fingers to secure them, so that 5 or 6 inches of floss extend between the fingers.
2. Press your thumbs against your index fingers to hold the floss loops in place. Extend your middle fingers to press against the rest of the floss so there is a short length of taut floss between them.
3. The upper teeth are harder to floss than the lower ones, and the back teeth harder than those in front. Start at one end of your upper jaw and work toward the center.
4. Open your mouth only slightly, so your cheeks are not taut against the teeth. At first, you may find a mirror helpful in determining your position. Insert the taut length of floss *behind* the rearmost upper molar, until it touches the gum. If the gum bleeds or hurts, you are probably pressing too hard. Pull the ends of the floss forward, until parts of the inner and outer surfaces of the tooth are covered. Rub the floss two or three times *up and down* the tooth surface (*not* back and forth), to dislodge plaque.
5. Insert the floss between the last molar and the next tooth. You will encounter resistance at the contact point between the teeth. Pull the floss *gently* back and forth until it passes through the contact point. Press the floss against the last molar, and rub the floss up and down two or three times between the gum and the contact point. Next, press the floss against the other molar, and repeat the process. Finally, remove the floss, again pulling gently back and forth as you pass through the contact point.
6. Move forward to the next interproximal space between the teeth, and continue until you reach the central incisors. Then go to the rear molar on the other side, and floss from there to the center.
7. If the floss begins to fray, or if plaque builds up heavily upon it, you can release a loop from one index finger and take up the slack on the other.
8. Floss the teeth of the lower jaw the same way as those of the upper jaw, starting at the rearmost molar at each end, and working toward the center.
9. Rinse thoroughly to flush away the loosened plaque. If the debris is heavy, you may find it helpful to brush the teeth first, or to use a mechanical irrigator.

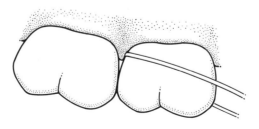

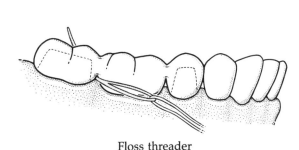

Floss threader

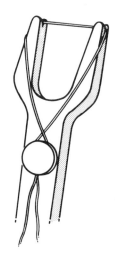

Floss holder

Flossing isn't as easy as brushing. It may seem awkward and tedious, especially at first. But eventually the procedure becomes routine. Step-by-step instructions are on page 31.

INTERDENTAL STIMULATORS

Interdental stimulators, sometimes called *gum massagers* or *gum cleaners*, come in various forms, such as soft wooden sticks and rubber or plastic cones. They stimulate and toughen the gum between the teeth, and help clean the proximal surfaces. But they have a more important function: They loosen the plaque inside the sulcus around each tooth, especially in areas not reached by flossing. After flossing, you should run the stimulator along all the gumlines, and press it gently but firmly against the triangular gum tissue between the teeth.

Some people—older people especially—have relatively large interproximal spaces between their teeth near the gumline. Flossing and interdental stimulators may not be as efficient for cleaning such spaces as *interproximal brushes*. These small, cone-shaped brushes, which are rather like miniature bottle brushes, are used in conjunction with a toothbrush.

PLAQUE-DISCLOSING AGENTS

Plaque-disclosing agents are available either in tablet or liquid form. Most contain a vegetable dye; some glow, or *fluoresce*, under ultraviolet light. When applied to the teeth, they combine with otherwise invisible plaque, and *disclose* the surfaces from which it hasn't been properly removed. They are especially useful in the early stages of a self-care program, and for periodic checks thereafter.

IRRIGATING DEVICES

Irrigating devices, powered by electric pump or by water pressure from the tap, drive pulsing jets of water through a narrow tube, dislodging food particles and other debris between teeth and along the gumlines. Because air is mixed with the jets of water, claims have been made that irrigation reduces the number of plaque-forming bacteria. Irrigating devices are especially useful for people who wear orthodontic appliances or prosthetic restorations. They do not remove plaque, however.

People who have periodontal disease or a heart-valve disorder must be cautious in using irrigation devices. Some dentists believe that, at high power, such devices may drive bacteria more deeply into the gums, extending the inflammation of the tissues and risking the spread of infection through the blood (see page 220).

MOUTHWASHES

Despite advertising claims, mouthwashes sold over the counter do not prevent either tooth decay or periodontal disease. Some antiseptic mouthwashes are said to weaken plaque so that it is more easily brushed away, but their effectiveness is still somewhat controversial. Mouthwashes that contain fluoride may provide a little added protection against decay, but fluoride-containing toothpaste usually gives adequate protection.

As a refreshing rinse, a little salt or baking soda (¼ teaspoon) dissolved in a glass (8 ounces) of water is likely to do as well as any commercial mouthwash. If you are on a low-sodium diet for medical reasons, consult your physician before using such a rinse.

Mouthwashes may even be harmful. They can cover up the foul taste and bad breath that often accompany tooth decay and periodontal disease. Concealing these symptoms can lead to delays in seeking professional treatment.

Mouthwashes containing a large amount of the antiseptic chlorhexidine are sometimes prescribed for the relief of gum inflammation (gingivitis). They are not for general use, have an unpleasant bitter taste, and stain the teeth.

THE INFLUENCE OF DIET

One way to reduce tooth decay and periodontal disease is to reduce the food supply of the bacteria that form plaque. The most important part of that food supply is sugar. The more you reduce sugar in your diet, the better chance you have of avoiding decay and periodontal disease.

Certain sweets are especially harmful. They include the following:

- Sweets that are retained in the mouth for a long time, such as hard candy, cough drops, and ordinary (non-sugarless) chewing gum.
- Sweets that stick to the mouth, such as caramels and other chewy candy, cookies and pastries, presweetened cereals, and dried fruit.
- Sweets that are eaten often, and between meals, such as sugar-sweetened drinks.

Certain sweet foods, however, are relatively harmless—these include fresh fruit and pure fruit juice, in which the concentration of sugar is low.

Raw fruits and vegetables actually contribute to dental health. They require vigorous chewing, which stimulates salivation and cleanses the teeth and gums.

TOBACCO

If you value the health of your mouth, avoid tobacco in any form. It doesn't cause the teeth to decay, but it does stain them. It also irritates all the soft tissues of the mouth and can lead to several disorders, including oral cancer (see pages 258, 260, and 262).

Nicotine is especially harmful to the gums. It constricts the blood vessels, which limits the blood supply to the tissues and lowers their resistance to infection. Tobacco users are more likely to contract periodontal disease and to suffer from it severely.

THE NEED FOR PROFESSIONAL CARE

The program of self-care outlined here will go far toward maintaining dental health. But it isn't complete. There is one other crucial part: making and keeping regular, semiannual appointments with your dentist. Only your dentist can identify early stages of tooth decay and gum inflammation, when they are still relatively easy to treat.

Only your dentist, moreover, can give your teeth the thorough cleaning they periodically need. No one is capable of removing absolutely all the plaque from his or her teeth. If plaque remains more than two days or so, it absorbs minerals from saliva and forms a hard, rough substance called calculus. Calculus doesn't cause decay, but it is unsightly and contributes significantly to gum inflammation. Brushing won't remove it—a dentist must scrape it off.

F I V E

FIRST AID FOR DENTAL EMERGENCIES

The most common dental problems—tooth decay and periodontal disease—develop gradually, and are treated with regular, ongoing care at home and in the dentist's office. But some situations come on suddenly; an accident may happen, or an acute symptom may unexpectedly appear. In such cases, it is usually best to get to your dentist for treatment as soon as possible. Nevertheless, first-aid measures can help to make you more comfortable and to assure the effectiveness of treatment. Just as important, there are some things you should *not* do in emergencies, so as not to make them worse.

A DENTAL FIRST-AID KIT

A few supplies are worth having at home in case of dental emergencies. Many of them are standard household items.

- Table salt or baking soda, to dissolve in warm water as a soothing mouthwash.
- Ice, to reduce pain and swelling. A sim-

ple cold pack can be improvised by placing ice in a plastic bag, wrapped in a moist cloth. An alternative is a commercial *snap-pack*. Striking it against a hard surface sets off a chemical reaction that quickly makes it cold.
- An over-the-counter topical anesthetic ointment or liquid (such as Anbesol, Orajel, Campho-Phenique, or Lidocaine Viscous Solution) to apply to mouth sores.
- A mild analgesic (pain reliever), such as aspirin or acetaminophen (Tylenol). If aspirin upsets your stomach, you may find a coated form less irritating.
- Sterile gauze pads to control bleeding.
- A small quantity of dental wax, supplied by your dentist. This soft, easily shaped material is most often used by orthodontic patients, to cover protruding parts of braces that are newly installed, or that have become bent or broken. The wax helps to prevent irritation of the adjacent soft tissue. It can sometimes be used to prevent irritation from a damaged fixed prosthetic bridge. It can also be placed

temporarily over a broken tooth, to help prevent irritation and contamination of the dentin and pulp (see below).

Another important resource is the address and the telephone number of your dentist. If your dentist has a colleague as a regular backup or standby, it would be wise to have that number as well. The address and number of the nearest hospital emergency room may also be helpful, but not all hospitals provide dental service. If you don't have a regular dentist, or if you are away from home, the local dental society may be able to make a referral. Look up "Dental Society" in the white pages of the telephone directory.

TOOTHACHE

An aching tooth is perhaps the most common dental emergency, and is certainly one of the most unpleasant. The usual cause is tooth decay, but other conditions may be responsible as well.

The pain will sometimes be reduced by analgesics such as aspirin. Ice may give relief, but inflamed tooth nerves sometimes don't respond to it, and occasionally become even more painful.

Don't apply a hot pack. Toothache often involves a bacterial infection, and heat can cause it to spread. Don't put an aspirin tablet against the tooth or gum; the acid can burn the soft tissue of the mouth (see page 263).

Until you can get treatment, try not to chew on the tooth, and avoid hot or sweet foods.

Remember that pain is the body's way of telling you something is wrong. Even if the toothache "goes away," you should go to your dentist for an examination as soon as possible.

IMPACTED FOOD PARTICLES

Sometimes a bit of fibrous food may become caught, or *impacted*, between two adjacent teeth and may resist being dislodged by the tongue. Try getting it loose by flossing between the teeth. You can exert extra force by first tying a small knot in the floss.

Such impactions may be evidence of tooth decay between the teeth, or of a rough or broken restoration such as a filling or a crown. If they recur between the same teeth, see your dentist.

If you wear a fixed bridge, and food particles become trapped under it, flossing is usually the best remedy. Use a *floss threader* (see page 31) to slip the floss under the bridge.

Food fragments may also be driven between the teeth and the gums, causing irritation. Popcorn is a common culprit. Try removing it with the soft, pointed end of an interdental stimulator (see page 32). If you cannot easily dislodge it without damaging the gum, go to your dentist. Don't count on it "working itself out."

A BROKEN TOOTH

Part of a tooth may be broken off in an accident or a fight, by chewing on a hard object, by the wedging action of a filling, or just spontaneously, for no apparent reason. Rebuilding the tooth with an inlay, onlay, or crown is the usual long-term remedy. Until you can get to your dentist, however, press a protective cover of dental wax over the broken tooth. If there is any pain, take an analgesic. Don't apply either heat or cold to the area. Switch temporarily to a soft diet, and try not to chew on the tooth. Avoid hard, crunchy, or very hot foods.

It is usually not possible to reattach the broken part. Nevertheless, save it if you can and take it to your dentist. If by any chance it is *not* a piece of tooth, but rather a tooth-colored restoration (such as a porcelain filling), it may be salvageable. Let your dentist make the decision.

A BROKEN OR LOST FILLING OR CROWN

Fillings and artificial crowns, like teeth, may become cracked or broken. They are, however, more likely to fall out completely. Temporary fillings and crowns are especially likely to come loose. First aid is much the same as for a broken tooth.

An artificial crown can sometimes be temporarily reattached with an over-the-counter denture adhesive (such as Fixodent) until your dentist can do a more permanent job.

If possible, save the filling or crown for examination by your dentist. Some restorations (crowns, in particular) can be salvaged for reuse.

Prompt professional treatment is very important. When a filling, or another restoration, has fallen out, it is often a sign that decay has worked its way underneath. If taken care of promptly, a cavity under a filling can often be treated with another, somewhat more extensive filling. If the decay is left untreated, root canal therapy may be necessary, or the entire tooth may be lost.

KNOCKED OUT (AVULSED) TEETH

Teeth that are completely knocked out of their sockets can often be reimplanted—if they are treated *promptly*. Since this injury tends to be most prevalent among young people, it is discussed in detail in Chapter 10 (page 101).

BENT OR BROKEN BRIDGES, DENTURES, OR ORTHODONTIC APPLIANCES

Dental restorations and appliances are fairly sturdy, but sometimes they may become bent or broken. Removable dentures are especially susceptible to damage.

Broken devices can often be put back together, at considerable savings compared with complete replacement. So save all broken pieces, even small ones, for your dentist. Put them in an envelope or a small plastic bag for safekeeping. *Don't* wrap them in a piece of tissue, which is all too easily mistaken for waste, and thrown away.

Do not undertake repairs yourself. Don't try to glue broken pieces back together—the glue can ruin them.

If a wire or a clasp of an orthodontic appliance is bent so that it irritates your mouth, bend it back only enough to reduce the irritation. You can also cover it temporarily with a small lump of dental wax, which your dentist can supply for such an emergency.

By contrast, if the wire clasp of a partial denture becomes bent, *don't* try to bend it back. It's too likely to break. Simply remove the denture until you can get to the dentist. Don't delay; without the support of the denture, the remaining teeth are likely to begin drifting out of place.

MOUTH SORES

Painful lesions may appear on the lips and the soft tissues inside the mouth. The most common are canker sores and cold sores (see pages 254 and 256) and local irritations from rough, hot, spicy foods ("pizza mouth"). If they persist for a week or more, your dentist should examine them—they may be symptoms of some serious disorder.

Ordinarily, these sores must be allowed to heal by themselves; there is no quick, effective treatment for them. Meanwhile, certain home remedies may make you more comfortable. Rinsing with warm salt water may reduce the irritation. So may applying a paste of baking soda to the lesions for a few minutes or pressing pieces of ice against them. Temporarily avoiding hot or spicy foods will help keep the irritation from getting worse. Over-the-counter topical anesthetics (see page 35) can give temporary relief. Analgesics will, at least, reduce the pain, though they aren't likely to kill it completely.

More important are remedies *not* to use. Don't put aspirin on the sores. It may anesthetize them, but the acid can seriously burn the soft tissue of your mouth. Don't take antibiotics unless they are specifically prescribed. They don't work on many of these conditions, and may have undesirable side effects. Don't use topical steroid ointments either, unless they are prescribed. They can cause certain infections to spread. Don't apply hot packs. These, too, can encourage the spread of infection.

A BITTEN TONGUE OR CHEEK

Occasionally you may bite your tongue or cheek by mistake, causing a temporary but often painful swelling and inflammation. Unless the bite is severe enough to cause bleeding, treat it as you would other mouth sores. But don't use a topical anesthetic. The loss of sensation increases the chance that you will bite the cheek again.

GUMBOILS

Painful, pimple-like swellings, called *gumboils*, may appear on your gums. They are usually formed by pus from an abscess (see page 62), working its way to the surface. Gumboils should be treated a little differently from other mouth sores. Rinse with warm salt water to relieve irritation and to encourage the boil to form a "head," which may eventually break to release its contents.

Since a gumboil is likely to be a symptom of a serious infection or gum disease, be sure to consult your dentist promptly if one appears.

GUM INFLAMMATION NEAR WISDOM TEETH

Sometimes the gum near an erupting third molar or "wisdom tooth," becomes inflamed and painful. This condition, called *pericoronitis* ("inflammation around the crown"), is especially likely if the molar is not erupting normally but rather is tipped or partially *impacted* (see page 152). Food particles and bacteria trapped between the gum and the malposed tooth cause the inflammation.

The long-term solution is likely to be the extraction of the offending tooth. Meanwhile, the infection should be treated the same way other mouth sores are (above). Carefully rinsing the mouth after eating may help prevent food particles from being trapped in gum crevices.

BLEEDING

For many people, bleeding is an alarming symptom. If bleeding occurs inside your mouth, first try to discover its source and how extensive it is.

To locate the source (if you don't already know it), rinse out your mouth with water, and use a mirror to determine whether the bleeding comes from the gums, the tongue, the palate, the floor of the mouth, or the lining of the cheeks or lips.

Then determine how severe the bleeding is. Even a little blood, when mixed with saliva, may seem to indicate extensive bleeding. Again, rinsing the mouth first and locating the source of the bleeding will help you determine its extent.

BLEEDING GUMS

Gums that are tender and that ooze blood readily sometimes indicate systemic disease (see page 272). Much more often, however, tender gums are a sign of chronic periodontal disease. In either event, they should receive prompt professional attention.

Meanwhile, rinsing with warm salt water may reduce soreness. But don't stop regular brushing—it helps protect, rather than injure, the gums. Also try to continue flossing and using an interdental stimulator, gently and carefully, to avoid further injury.

BLEEDING AFTER A TOOTH EXTRACTION

Slight bleeding immediately after an extraction is normal, and a clot usually forms within an hour or so. This clot should be left undisturbed until the wound starts to heal—usually after a day or two.

If bleeding doesn't stop promptly after an extraction, or starts again, try pressing a gauze pad over the area for 20 minutes or so to control the flow. You can often hold the pad in place simply by biting down on it. An alternative is a wet tea bag; the tannic acid in tea helps a new clot to form.

BLEEDING FROM LACERATIONS
INSIDE THE MOUTH

Bleeding from lacerations (wounds) of the tongue, gums, palate, or other soft tissue inside the mouth can often be temporarily controlled by pressure. Place an ice cube or a gauze compress moistened with cold water directly over the wound. Hold it firmly in place with your fingers or with your tongue until the bleeding stops. Seek professional treatment without delay, such wounds can easily become infected.

BLEEDING FROM LACERATIONS
OUTSIDE THE MOUTH

Bleeding from lacerations of the lips or cheeks can often be stopped by pressure as well. If dirt, a splinter, or other foreign matter has gotten into the wound, don't try to remove it yourself. You may drive it further under the surface, making it harder to remove and risking a permanent scar.

Get professional help right away. You may need an antibiotic or a tetanus shot to ward off infection, and stitches to close the wound.

BRUISED LIPS OR CHEEKS

Tissues of the lips and cheeks are easily bruised by blunt trauma, and they quickly swell, causing a "fat lip" or the like. To minimize the swelling and discomfort, place ice against the area as soon as possible, and hold it in place for about 20 minutes. Repeat if necessary, but don't apply the ice for more than 20 minutes in each hour, since excessive chilling can seriously damage the skin.

DISLOCATED JAW

By accident, the lower jaw (*mandible*) may be dislocated at the temporomandibular joints on one or both sides. Whiplash injury from an automobile collision is a common cause, but even yawning too wide, or taking too big a bite of food, can do it.

If you suddenly find that you can't close your mouth, try to stay calm. Nervous agitation makes it harder to relax the jaw muscles. Try, gently, to work the jaw loose, by moving it from side to side. But don't try to force it shut, and be careful to keep your fingers out of your mouth, in case it shuts suddenly. Generally it is better to seek immediate help from your dentist or physician. Reducing a dislocation isn't hard, but it is best done by a professional (see page 155).

BROKEN JAW

If, after a blow, you find that you cannot move your jaw without great pain or if you can feel a rough, uneven spot along the bones of either jaw or if your upper and lower teeth no longer meet in the same positions as before, you may have fractured your jaw. Seek help immediately, either from hospital emergency room staff or from an oral surgeon. Your jaws may have to be immobilized with wire splinting, not only to make sure the bones knit properly but also to protect loosened teeth (see page 155).

SIX

OVERCOMING DENTAL FEAR

Only about 50 percent of all Americans receive regular professional dental care. There are several reasons for this low figure, but one of the main reasons is that many people are afraid to go to the dentist. Studies indicate that between 8 to 15 percent are so fearful of dental treatment that they avoid it altogether.

The consequences are obvious. It is all but impossible to assure dental health without regular professional attention. Tooth decay and gum disease become virtually inevitable, and they lead to painful infections and eventual tooth loss. Yet many people avoid the routine treatment that could prevent or halt these problems at an early stage. Some seek help only when the pain of toothache or gum inflammation is severe enough to outweigh their fear. Some respond only to strong social pressures: the bad breath that often accompanies these conditions becomes so offensive, or the decay and loss of teeth become so disfiguring, that they seek belated assistance. But a few remain so terrified of dental treatment that they will avoid it even when suffering extreme pain. We have encountered exceptional cases in which patients have attempted to pull their own aching teeth rather than go to a dentist.

Moreover, even patients who are not so frightened of dental treatment may suffer anguish from dental fear. As any dentist can attest, most patients are at least mildly apprehensive about treatment. In fact, no one who feels such fear, either before or during treatment, need feel alone.

Overcoming fear of treatment is an essential part of dental care. If you or someone in your family suffers from such fear, there are several methods of combating it. A collaboration between dentists and psychologists has produced effective techniques of behavioral therapy to help you reduce dental fear to a minimal level and cope with any fear that remains.

SOURCES OF DENTAL FEAR

Dental fear generally can be divided into three categories: fear of pain, fear of gagging or choking, and fear of loss of control.

The fear of pain often centers on particular dental instruments: the dental drill, the hypodermic syringe used to inject anesthetics, and hand instruments such as probes and curettes. Anesthetics and other modern techniques of dentistry now make most such fear unnecessary. Nonetheless, you may have become fearful as a result of unpleasant experiences in the past, before these techniques were developed. It is quite natural to dread and avoid whatever has caused pain previously.

The fear of gagging or choking also has a realistic basis. Some people have especially sensitive mouths and throats, and the instruments and liquids used in treatment can trigger muscle spasms. For others, the feel of foreign objects in their mouths gives them the impression that they are drowning or strangling. Again, though, modern techniques minimize these effects.

The fear of loss of control has two aspects. The first is the fear of losing control to the dentist and of being a helpless victim during treatment. You may, for instance, become anxious at the prospect of having your mouth invaded, or made numb with an anesthetic. This anxiety may be reinforced by the environment of the dental office, especially the dental chair, which customarily puts the patient in a semirecumbent position. And your anxiety may be intensified by a general fear of the unknown—of not being quite sure what the dentist is going to do, and how it will feel.

You may also fear losing *self*-control. You may be afraid of fainting, vomiting, or suffering a panic attack. As we will explain shortly, dentists have several ways to reassure you in such situations and to give you a sense of control over your feelings and your treatment.

In addition, you may feel anxious when you smell the distinctive odor of the dentist's office, or when you see a typical dental uniform, especially since nowadays it often includes a mask and surgical gloves.

Finally, you may avoid seeking treatment out of embarrassment. You may be afraid of what the dentist might discover—teeth or gums in such poor condition that extensive further treatment is required. You may not only fear the discomfort and cost involved, but also dread the dentist's disapproval and criticism for having neglected your dental health.

Unfortunately, these fears are powerfully reinforced by a tradition that no longer has any basis at all: the popular myth that dental treatment must of necessity be unpleasant, frightening, and painful. It goes back to the mercifully distant past, when dental treatment was all three. Modern techniques have made such a view obsolete, yet the myth lingers on. It is kept alive in the jokes of cartoonists, columnists, and television comedians. It is transmitted to children by parents who threaten to punish misbehavior with "a trip to the dentist." It is also transmitted by parents who unwittingly infect children with their own fear. This persistent folklore causes much unnecessary anguish, and does great harm, but it is regrettably slow to die.

ASSESSING DENTAL FEAR

If your fear is strong enough to cause emotional distress and to lead you to avoid treatment, it is often advisable to treat the fear itself before any actual dental procedures are begun. Your dentist may provide such treatment unassisted, or may collaborate with a psychologist.

The first step is to assess your fear—to discover how intense it is, and what its sources are. For this purpose, the two questionnaires on pages 44 and 45 can be very helpful. The first, called the *dental anxiety scale*, measures the general level of dental fear. The second, called the *dental fear inventory*, is designed to pinpoint aspects of treatment that are especially frightening.

The items in the dental fear inventory range from mild ("sitting in the dentist's office") to intense ("having a tooth drilled"). Knowing the sources of your fear is very helpful in *desensitization* treatment, as will be explained shortly.

PATIENT REASSURANCE

Because dental fear is so prevalent, dentists routinely use several strategies for *all* patients, regardless of whether or not they are identifiably fearful. These strategies include the following:

- *The dentist will avoid inflicting pain whenever possible.* This may seem obvious, but it requires the dentist's constant attention. Pain can be avoided, but doing so requires care and patience. And there is nothing like past pain to increase future fear.
- *If pain does occur, it should be ended immediately.* The dentist should resist the temptation to "keep going," or to "finish up," but rather should take immediate steps to provide relief.
- *If there is any possibility that a procedure will cause discomfort, the dentist will warn the patient first.* Pain that you expect, and are prepared for, is much easier to tolerate than sudden pain. The converse of this rule is also true: If you are told that a procedure won't hurt, the dentist must be sure that it won't.
- *Diagnosis and treatment will be put in a positive light.* In discussing diagnosis and treatment, the dentist should emphasize the desirable ends to be achieved—relief from pain, better appearance, etc.—over the potentially frightening means required (drilling, extraction of teeth, surgery, etc.).

- *The dentist will minimize the stress of new procedures.* The dentist should avoid abrupt, fast movements, especially when beginning a procedure you are unfamiliar with.
- *The dentist will not adopt a negative, judgmental attitude.* You should be praised for desirable behavior, not criticized for undesirable behavior. You should be encouraged to practice self-care, but not blamed for negligence. Above all, you should not be blamed or ridiculed for being fearful.
- *The dentist will provide a "stop" signal.* You and your dentist agree upon a simple signal, such as raising one hand, to halt treatment, at least temporarily, if it becomes intolerably painful or frightening. You should also be able to "take a break" during an extended procedure, if only to rest your tired jaw muscles. This is crucially important in creating a sense of control over treatment and in reducing feelings of helplessness.

DISTRACTION

In addition, one approach to reducing patient anxiety is used by virtually every dentist: pleasant surroundings that distract your attention from the possibly unpleasant aspects of treatment. Distraction can take many forms. Some are very simple and obvious, such as painting the office walls soothing pastel colors, decorating with attractive pictures and posters, or playing relaxing music. Some dentists install aquariums in their waiting or treatment rooms; many patients find that watching fish swim to and fro has a calming, relaxing effect.

Some dentists go even further. They provide patients with headphones and a choice of recorded programs. Or they install video sets, or even video games, that can be played

HOW AFRAID ARE YOU?

Dental Anxiety Scale

Directions: After each of these questions, circle the number of the answer that corresponds most closely to your feelings. Then add up the numbers to arrive at a total score.

A. If you had to go to the dentist tomorrow, how would you feel about it?
  1. I would look forward to it as a reasonably enjoyable experience.
  2. I wouldn't care about it one way or the other.
  3. I would be a little uneasy about it.
  4. I would be afraid that it would be unpleasant and painful.
  5. I would be very frightened of what the dentist might do.

B. When you are waiting in the dentist's office for your turn in the chair, how do you feel?
  1. Relaxed.
  2. A little uneasy.
  3. Tense.
  4. Anxious.
  5. So anxious that I sometimes start to sweat or feel almost physically sick.

C. When you are in the chair waiting while the dentist gets the drill ready to begin working on your teeth, how do you feel?
  1. Relaxed.
  2. A little uneasy.
  3. Tense.

  4. Anxious.
  5. So anxious that I sometimes start to sweat or feel almost physically sick.

D. You are in the dentist's chair to have your teeth cleaned. While you are waiting, and the dentist is getting out the instruments used to scrape your teeth around the gums, how do you feel?
  1. Relaxed.
  2. A little uneasy.
  3. Tense.
  4. Anxious.
  5. So anxious that I sometimes start to sweat or feel almost physically sick.

The lowest possible score on this scale is 4. Scores of 5 through 8 suggest a "normally reluctant" patient, who undergoes treatment willingly but with some trepidation. A score of 9 through 12 indicates that you are a moderately anxious patient and that you may habitually forget appointments, arrive late, or use minor excuses to cancel. A score of 13 to 15 reveals an anxiety so extreme that you are likely to avoid regular treatment. A score above 15 is evidence of anxiety or phobia so severe that you would probably consent to treatment only in an emergency.

WHAT MAKES YOU AFRAID?

Dental Fear Inventory

Directions: On a scale of 0 to 10, where 0 is a state of mind when you are so relaxed you could fall asleep, and 10 is the point at which you're fearful that you might faint, become sick, or run out of the treatment room, rate the following situations. If there is a situation not on the list that makes you fearful, write it down and rate it.

_____ 1. Sitting in the dentist's waiting room.

_____ 2. Smelling the odor of the dentist's office.

_____ 3. Sitting up in the dentist's chair.

_____ 4. Reclining in the dentist's chair.

_____ 5. Seeing the dentist enter the treatment room.

_____ 6. Having dental X-rays taken.

_____ 7. Seeing the dental probes and other instruments.

_____ 8. Having the dental instruments manipulated in my mouth.

_____ 9. Having my teeth cleaned.

_____ 10. Seeing the needle and syringe for anesthesia.

_____ 11. Receiving an anesthetic injection.

_____ 12. Hearing the noise of the dentist's drill.

_____ 13. Having a tooth drilled.

_____ 14. (Other)

(You are advised to discuss the results of this inventory with your dentist.)

from the chair. Most dentists, however, do not find such extreme methods necessary.

LEARNING TO RELAX

Anxiety is always accompanied by physical tension. Conversely, it is impossible for a person to be both anxious and physically relaxed at the same time. Therefore, one of the best ways to combat dental fear is by learning to relax. Many dentists and psychologists use relaxation training to reduce their patients' general level of anxiety, before trying to deal with their fears.

Relaxation techniques, however, don't require a teacher or a therapist. You can easily learn them, and master them through practice. One of the simplest is a breathing exercise, which you can use as an "instant tranquilizer" just about anywhere, any time:

- Inhale slowly and deeply, counting to five at one-second intervals. Between each count, think of a single word, such as "calm," or "peace," to help free your mind of distracting or stressful thoughts.
- Hold your breath for one second, and then exhale slowly, counting backward from five to one, and silently repeating your chosen word. At the same time, let your chest and stomach muscles relax, and drop your shoulders.
- Repeat this cycle three times.

You can follow this exercise with a more extended series of exercises called *progressive relaxation.*

In these exercises, you simply tense and then relax groups of related muscles in progression, over the whole body. There is no set order, but you might start at the feet (curling your toes), and end at the head (wrinkling your forehead). Tensing muscles before relaxing them produces a greater degree of relaxation than simply trying to relax them. A typical series is summarized on page 47.

For best results, you should perform these exercises daily, for 15 to 30 minutes. Eventually, they become a habit. You can then perform them quickly, in abbreviated form, in any stressful situation, including dental treatment. Just as important, once these exercises become a habit, you are likely to experience a generalized reduction in your level of anxiety. Many people, in fact, use them to help manage the inevitable stresses of everyday life.

GUIDED IMAGERY

You can supplement and reinforce relaxation exercises with a widely used technique called *guided imagery.* It is designed to train the mind, just as progressive relaxation is designed to train the body. Though it is often a part of formal programs of anxiety reduction, anyone can master it, with or without assistance.

You begin by developing an image in your mind—a mental image of a pleasant, tranquil experience—and then concentrate your attention upon that image, trying to block out all other thoughts and sensations. You should repeat this procedure as an exercise, until it becomes a habit. You can then use it to relieve stress in a variety of situations, including dental treatment.

The choice of imagery will vary from person to person. Because so many people find it enjoyable and relaxing to go to the beach, a beach scene is a very common choice. It should be full of specific, concrete details, as in the following:

The scene is a quiet beach, on a sunny summer day. The weather is warm, but not hot, because of a gentle, cooling sea

PROGRESSIVE RELAXATION EXERCISES

You can perform these exercises sitting or lying down. Before starting, try to become as relaxed as you can. Take a deep breath, hold it about three seconds, and let it out very slowly for seven seconds more. As you exhale, think of a single word, such as "calm," or "peace," to help free your mind of distracting, stressful thoughts. Repeat this 10-second cycle three times.

Then perform the exercises, using the same procedure for each. While reciting the instructions slowly to yourself, devote about 10 seconds to tensing each group of muscles, and 20 seconds to relaxing. Repeat the exercise, and go on to the next.

The instructions for the first exercise provide the formula for the rest.

1. Curl the toes of your left foot downward. Hold this tense position. Feel the cramped tightness in your muscles. [10 seconds.]

   Now, relax. Let the tension drain from your muscles. Feel the warm, comfortable sensation of relaxing. [20 seconds.] [Repeat the exercise.]
2. Curl the toes of your right foot downward . . .
3. Pull the toes of your left foot toward your face . . .
4. Pull the toes of your right foot toward your face . . .
5. Tense the muscles in your left thigh, by pressing it against your other leg . . .
6. Tense the muscles in your right thigh, by pressing it against your other leg . . .
7. Tighten the muscles of your buttocks, by pulling them together . . .
8. Tighten the muscles of your stomach . . .
9. Pull your shoulder blades toward each other . . .
10. Hunch your shoulders toward your ears . . .
11. Press your left arm hard against your side . . .
12. Press your right arm hard against your side . . .
13. Make a tight fist with your left hand . . .
14. Make a tight fist with your right hand . . .
15. Push the back of your head hard against the floor or chair . . .
16. Clench your teeth, push your tongue against the roof of your mouth, and smile broadly . . .
17. Squint your eyes tightly shut, and wrinkle up your nose . . .
18. Raise your eyebrows as high as you can, and wrinkle your forehead . . .

Finally, let your whole body relax. Breathe deeply but naturally. Think of sinking . . . going limp . . . letting go. Enjoy the sensation of complete relaxation.

breeze. The sand feels warm and soothing between the toes. Overhead, a few fleecy clouds drift through a brilliant blue sky. In the distance, near the horizon, two small sailboats tack back and forth, so far away that they barely seem to be moving at all. The waves break upon the shore in a slow, regular rhythm. They send shallow flows of foamy water up the sloping sand, and carry the scent of salt and seaweed. As they ebb and flow, small shore birds dart back and forth along the water's edge, searching for food in the glistening wet sand. . . .

A session of guided imagery can take place either before or after progressive relaxation. One reinforces the other. Some dentists, especially those working in collaboration with clinical psychologists, reinforce relaxation training with a mechanical monitoring system, *biofeedback*. This technique is also used in the treatment of stress-related temporomandibular disorders.

DESENSITIZATION

Dental fear is learned behavior—no one is born with it. Almost any learned behavior can be unlearned, or rather, some other behavior can be learned in its place. One of the ways you can learn to overcome dental fear is by gradual exposure to the sources of your fear. This step-by-step process of learning not to fear what you have previously feared is called *desensitization*.

Here is how a typical course of desensitization proceeds. Suppose that your dental fear inventory reveals a particular aversion to the needle and syringe used to inject anesthetics. Fear of needles is, in fact, quite common. Your dentist might begin by showing you, at a distance, the syringe without the needle attached or with the needle still in its protective sheath. If this sight makes you anxious, you will be encouraged to perform a series of relaxation exercises, or a brief session of guided imagery, to help you regain your composure. Only when you are calm and relaxed will the dentist bring the syringe closer to the chair.

You will be encouraged to touch and handle the syringe, first with the needle covered, and then with it uncovered. The dentist will show you how fluid is drawn up into the syringe, and how it is squirted out of the needle. You will perform this operation, using water from a cup. If at any point you find yourself becoming frightened and uncomfortable, the session will halt, and you will again

be encouraged to use relaxation techniques until you are ready to continue.

In the next step, the dentist will touch the needle lightly to your gum. If this provokes too much anxiety, a cotton swab may be used instead. The dentist first touches the gum with the padded swab. Then, the swab is broken in two, and the gum is touched with the bare wood.

Next, the dentist places a dab of topical anesthetic on your gum, so you can become used both to the numbness and the sour, bitter taste. The needle is touched to the same spot, to demonstrate the lack of sensation. Finally, the dentist actually injects the anesthetic, a few drops at a time, with pauses in between.

During this process, you shouldn't feel pressured to go on to actual dental treatment. However, once desensitization has made injection possible, most patients choose to continue. Furthermore, when desensitization has once been successful, it needs little reinforcement. The results are likely to be lasting.

FLOODING, OR IMPLOSION

Some dentists and psychologists use a strategy that, like desensitization, aims to overcome fear by exposing you to whatever causes your fear. But unlike desensitization, this strategy isn't gradual or gentle. Instead, the therapist will direct you to imagine or recall the feared experience in detail—to *flood* your consciousness with the frightening memory. It is believed that such an intense recapitulation, however unpleasant, will cause the fear to collapse upon itself—to *implode*.

Flooding or implosion therapy is most commonly used when dental fear has arisen from past dental treatment that has been painful or frightening or both. Therapists maintain that patients achieve quick and lasting relief. However, it takes great skill to lead a patient through such a traumatic reenactment without producing panic or simply reinforcing the fear. The method is usually best employed by a highly trained mental-health professional—a psychologist or a psychotherapist—rather than by the average dentist.

MODELING

One method of desensitization training has proved especially effective with children. It is called *modeling*, and it consists simply in having the child watch the successful experience of another patient, usually an older child. The fearful child is thus encouraged to learn and imitate the fearless, relaxed behavior of the model.

In the past, dentists used actual children, often older siblings, as models. But since the behavior of children (and of adults, for that matter) is not entirely predictable, this method wasn't always satisfactory. The videocassette has provided dentists with a tool that is just about ideal for the purpose. Using video recordings, dentists can demonstrate in advance virtually any aspect of treatment.

Incidentally, there is no need for children to be afraid of dental treatment. Modern procedures can and should be painless, and dentists, especially those trained in pediatric dentistry, are taught effective methods of reassuring young patients. Nonetheless, under certain circumstances, children do learn dental fear. Their first dental experience may result from a painful traumatic emergency—a broken tooth or a cut mouth. They may be the victims of teasing siblings or playmates who tell them that "going to the dentist" is frightening and painful. Their parents may themselves suffer from dental anxiety, and may communicate this anxiety, despite the best of intentions.

Finally, their dentist just may not have the training, the experience, or the sensitivity to deal with children's natural apprehensions about the uncomfortable and the unknown.

For all these reasons, it is very important for parents to devote as much care in selecting a dentist for their children as they would in selecting a pediatrician. And if your child does show signs of marked dental anxiety, it is important to seek prompt treatment before it becomes deep-seated and habitual.

MEDICATION AND ANESTHETICS

Most dentists prefer to use psychological methods to overcome the psychological problem of dental fear. But sometimes pharmacological methods—medications and anesthetics—are not only appropriate but also unavoidable. There may be no other way of inducing a very fearful patient to accept treatment. Dental emergencies in particular—toothaches, fractures, severe gum inflammation, and the like—may impel the dentist to use these methods not only to control physical pain but also to overcome the patient's terror.

In general, the same medications and anesthetics that are used against pain (see pages 51 and 52) are also used against fear. They range from antianxiety medications such as diazepam (Valium), taken in small doses before treatment, to powerful sedatives, administered intravenously. One of the most widely used is the familiar nitrous oxide—"laughing gas." General anesthesia, however, is seldom used for this purpose; the additional risks don't justify it.

There are several reasons not to use pharmacological methods for treating dental fear or, at least, to use them only sparingly. They do entail certain risks, and often have undesirable side effects. But more important, they offer only temporary relief, and do not attack the problem directly. They enable patients to

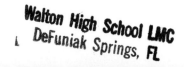

avoid confronting their fear, whereas there is evidence that directly confronting fear is the only sure way to overcome it. Consequently, many dentists will use pharmacological methods only to supplement behavioral techniques such as relaxation training and desensitization.

THE BENEFITS OF FEAR CONTROL

Learning to overcome dental anxiety offers you several benefits. First, of course, it is cru-cially important to your dental health, since fear so often leads to the avoidance of treatment. Overcoming fear also makes treatment itself a far less painful experience, emotionally.

But you may find that the benefits go further. People who suffer dental anxiety are often ashamed of the condition of their teeth, and ashamed of their fear as well. If you are one of these people, overcoming your fear and getting proper dental treatment may significantly improve your self-confidence and self-image. You may not only feel better about your teeth but about yourself as well.

S E V E N

DENTAL ANESTHESIA: THE CONTROL OF PAIN

Many people fear dental treatment because they believe it will be painful. For some, the fear is reinforced by the memory of painful treatment. But there is now no reason for fear—there is no reason for dental treatment to hurt. Modern dentistry has available a wide variety of anesthetics that can prevent pain during virtually any procedure. They range from mild *topical* anesthetics that are applied to specific surfaces, to *general* anesthetics that cause complete unconsciousness.

TOPICAL ANESTHETICS

The "first line" of anesthesia is topical anesthetics. For dental treatment, they are applied to small areas on the surface of the gums, the lining of the mouth, etc., to make them insensitive to pain for a brief period.

Topical anesthetics may take the form of a liquid, a gel, or an aerosol spray. *Lidocaine* and *benzocaine* are the two most widely used. They are absorbed through the surface and

into the soft tissue, where they affect the nerve cells and temporarily block the transmission of sensory impulses to the brain. The area feels numb. Then, as the anesthetic diffuses and dissipates, the effect "wears off," and sensation returns.

Topical anesthetics work only in the immediate area of application. Dentists use them to prevent discomfort from such simple procedures as cleaning the teeth, examining the gums, and treating mild gum inflammation. They can also be applied to block the sensation of the needle prick for *local* anesthesia (see below). And you can apply them yourself to relieve the pain of oral lesions such as canker sores and cold sores.

LOCAL ANESTHETICS

The most widely used anesthetics in dental treatment are *local* anesthetics. Traditionally, they are injected into the soft tissue through a fine, hollow needle. A more recent option is a thin, high-pressure jet, such as the Madajet, which impels the fluid anesthetic directly into the tissue. Dentists use a local anesthetic for such diverse procedures as filling cavities, cleaning out periodontal pockets, removing the pulp in root canals, preparing teeth for artificial crowns or other restorations, and performing minor oral surgery such as tooth extraction.

These anesthetics work in much the same way as topical anesthetics, to block the transmission of nerve impulses. The most widely used, *lidocaine, prilocaine,* and *mepivacaine* wear off fairly quickly. A longer lasting anesthetic, *Marcaine,* is sometimes used either during or after a procedure, for continuing pain control. All these names end in -caine simply because the first local anesthetic used in medicine was cocaine. *Novocaine* ("new cocaine") is a popular term for any local anesthetic, but Novocaine itself is rarely used.

Sometimes other substances are combined with local anesthetics to make them more effective. The most common of these is *epinephrine.* It constricts the blood vessels, minimizing bleeding, and slowing down the diffusion of the anesthetic so its effects last longer. But epinephrine can have side effects that make it an unsuitable choice for certain patients (see page 55).

Dentists inject local anesthetics to achieve either *infiltration* or *nerve block.* For infiltration, the anesthetic is injected into the immediate area to be treated—such as the gum around a single tooth. The numbing effect is largely limited to that area. To achieve nerve block, the anesthetic is injected near one of the major sensory nerves of the jaws. The anesthetic blocks impulses from the whole area served by that nerve—a group of teeth, or perhaps the whole side of a jaw, including the chin, lips, and tongue.

Infiltration generally takes effect faster and wears off sooner than nerve block. Dentists tend to use it for relatively simple, brief treatment such as filling a single tooth. Nerve block is often preferred for a longer, more extensive procedure, such as periodontal surgery or root canal treatment. It is also often used when the soft tissue around a tooth is infected, and the dentist wishes to avoid inserting a needle into it.

Nerve block may be the only possible option during treatment of the lower jaw (mandible). The bone structure, especially toward the back, is so dense that an anesthetic often won't diffuse through it.

Recently, a special form of infiltration, *intraligamental injection,* has come into use when an individual tooth is being treated. The anesthetic is injected under relatively high pressure into the periodontal ligament at one or more points around the tooth. The anesthetic reaches the nerves within the ligament, and numbs the area. This technique can be used to anesthetize even the teeth of the mandible.

For dental procedures, local anesthesia has several advantages: It can be administered easily and painlessly. It has a long record of safety and effectiveness, and the possible risks and side effects (see page 54) are relatively few. The patient remains alert, and needs little or no recovery time afterward. For all but the most extensive treatment, local anesthesia is the technique of choice.

The main drawback is psychological. Many people are afraid of dental treatment in general, and of needles in particular. Sedative medications can reduce this anxiety (see below), and general anesthesia can obliterate it entirely (see page 53). But learning to confront and manage dental fear is the better solution in the long run (see Chapter 6).

SEDATIVES

For long or extensive procedures, dentists often supplement local anesthetics with *sedatives.* These enhance the effectiveness of other anesthetic agents in several ways.

First and foremost, they reduce awareness

and anxiety. You are likely to feel light-headed and euphoric, in a state of "twilight" consciousness between waking and sleeping. They also alter your perception of time, making it seem to pass more quickly. Some sedatives can produce amnesia, so that you have little or no recollection of the experience afterward. And, finally, though they do not directly block pain sensations, they alter and reduce your *perception* of pain. This reduced perception of pain enables the dentist to reduce the amount of anesthetic used.

You can take sedatives orally, if only a small dose is needed. For long procedures, however, dentists often give them by intravenous injection. One of them (nitrous oxide) is inhaled. A wide range of agents is available, and they are often combined for maximum effectiveness and safety—a technique called *balanced anesthesia.* They fall into seven basic categories:

- *Barbiturates* are the active ingredients of many sleeping pills. In large enough doses, they will not only sedate you but also make you unconscious. They have a depressant effect on much of the central nervous system. A wide variety is available, under many brand names. Among those commonly used in dentistry are *methohexital (Brevital), pentobarbital (Nembutal),* and *thiopental (Pentothal).*
- *Nonbarbiturate hypnotics* differ chemically from barbiturates, but work in much the same way. At relatively low doses, they are sedatives. At higher doses, they are *hypnotic*—they put you to sleep. The most common are *chloral hydrate* and *glutethimide.* They are more frequently used in treating children than adults.
- *Antianxiety medications,* also known as *minor tranquilizers,* work more selectively than barbiturates, and affect the parts of your brain that control emotions. They directly reduce anxiety and induce muscle relaxation. The most common are the

benzodiazepines. Chlordiazepoxide (Librium) is generally taken orally to reduce anxiety before treatment. *Diazepam (Valium)* can be taken orally or it can be injected intravenously during treatment. *Midazolam (Versed)* is administered only by injection.
- *Narcotics* diminish the perception of pain. The best known is *morphine,* derived from opium. It is seldom used as a conscious sedative. The most common narcotic sedatives are *meperidine (Demerol)* and, more recently, *fentanyl (Sublimaze).*
- *Antihistamines* are best known as medications that relieve allergic reactions, such as hay fever. But some of them have significant sedative effects as well. The most widely used antihistamines are *promethazine (Phenergan), diphenhydramine (Benadryl),* and *hydroxysine (Atarax, Vistaril).*
- *Ketamine* is a powerful *dissociative* drug. It can make you feel totally detached from your surroundings. Like other sedatives, it also greatly reduces pain and produces amnesia. It is more often used for children than for adults.
- *Nitrous oxide,* a compound of nitrogen and oxygen, is probably the most common sedative used in dentistry—going back for more than a century. It is still among the safest and most popular. It is inhaled, along with oxygen, through an anesthetic mask. It causes giddiness and euphoria—hence the popular name "laughing gas." Nitrous oxide has two advantages over several of the other sedatives: it has few unpleasant side effects and it wears off quickly. Although not a true analgesic, it diminishes anxiety and has the effect of raising the pain threshold.

GENERAL ANESTHESIA

General anesthesia, producing complete unconsciousness, is customarily used for procedures such as major oral surgery, in which the patient must remain profoundly anesthetized and completely relaxed for a considerable period of time. It can, however, be used for any kind of treatment, and some extremely anxious patients cannot be treated without it.

But local anesthesia is safer and easier to manage. General anesthetics do more than just "put you to sleep." They also relax the muscles, and block many of your body's *autonomic reflexes*. These include the "gag" reflex that protects you from swallowing substances other than food, and the reflex that keeps you from "swallowing the wrong way"—drawing foreign matter into the passages to your lungs. Under deep general anesthesia, even your breathing reflexes may be affected, so breathing may have to be artificially assisted for the duration of the operation.

Only someone with special training—a medical or dental anesthesiologist or an oral surgeon—should administer a general anesthetic. And its administration should take place either in a hospital operating room or its office equivalent.

In larger doses, many of the agents used as sedatives could also serve as general anesthetics. But sedatives are used more frequently as preparatory, or "bridge," medications—to reduce anxiety and tension before general anesthesia.

Most general anesthetics are gases that are inhaled. The first ones to be used, chloroform and ether, are now obsolete. They have been replaced by *halothane (Fluothane), methoxyflurane (Ethrane),* and *isoflurane (Forane).*

General anesthetics are initially administered through an anesthetic mask, which covers your nose and mouth. Then, when you become unconscious, this mask is replaced by one that covers only your nose, or by a flexible tube passing through the nose to the throat. The anesthetics take effect quickly—in a minute or two—but because they are absorbed so widely into your system, they may take several hours to wear off.

NEUROLEPTIC ANESTHESIA

Some dentists use a technique called *neuroleptic* anesthesia. It includes the use of one of the *major tranquilizers,* or *neuroleptics.* The most common choice is *droperidol (Inapsine).* This is combined with a narcotic, usually *fentanyl* (page 53), and administered intravenously. You may be given nitrous oxide (page 53) as well.

The degree of anesthesia varies, depending on the amount of anesthetic used. Lighter doses produce a light sleep, in which you feel detached and free of discomfort, but are not completely unconscious. The effect is more powerful than that of local anesthetics, but your protective reflexes are not blocked.

Higher doses may produce general anesthesia—they make you completely unconscious. But recovering from neuroleptic anesthesia is likely to take less time than recovery from inhaled general anesthetics.

RISKS AND SIDE EFFECTS

Generally speaking, all anesthetics in current use are safe. The percentage of patients experiencing unpleasant or dangerous consequences is extremely low. Nevertheless, there are certain risks and side effects that you ought to be aware of in giving your informed consent to treatment.

These risks and side effects vary considerably. Local anesthetics cause fewer and less severe problems than sedatives. Sedatives, in turn, are less likely to have undesirable consequences than general anesthetics. Patients with certain medical disorders, such as heart disease, hypertension, asthma, sickle cell anemia, and diabetes (see Chapter 20) are more likely to experience difficulties, and may have to avoid particular anesthetics. Expectant mothers should avoid anesthesia except in emergencies—especially during the first three months and the last three months of their pregnancies. Sedatives and general anesthetics should not be given to patients who have a fever, a cold, or other acute upper respiratory infections.

Certain precautions are taken to prevent accidents and other complications. For example, a pack of gauze or similar material may be placed in the back of your mouth, to keep foreign matter from being swallowed or (worse) inhaled into your lungs. Contact lenses are generally removed, and your eyes may be covered.

LOCAL ANESTHETICS

Perhaps the most common risk in local anesthesia is fainting (*syncope*). It is essentially a response to stress—either emotional stress from anxiety or physical stress from the actual administration of the anesthetic. In either event, the body's reflexes reduce the output of blood from the heart, thus lowering blood flow to the brain. You may temporarily lose consciousness, or you may just feel chilly, clammy, dizzy, or nauseated.

Fainting is less likely to occur if you are lying down so the blood can flow more easily to your head. Reducing anxiety can also be helpful, either with sedatives or by measures to overcome dental fear (see Chapter 6).

There is one risk that the design of modern injection syringes has greatly reduced—the risk of inadvertently injecting the anesthetic into a blood vessel. When that happens, the anesthetic may disperse too fast from the area to be treated, reducing its effectiveness. Or the anesthetic may be carried into your system, where it may cause fainting, irregular

heartbeat, headache, or temporary mental confusion.

Rarely, the needle used for injection may contaminate tissue with bacteria from the mouth, and an infection may result. The needle may also cause bleeding or bruise the soft tissue. And either the needle or the injected anesthetic can irritate nearby muscles, causing a condition called *trismus*—the muscles are sore, and you may find it difficult to open your mouth. All these complications are usually temporary, and more annoying than dangerous.

Sometimes the anesthetic will affect nerves other than those it is intended to affect. The tongue and lips may be numb and immobile, or one eyelid may droop. In rare instances, a patient may suffer blurred or double vision, or even temporary blindness. If the anesthetic is injected into the roof of the mouth (the *palate*) the sensation of swallowing may be lost, and gagging may result. These conditions, too, are temporary, and usually require no special treatment.

Even more rarely, negative reactions to the anesthetic itself may occur. Some patients may be allergic to the agent, or to other ingredients in the solution. Epinephrine, which is often added to local anesthetics to augment their effectiveness, may temporarily make the heart race, or beat irregularly. Patients with heart disease or hypertension may need a formulation that doesn't contain this stimulant.

Your dentist is likely to instruct you not to eat or chew until the anesthetic has completely worn off. There's a good reason for this. Without the protection of sensation, there's a good chance that you may accidentally chew your cheek or tongue.

SEDATIVES

With the possible exception of nitrous oxide, sedatives have much more powerful and more lasting effects on the central nervous system than local anesthetics have. You may have symptoms no more severe than drowsiness and lack of alertness, which make certain activities (such as driving) unwise until the effects of the medication have completely worn off. In more extreme instances, some sedatives may produce temporary mental confusion, or even hallucinations. If a patient is anxious about treatment, the anxiety is likely to return as the effects of the sedative wear off.

Some sedatives, such as narcotics, and nitrous oxide in high doses, may upset the stomach and cause nausea and vomiting. Some of them depress the functions of the body sufficiently to produce dizziness and fainting.

During treatment, sedatives are often given by continuous intravenous injection. Sometimes blood from the vein may leak into nearby tissues, creating an unsightly but temporary bruise (a *hematoma*). The needle may also produce small blood clots in the vein, causing painful inflammation. This is usually mild, and can be treated with minor analgesics or a topical anesthetic ointment until it subsides. In rare instances, however, the inflammation is more severe and persistent, and affects a larger portion of the vein. This condition, called *thrombophlebitis*, may require more extensive treatment, such as an *anticoagulant*, a drug that dissolves clots.

Perhaps the most serious risk of sedatives, especially when relatively large doses are administered, is that they may not simply produce sedation but also general anesthesia—they may make you lose consciousness, and block your body's protective reflexes (see page 54). There is then a danger that foreign material will be drawn into the breathing passages, or even into the lungs. Neuroleptic anesthesia carries the same risk.

GENERAL ANESTHETICS

Because general anesthetics affect the body so profoundly, they pose more risks, and re-

quire a much longer recovery period. Patients often suffer mild sore throats after anesthesia, either because the nasal tube has irritated the throat lining, or the inhaled anesthetic has dried it out. Headaches and nausea may occur, as may faintness, dizziness, and heart palpitations.

The physical position of the patient and the equipment during general anesthesia is very important. Improper positioning can place undesirable pressures on nerves in the arms, legs, or head, resulting in temporary numbness or even paralysis. Moreover, the mouth should not be kept wide open for a long period of time while the muscles are relaxed—damages to the temporomandibular joints can result.

The greatest danger during general anesthesia is that the patient, for any of several reasons, may not get sufficient oxygen. For example, the tube supplying the mixture of anesthetic and oxygen may become kinked or blocked, or it may not be correctly placed to inflate both lungs. Also, the airway to the lungs may be blocked if the patient should vomit during the operation. That is why you are required to fast for up to 12 hours beforehand. Lack of sufficient oxygen, even for a period of minutes, can cause severe damage to the brain and other organs, or even death.

POSTOPERATIVE PAIN RELIEVERS

Anesthesia can prevent pain during treatment, but procedures such as root canal therapy, extraction, and oral surgery inevitably damage the tissues, and cause some measure of postoperative discomfort or pain. Thus, anesthesia is followed up by analgesics until healing begins. These vary according to whether pain is mild, moderate, or severe.

ANALGESICS FOR MILD PAIN

For mild postoperative pain, one of the best analgesics is ice. Cold tends to prevent or reduce swelling, which is a significant cause of pain. Cold also has an anesthetic effect on the nerves that transmit pain impulses to the brain. Ice is simply applied by putting it in a plastic bag, wrapped in a moist cloth. One precaution: apply ice for only 20 minutes in any hour. Longer contact can damage your skin.

After procedures like periodontal treatment, rinsing the mouth with a mild solution of salt or baking soda, or with an antiseptic mouthwash, can be soothing. Topical anesthetics (page 51) may also be prescribed, either as a mouthwash or an ointment.

The two most widely used analgesics are aspirin *(acetylsalicylic acid)* and *acetaminophen* (as, for example, *Tylenol, Datril).* Acetaminophen is considered to be the safer of the two. The acid in aspirin can upset the stomach (though coated forms reduce this effect). Aspirin also diminishes clotting of the blood, so it should not be used if bleeding is likely to be a problem. Finally, aspirin has recently been connected with a rare but serious childhood disease called *Reye's syndrome,* and pediatricians now recommend that aspirin not be given to children with any sort of respiratory infection, and especially influenza.

Some over-the-counter analgesics combine aspirin or acetaminophen with the stimulant caffeine. Some patients find these combinations more effective than aspirin or acetaminophen alone.

Nonsteroidal anti-inflammatory drugs (NSAIDs) are ordinarily used to relieve inflamed muscles and joints. But many people also find them effective as general analgesics. One of the most popular of these is *ibuprofen.* Mild formulations (such as *Advil* and *Motrin*) are available over the counter. Another common NSAID is diflunisal *(Dolobid).* Sometimes these medications are prescribed for use *before* treatment—a process called *pre-loading.*

Another relatively recent technique for relieving pain is *transcutaneous electrical nerve stimulation (TENS). Transcutaneous* means "across or through the skin." A TENS machine passes short pulses of mild electrical current through electrodes placed on the skin. These electrical signals "compete" with pain signals, and inhibit the nerves from transmitting them to the brain. Formerly, TENS treatment could only be provided in a professional office, but portable units are now available, for use at home.

ANALGESICS FOR MODERATE OR SEVERE PAIN

Most medications to relieve moderate or severe pain have a *narcotic* (page 53) as their most active ingredient. Narcotics are effective against pain, but they can cause psychological and physical dependence. They are available only by prescription, and should be used for only brief periods.

Narcotics vary in strength. Relatively mild ones usually contain *codeine,* often mixed with aspirin or acetaminophen. Moderately strong formulations, such as *Darvon* and *Dolene,* may be based upon *propoxyphene,* or they may contain *meperidine,* which is also used as a sedative. *Demerol* is a familiar brand. The strongest medications contain such narcotics as *oxycodone (Percodan, Percocet,* or *Tylox)* or *hydromorphone (Dilaudid),* which are almost as potent as morphine.

SPECIAL ANESTHETIC TECHNIQUES: HYPNOSIS AND ACUPUNCTURE

Some dentists make use of anesthetic techniques that are now considered unconventional but have long traditions behind them. Neither hypnosis nor acupuncture is completely understood, in terms of Western science, but both have been proven effective, at least for certain patients. Often they are not used by themselves, but as adjuncts to more conventional anesthesia. They appear to be especially useful as sedatives, to diminish anxiety and encourage relaxation.

Hypnosis artificially induces a state of consciousness that in some respects resembles sleep. The attention of the subject is heightened but narrowly focused, and is strongly affected by suggestions from the hypnotist. Thus, it can be used to produce feelings of relaxation and comfort and to block pain from consciousness.

Acupuncture follows a tradition in China that goes back thousands of years. Fine needles are used to pierce specific areas of skin and muscle, to prevent or relieve pain in other parts of the body. To stop pain in the teeth and mouth, for example, the needle is often inserted through the pad of muscle between the thumb and forefinger of one hand. The subject is said to feel hardly any pain from the needle itself, but merely sensations of tingling and numbness. There is experimental evidence that acupuncture works by stimulating the body's production of *endorphins*—chemicals naturally produced in the body that hinder the transmission of pain to the brain.

Neither hypnosis nor acupuncture is effective for everyone. And no one knows precisely how to predict which patients will be helped. Nonetheless, they have proved useful in many cases, including cases in which other anesthetics have failed.

EIGHT

TOOTH DECAY
AND OPERATIVE DENTISTRY

Teeth, like bones, are *hard tissues*—the densest, strongest tissues of your body. The outer layer of the crowns, the enamel, is the hardest substance of all, and can withstand many years of wear from chewing. Yet teeth have an often fatal weakness: under certain conditions, they will surely and quickly decay.

Restoration of decayed teeth is called *operative dentistry*. Along with preventive care, it is a basic component of the general dentist's practice.

CAUSES OF TOOTH DECAY

There are three necessary conditions for tooth decay. To minimize decay, you must pay attention to all three.

- *Bacteria in the mouth*. The warm, moist interior of your mouth is a rich environment for bacteria, and your mouth is full of them. Bacterial species that digest sugar, such as *Streptococcus mutans* and *Lactobacillus acidophilus*, are thought to be

especially responsible for tooth decay.
- *Food for bacteria*. To survive and reproduce, bacteria need food. Decay-producing bacteria need a particular kind of food: sugar, in any of its forms. The diet of modern society is rich in sugar, which is why tooth decay is sometimes described as a "disease of civilization."
- *Teeth susceptible to decay*. Susceptibility to decay depends, to some extent, on heredity. Also, the teeth of children and adolescents are generally more susceptible than those of adults. And certain diseases and other conditions that occur in childhood, when the teeth are developing, can make them more susceptible. But few people of any age have teeth that completely resist decay, and decay is especially likely to occur on certain tooth surfaces.

THE PROCESS OF TOOTH DECAY

Tooth decay is a gradual, step-by-step process, which ordinarily begins at the outer

STAGES OF TOOTH DECAY

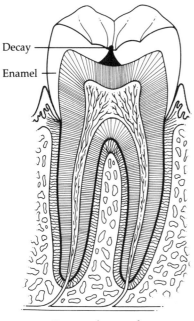

Decay

Enamel

Decay of enamel

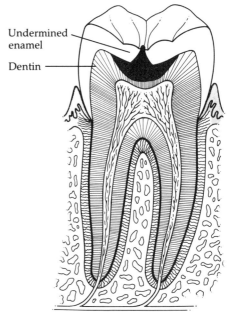

Undermined enamel

Dentin

Decay of dentin

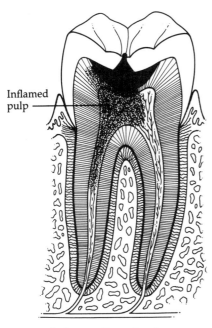

Inflamed pulp

Inflammation of pulp

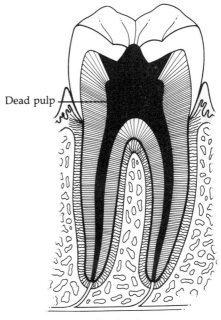

Dead pulp

Death of pulp

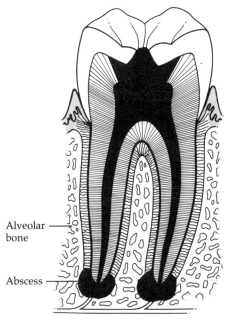

Alveolar bone

Abscess

Abscess formation

face. There the acids react chemically with the minerals in the enamel, and dissolve them. Decay usually begins with a tiny pit on the surface, which enlarges to become a cone-shaped "soft spot" of partly dissolved enamel.

Since enamel is made up almost entirely of minerals and contains no living cells, this stage of decay is usually painless. It is also likely to be invisible—at least to you. During a routine examination, your dentist may find evidence of it with the fine end of an explorer. It may also show up as a small "shadow" of reduced density on a tooth in a dental X-ray.

The process of decay is kept going by giving the bacteria additional food—more sugar. The longer and more often sugar is fed to the bacteria, the more acid will be produced, and the faster the decay. Untreated, it will eventually reach the dentin that forms the main substance of the tooth.

layer of enamel, penetrates the dentin, and may finally reach the pulp. Although various theories have been advanced, there is general agreement that the process starts with the formation of *plaque*.

PLAQUE FORMATION AND ENAMEL DECAY

As noted above, your mouth normally contains large numbers of bacteria, and many of these bacteria digest sugar. Among the by-products of sugar digestion are acids, particularly *lactic acid*. As long as the bacteria float freely in the saliva, they do little harm. But if they remain undisturbed on your teeth, they tend to combine with food debris and their own digestive products, to form a sticky, concentrated film. This film is called *dental plaque*, or simply *plaque*.

Plaque holds the acids released by bacteria in firm, prolonged contact with the tooth sur-

PENETRATION OF THE DENTIN

Dentin is part minerals and part slender, tubular extensions of living cells called *odontoblasts*. Both can decay. The minerals can be dissolved by acids, and the odontoblasts can be infected by bacteria. Damaged odontoblasts can "communicate" chemically with the nerve cells of the pulp. Thus, at this stage, you may begin to sense decay—your tooth may become sensitive in various ways, or may begin to ache. However, it must be emphasized that decay in the dentin may cause no symptoms that you're aware of.

Decay spreads faster in dentin than in enamel. It tends to form a second, soft "cone" of disintegrated material under the enamel. Even if there is sound enamel above this decayed dentin, it becomes undermined, and is likely to collapse. At this stage, the damage may become an observable hole, or *cavity*.

PENETRATION OF THE PULP

Eventually, decay may reach the pulp of the tooth, which contains the blood vessels and nerves. At this stage, the tooth is likely to ache. Inflamed soft tissues attempt to swell, but are restricted by the hard tooth, a process that often causes intense pain. Even at this stage, though, there may be no symptoms, which is one reason why regular checkups are so important.

The survival of the tooth is now at stake. Irritation or infection may cause the pulp to die, and may also lead to the formation of a severely inflamed hollow, called an *abscess,* under the root. Usually these conditions can be remedied by *endodontic* treatment (see Chapter 12), but sometimes the tooth must be extracted.

Moreover, infection from abscessed teeth may spread through the bloodstream to other parts of the body, causing serious illness. For some patients, especially those with certain heart diseases or conditions, such infections can be quite dangerous (see page 219).

PREVENTION OF TOOTH DECAY

The best "cure" for tooth decay is to prevent it. All three of the conditions necessary for decay should be considered. The best way to reduce susceptibility to decay is through the use of fluorides (see page 86). You can reduce the food supply for bacteria by minimizing sugar in your diet. And the buildup of bacterial plaque can be controlled by a twofold program of conscientious home care and regular professional care.

LOCATION OF CAVITIES

Tooth decay tends to occur most often on certain surfaces of the teeth, here listed in order of prevalence:

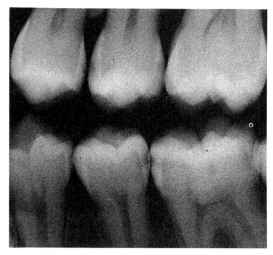

Evidence of decay on X-ray of teeth (lower center)

- Grooves of the back teeth—molars and premolars—readily trap food particles and bacteria. Some may have *fissures:* deep, narrow crevices that are virtually impossible to keep clean.
- *Proximal surfaces*—surfaces between adjacent teeth—also require a special effort to keep clean, especially at the *contact points* where one tooth actually touches another.
- Around the neck of each tooth, at the base of the crown, the edges of the gums form a loose "cuff." In this cuff is a shallow, V-shaped depression called a *sulcus,* where food and bacteria are likely to collect. Moreover, in later life, the gums tend to recede, exposing some of the relatively soft *cementum* that covers the root of the tooth.

DETERMINING THE EXTENT OF TREATMENT

Once your dentist has identified decay in a tooth, the severity of the damage is likely to determine how extensively it must be treated.

If the decayed area is very small, and extends only slightly into the enamel, the dentist may choose to leave it alone. Sometimes the enamel will absorb minerals from saliva and repair itself. The dentist will note any such tooth on your chart, for examination at the next regular visit.

If decay extends only into the enamel, the dentist may nonetheless choose to treat it. Early repair of the enamel is relatively easy to accomplish and gives the dentist a wider choice of materials to use. It also helps keep the decay from proceeding further.

If decay has penetrated the dentin, the dentist will almost surely choose to treat it, if only to make sure it doesn't reach the pulp. If possible, the dentist will simply remove the decay and insert a filling. But sometimes the decay is so extensive, and the tooth so fragile, that it must be restored with an artificial crown.

If decay has reached the pulp, the survival of the tooth is at stake, and may require root canal therapy. In very severe cases, the tooth may have to be extracted.

PREPARATION OF CAVITIES

The first step in treating a decayed tooth is to prepare the cavity (or cavities) for restoration. The decay must be removed, along with any enamel that is not supported by sound dentin underneath. The cavity must also be shaped so the filling can be snugly fitted and securely anchored in place.

There is no reason for the process to hurt. The dentist should use whatever method is appropriate to prevent pain. In most instances, this will include the application of a topical anesthetic, followed by a numbing injection of a local anesthetic. If you are especially apprehensive about treatment, you may benefit from special treatment for dental fear (see Chapter 6).

Once anesthesia is administered, the dentist tries to minimize contamination from the bacteria in saliva. The dentist may insert rolls of absorbent cotton or gauze near the tooth, or may surround it with a *rubber dam*—a thin rubber sheet that forms a kind of protective apron around the base of the crown.

The dentist may also place a *saliva ejector*— a tube attached to a suction pump—in your mouth, and may ask you to hold it in place. And the dentist's assistant may periodically use stronger, high-speed suction to keep saliva, water, and debris out of the working area.

Cleaning out decay and shaping the cavity is performed mainly with *handpieces* fitted with a variety of cutting *burs* (see page 21). Handpieces may also direct air, water, or a mixture of both into the cavity, to control heat caused by friction and to flush away debris.

A high-speed handpiece is generally used to cut through enamel. This may be supplemented by a lower-speed handpiece, to clean out decayed dentin. Manual instruments, such as spoon-shaped scrapers, may also be used.

In recent years, traditional handpieces have been supplemented with special machines that impel thin jets of chemicals into

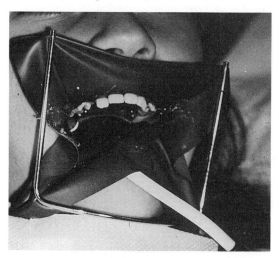

Teeth isolated by rubber dam

the cavity, dissolving the decay. These machines seldom replace a handpiece entirely, but are most often used in the same way a low-speed handpiece is, to remove decayed dentin. In the future, laser energy may be harnessed for this function.

If possible, the dentist will avoid penetrating the dentin completely, since the pulp can be easily and fatally damaged by infection or trauma. If the pulp is indeed exposed, the dentist will have to use special procedures to protect it (pages 67–68).

Once the cavity is shaped, it is cleaned and dried. It should now be free of contamination, and ready for restoration. The remaining steps of the process will vary considerably, depending upon the specific materials used for the filling.

FILLING MATERIALS

There is no single, ideal material for dental fillings. Each type has advantages and disadvantages, which you and the dentist should weigh in making a choice. The materials most dentists now use are *silver amalgam, gold, composites,* and *porcelain.*

SILVER AMALGAM

The most common filling material is a mixture, or *amalgam,* of silver with mercury, alloyed with small amounts of other metals. When first prepared, it has a soft, putty-like consistency, which can be readily shaped to fit the cavity and carved to match the original tooth surface. It then gradually hardens, like concrete, to a stable, solid filling.

Silver amalgam is most often used to fill cavities in relatively inconspicuous teeth, such as molars. It is the quickest, easiest, and most cost-effective filling material the dentist can use; and it has a record of effectiveness

and safety going back more than a century. It is long-lasting, wear-resistant, and *biocompatible*—that is, it is relatively unlikely to irritate living tissue such as the dentin or pulp of the tooth or the adjacent ligament and gums. If properly used, it completely seals the cavity, and this seal remains stable over time.

Silver amalgam does have disadvantages. It is brittle, and requires support from the surrounding tooth to keep it from chipping or shattering. Thus, it is not suitable for extensive restorations, or for surfaces, such as biting edges, that are subjected to heavy chewing pressure.

Another potential disadvantage is that silver amalgam isn't actually cemented to the cavity walls. It is held in place by a close frictional fit, plus *undercutting* the cavity to "lock in" the filling when it hardens. Occasionally an amalgam filling becomes loose and falls out, or allows bacteria to invade around its edges.

For many people, the chief disadvantage of silver amalgam is how it looks. It has a

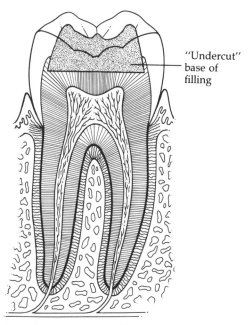

"Undercut" base of filling

Silver amalgam filling

naturally dark, very conspicuous color that contrasts sharply with the natural color of tooth enamel. Furthermore, over time, it may discolor the enamel around it. Most people don't like it on any visible tooth surface. Thus its use tends to be limited to the back teeth—particularly their tops and inside surfaces.

In recent years, the safety of silver amalgam has been questioned because it contains mercury. Mercury is indeed a dangerous poison—but no danger has been shown to result from dental fillings. You need not fear having cavities restored with this material. Even more important, as long as your present amalgam fillings are basically sound, you should not have them removed and replaced with some other material.

GOLD

This durable, corrosion-free metal also has a long record of successful use in dental restorations. In the past, it was often applied in the form of *gold leaf*—thin, flexible sheets worked into the cavity, and compacted there with hand instruments. Today, most gold fillings are solid—cast in a mold of the cavity, and cemented in place.

Even more than silver, gold is long lasting, wear resistant, and biocompatible. It is *not* brittle. Rather, it is so strong that it can actually reinforce the tooth to which it is attached, and can be used to restore exposed biting surfaces. It has a lighter, less conspicuous tonality than silver, and does not discolor the surrounding enamel.

However, gold fillings look unquestionably artificial. Many people prefer not to have them used on highly visible tooth surfaces. They are also expensive—because of the cost of the metal and because of the time and skill it takes to fabricate and insert them properly. Finally, some patients object to gold fillings because the insertion process requires at least two office visits.

COMPOSITES

Composites are a varied group of materials that have two main ingredients: a *binder* of plastic resin and a *filler* of finely ground, glass-like particles. These ingredients are mixed together and applied to the tooth in thin layers, which are then chemically hardened, or *cured.*

The most outstanding characteristic of composites is their color. They are naturally white, and can be toned to make a reasonably close match with any tooth color. Thus, dentists often use them to restore cavities on the highly visible tooth surfaces toward the front of the mouth.

Used with the proper bonding agents, composites form (at least initially) a strong attachment with the adjacent tooth surface, and require a minimum of support. Like silver amalgam (but unlike gold or porcelain), composite fillings can be inserted in a single office visit.

Composites, however, are not as strong as metal fillings. They are somewhat brittle and subject to abrasion. Thus, many dentists do not consider them suitable for areas that receive heavy wear, such as the biting surfaces of the molars and premolars, unless the cavities being filled are very small and shallow.

Composites are not as biocompatible as silver amalgam or gold, and must be carefully separated from dentin and pulp with *bases* or *liners* (page 66). Though they match teeth closely when they are first inserted, their color may change, and they are easily stained.

The main drawback of composites is their impermanence. Over time, boundaries between the tooth and the filling tend to open up. These "leaky" boundaries invite renewed invasion by bacteria. As a result, composite fillings are likely to require periodic replacement.

Incidentally, composites are sometimes mistakenly described as "porcelain." They do resemble porcelain but are very different in composition.

PORCELAIN

Porcelain is a ceramic material, like that used for fine china. Porcelain fillings are customarily formed in a mold of the prepared cavity, hardened by baking and then cemented in place. Like composites, porcelain restorations can be colored to match adjoining teeth, and are considered especially suitable for restorations on visible tooth surfaces.

Porcelain has the same main advantage as a composite: it can be made to look like tooth enamel. But it is longer lasting and more resistant to wear than any composite, it forms a better boundary with the tooth, and it resists staining.

Porcelain has certain disadvantages as well. Unlike gold, it is brittle—somewhat more so, in fact, than silver amalgam. Like gold, and unlike silver or composites, porcelain fillings require at least two office visits. And like gold fillings, they require time, skill, and special equipment, which make them relatively expensive.

PREPARATIONS FOR RESTORATION: BASES AND LINERS

Before inserting any filling material into a prepared cavity, the dentist may have to place a *base* or a *liner* on the cavity surface. The main difference between bases and liners is thickness. Bases are applied fairly thickly; liners are more like paint, and are applied thinly.

The main function of bases and liners is to insulate the pulp from irritation (especially heat and cold, and the chemicals in composites), which could kill the nerve. The deeper the cavity, the more protection is required. Bases and liners act to separate the filling from the cavity surface and to seal off the dentin tubules that might carry contaminants to the pulp.

The most common liner has *calcium hydroxide* as its main ingredient. It is used especially

in cavities that are close to the pulp, for it not only protects the pulp but also encourages the formation of dentin.

Even after it hardens, calcium hydroxide is not very strong. It is often supplemented with layers of other materials, which provide more support to the overlying filling. These other bases and liners may be used by themselves in cavities that are relatively shallow. But if the cavity is close to the pulp, calcium hydroxide must be inserted first—no other base or liner leads to the formation of new dentin.

Other commonly used bases include *zinc phosphate,* and *zinc oxide* mixed with *eugenol.* These provide more support than calcium hydroxide; zinc phosphate is particularly strong. The zinc oxide mixture is often useful if the tooth is sensitive. Eugenol (oil of cloves) has a long record of effectiveness as a sedative for inflamed nerves. (Incidentally, it is responsible for the characteristic odor of dental offices.)

At present, dentists are making more frequent use of *glass ionomer cements,* both as bases and liners. Their main advantage is that they *are* cements and thus adhere to the cavity surface. They also release tooth-protecting fluorides. But the chemicals in them are somewhat irritating to the pulp, and they are primarily used with a calcium hydroxide liner.

A material in long use as a liner is *dental varnish,* copal resin dissolved in ether. It seals off the dentin tubules and helps desensitize the nerve. It is most often used under silver amalgam fillings.

Some bases and liners can only be used with certain kinds of fillings. For example, zinc oxide and eugenol cannot be used with composites because they react chemically with the plastic binders and keep them from hardening properly.

Sometimes a dentist will choose not to use a base or liner. Silver amalgam, for example, is relatively inert, and not as likely as some other fillings to cause irritation.

PULP CAPPING

If decay extends to the pulp of the tooth, it is likely that the nerve will die, and that root canal therapy will be necessary. But the dentist may try to keep the nerve alive with a *pulp cap*. There are two basic pulp capping procedures: *direct* and *indirect*.

Direct pulp capping is used when the removal of decay actually exposes the pulp. The dentist places a protective layer of calcium hydroxide over the pulp, and may apply a sedative layer of zinc oxide and eugenol over that. The dentist may then choose to insert either a *permanent* filling, or a *temporary* filling of zinc oxide and eugenol.

If the pulp cap is successful, the nerve should slowly pull away from the calcium hydroxide, forming a small gap in which new dentin forms. After a few weeks or months, the dentist will determine whether the pulp is alive and healthy. If it is, the temporary filling (if used) will be replaced. But if the nerve is inflamed or dead, root canal therapy will be necessary.

Indirect pulp capping may be appropriate if the dentin next to the pulp is softened but not completely destroyed by decay. The dentist leaves at least some of this softened dentin on the floor of the cavity. Again, calcium hydroxide is applied as a liner, and covered with a temporary filling of zinc oxide.

After a few weeks or months, the dentist removes the temporary filling. Sometimes, not only has new dentin formed, but the softened dentin has also remineralized. A permanent filling can then be inserted. If remineralization has not occurred, the remaining decay is removed, and a direct pulp cap is applied. But if there is evidence that the nerve has died, root canal therapy will be necessary.

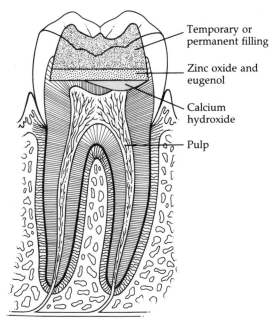

Direct pulp capping

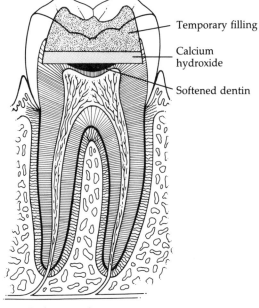

Indirect pulp capping

RESTORATION PROCEDURES

Once a cavity has been completely prepared, the procedures for restoration will vary considerably, according to the materials used (silver amalgam, composite, gold, or porcelain).

SILVER AMALGAM

Silver amalgam is the quickest and easiest material to insert into a cavity. Since the amalgam does not adhere to the tooth, and since no cement is used, the cavity requires special preparation—it must be slightly *undercut*, to "lock" the filling in place (see illustration page 64).

If the cavity is very extensive, undercutting alone may not suffice. The dentist may drill small holes into the sound tooth around the cavity, and then insert reinforcing pins (rather like reinforcing rods in concrete) to help fasten the filling in place.

Shortly before the amalgam is to be used, its components are mixed together in an *amalgamator*—a machine like a miniature paint shaker. The dentist picks up the putty-like amalgam in a tubular *carrier*, and transfers a little of it at a time to the cavity. A *plugger* or *condenser* is used to drive the material firmly into all parts of the cavity and to form it into a homogeneous whole. This may be a blunt-ended hand instrument, or a small mechanical hammer attached to a handpiece.

The cavity is overfilled, and the still soft amalgam is then carved back to match the original contours of the tooth. If the filling is on a biting surface, the dentist will use *articulating paper* to check the mesh with the opposing teeth. When you bite on the paper, it transfers marks to the teeth and to the filling at the points of contact. If the filling is too high, it can be reduced.

The dentist must sometimes use a special technique to fill a cavity on the side of a tooth—especially a cavity on a *proximal surface* next to an adjacent tooth. A *matrix* of very

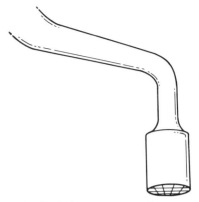

Head of plugger, or condenser

thin sheet metal is wrapped around the crown of the tooth, and a small triangular wedge is pushed into the interproximal space at the gumline. The matrix and wedge create a kind of mold or form, which replaces the missing wall of the tooth while the amalgam is being inserted. They are then removed, and the surface is carved as usual.

The amalgam must be inserted quickly; the material begins to harden after a few minutes. And once it has hardened, no further amalgam can be added to it.

Amalgam becomes solid within an hour or so, and reaches its full strength after 24 hours. After treatment, the dentist will probably advise you not to eat anything for an hour and

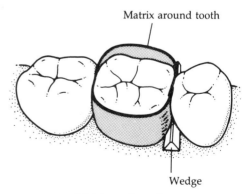

Matrix around tooth

Wedge

Matrix and wedge

a half, and certainly not until the anesthetic has completely worn off. You should also try not to chew on that side for 24 hours.

The dentist may have you return a day or so later, to have the filling polished. This procedure helps keep plaque from sticking to the surface. But many dentists (and many patients) don't find it worth the bother of a special visit, and postpone it until the next regular cleaning appointment.

COMPOSITES

Unlike other types of fillings, composites actually adhere to the walls of cavities, and no particular cavity shape is required. The final step in cavity preparation is etching the enamel surface with acid to make it rougher and more adhesive.

Next, the dentist brushes one or more coats of a liquid plastic *bonding agent* onto the cavity surface. The bonding agent is then chemically hardened, or *cured*. Some bonding agents self-cure; others are cured by shining a very bright light on them for up to 30 seconds.

Then the dentist applies the doughy, tooth-colored composite. It tends to shrink as it dries, and the more thickly it is applied, the more it shrinks. It is therefore laid on in successive thin layers, which readily stick to one another before they fully harden.

When the layers of composite are built up to the desired level, they, too, are cured to harden them. Their outer surfaces are then carved and polished.

Composites are often used to restore cavities on the proximal surfaces of visible teeth. A matrix somewhat similar to that used for silver amalgam may have to be placed around the tooth, to shape the restoration and hold it in place until it hardens. Since composites are often cured with light, the matrix used is transparent mylar plastic, rather than metal.

Once composite fillings have been cured, they are as hard as they will ever be. When the anesthetic wears off, you don't have to delay chewing on the restored tooth.

CAST GOLD AND PORCELAIN

Procedures for cast gold and porcelain fillings are similar, since both must be fabricated outside the mouth, and then inserted and cemented in place.

Cast fillings require at least two visits. At the first, the dentist prepares the cavity. The cavity for a cast restoration, unlike that for amalgam, must not be undercut, but rather must taper slightly toward the bottom, so the solid filling can be slid into place.

The dentist then takes an impression of the tooth and cavity. The procedure is much the same as for a diagnostic impression (see page 24), but a material that makes a more highly detailed impression is used, and it takes longer (five to seven minutes) to become firm. A temporary filling, which is sometimes made of a base such as zinc oxide (pages 66 and 67), or sometimes an acrylic plastic, is then inserted, to protect the cavity from contamination and fracture until the next visit.

In a dental laboratory, a plaster mold is cast from the impression, and the filling is fabricated to fit the cavity. The fit is crucial; it must be snug, yet not so tight that the filling cannot be inserted.

During the second visit, the temporary filling is removed. The dentist places the permanent filling in the cavity and checks it for fit and for its effect on the bite. The outer surface of the filling is ordinarily fabricated a little "high," so it can be trimmed to an exact fit.

The procedures for gold and porcelain fillings differ slightly. A gold filling is usually removed for trimming, and then replaced and cemented in place. A porcelain filling is brittle, so any recontouring should be done *after* it is cemented to the supporting tooth.

Both gold and porcelain fillings are cemented in place. For gold, any of several permanent cements, such as zinc phosphate, may be used. Porcelain fillings are now customarily cemented with a composite. The procedure is very similar to that used for a composite filling. The dentist roughens the cavity surface lightly with acid, and coats it with a bonding agent. Then a layer of composite is applied, the filling is slipped into place, and the composite is cured until it hardens.

RECOVERY FOLLOWING TREATMENT

A restored tooth may be temporarily sensitive to cold or other stimuli, especially if the cavity was extensive and close to the pulp. It may take several days to a few weeks for the nerve to calm down.

Occasionally a metal filling will produce a metallic taste or even a tingling sensation in your mouth. This could mean that the metal is reacting chemically with other substances and acting as a kind of weak battery. Soon, though, the "battery" will run down, and the symptoms will disappear.

When first inserted, the filling may feel tight or high. This sensation often goes away when the anesthetic completely wears off. If it persists more than a day or so, report it to your dentist. The filling may need reshaping.

The restoration of decayed teeth is still a major part of general dental practice. It shouldn't have to be, and in the future, as preventive care is practiced more widely, it should become less common. Dentists would not mourn the loss of this kind of work. On the contrary, they would be quite happy if tooth decay became as rare as smallpox.

N I N E

PERIODONTICS: TREATING THE SUPPORT STRUCTURE

Just about everyone knows about decay, and how it can lead to the destruction and eventual loss of teeth. Yet, if you're an adult, you're more likely to lose teeth for another reason. Periodontal disease—a disease of the supporting tissues *around* the tooth—can be so severe that the teeth loosen and fall out. In our society, periodontal disease is at least as prevalent as tooth decay, but relatively few people know exactly what it is or what they should do about it.

The prevention and treatment of periodontal disease is called *periodontics*, and it is the special province of *periodontists*. But virtually all general dentists devote attention to periodontal health, and many now perform extensive periodontal treatment. Periodontal care is basic care—as essential to dental health as the prevention and treatment of tooth decay.

THE PERIODONTIUM

To understand periodontal disease, it will help to be familiar with the basic periodontal tissues, the *periodontium*.

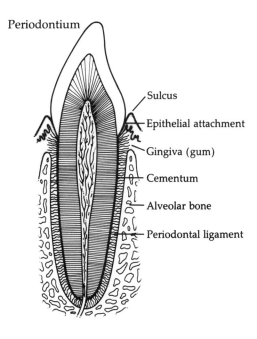

Periodontium

Sulcus

Epithelial attachment

Gingiva (gum)

Cementum

Alveolar bone

Periodontal ligament

The teeth are seated in sockets in the alveolar bone of the upper and lower jaws (*alveolar* comes from the Latin word *alveolus*, meaning "hollow"). But the bone itself doesn't grip the teeth; they are stabilized by fibers of connective tissue—*periodontal ligament*—that extend between the tooth roots and the bone sockets.

The periodontal ligament can be compared to an elastic hammock. Its many fibers hold each root firmly; however, it also acts as a shock absorber to protect the tooth against heavy chewing pressure. Additional shock absorption comes from a network of blood vessels running among the ligament fibers.

The outermost layer of the root, the *cementum,* is relatively soft, compared with the hard enamel of the crown. Part of the root extends out of the bone socket, and is particularly vulnerable to wear and decay if exposed. Normally, it is covered and protected, as is the surface of the adjacent bone, by a thick layer of soft tissue known formally as *gingiva* and familiarly as the gum.

When a tooth first erupts, the gum covers the whole root and even overlaps the enamel. Thereafter, for a variety of reasons, the gum gradually recedes. In old age, it is common for at least a portion of the root to be exposed.

The gum isn't attached to the tooth at its highest visible point. Instead, it forms a short "cuff" around the tooth, and between the tooth and the cuff is a shallow, V-shaped groove, called the *sulcus.* Normally, it is no more than a couple of millimeters deep. At the bottom is an *epithelial attachment* between the gum and the root.

PLAQUE: THE PRIMARY CAUSE OF PERIODONTAL DISEASE

The part of the tooth next to the sulcus is particularly hard to keep free of bacterial plaque (see page 61). Even if you conscientiously brush and floss, you may fail to remove plaque from this area, or to prevent bacteria and their products from irritating your gums.

Moreover, when plaque remains undis-turbed for more than a couple of days, it absorbs minerals from saliva and forms *calculus,* or *tartar*—a rough, hard material that sticks fast to teeth. You can't brush it off; only your dentist can remove it, using dental instruments. Calculus in and around the sulcus serves as a "plaque trap," which further inflames the gums.

The gum tissue constantly resists these attacks by plaque and calculus, but its natural defenses may not fully protect it from inflammation and infection. Thus, plaque and calculus constitute the primary cause of the most common disorder of the periodontium: *chronic periodontal disease.*

STAGES OF CHRONIC PERIODONTAL DISEASE

Chronic periodontal disease begins with mild gum inflammation and tends to become more severe over time. Its course can be divided into four basic stages.

GINGIVITIS

The first stage is the inflammation called *gingivitis.* It may occur in one or more localized areas, or more generally. The edges of your gums, normally coral pink, may become reddish or purplish, and slightly swollen. They may feel tender when you touch or brush them, and they may bleed easily. Your mouth may taste stale and sour, and your breath may be foul.

But gingivitis often produces no noticeable symptoms. That is the chief danger of chronic periodontal disease—it can develop gradually and painlessly without you being aware of it, until it becomes serious enough to threaten the stability of your teeth.

STAGES OF PERIODONTAL DISEASE

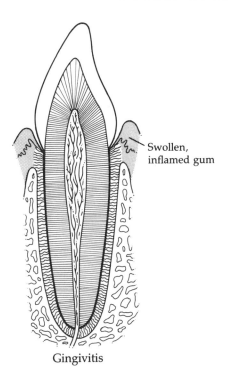

Swollen, inflamed gum

Gingivitis

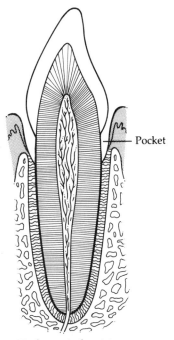

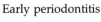

Pocket

Early periodontitis

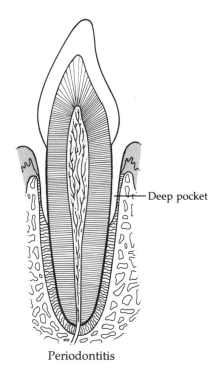

Deep pocket

Periodontitis

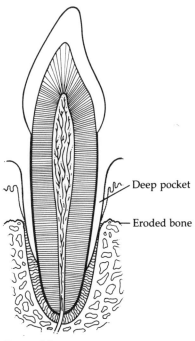

Deep pocket

Eroded bone

Loss of bone support

PERIODONTITIS

In the second stage, *early periodontitis*, the tissue lining the sulcus becomes more inflamed and swollen, and can no longer heal itself. The epithelial attachment migrates down the root of the tooth, and the sulcus becomes deeper, forming one or more *pockets* between gum and root.

These pockets provide an even better environment for bacteria. The inflammation spreads and worsens, not only damaging the gum tissue but also starting to attack the periodontal ligament and the alveolar bone that hold the tooth in place.

You may still have no obvious symptoms, but a professional examination will reveal the damage. Your dentist will use a *periodontal probe*—essentially a narrow ruler (see page 20)—to measure the depth of each periodontal pocket, and will take *periapical* X-rays (see page 23) to assess the extent of bone destruction. At stage two, pockets can be four to five millimeters deep. Bone resorption, if any, will be slight.

MODERATE PERIODONTITIS

Periodontitis does not progress steadily but rather intermittently. The symptoms and rate of destruction vary. At stage three, the gum continues to erode, and the epithelial attachment retreats still further down the root. The pockets deepen, to about five to six millimeters. In these deeper pockets, new and more virulent forms of bacteria grow and thrive. The periodontal ligament and alveolar bone are inflamed, and resorption becomes severe.

TOOTH MOBILITY AND LOSS

In the fourth stage, so much ligament and bone are lost that the tooth, no longer stable, becomes loose in its socket. The bone loss also magnifies pressures exerted by chewing, and makes the tooth even looser. Eventually the tooth will be completely deprived of support. It will fall out, or require extraction.

PREDISPOSING CONDITIONS OF PERIODONTAL DISEASE

Chronic periodontal disease is thought to be triggered, or at least made more severe, by several *predisposing* factors. Some of these may be inherited: a tendency toward periodontal disease seems to run in families. Other factors include various irritants, hormonal changes, nutritional deficiencies, and certain medications.

Moreover, several other disorders produce gum inflammation (see below, page 80). They may occur alone, or they may accompany chronic periodontal disease. The interrelationships between chronic periodontal disease, its predisposing factors, and other gum disorders are complex and not completely understood.

IRRITANTS

Substances that irritate your gums—either mechanically or chemically—may not in themselves cause periodontal disease. But they can often provoke periodontal inflammation, or make it worse.

• *Food fragments* can become wedged between the teeth, or between a tooth and the gum. You can usually remove these from the gum margins by careful brushing. Flossing, and the use of a mechanical irrigator, also help remove particles between the teeth. But if fragments have been driven deep into the gum, they may cause local infections that must be professionally treated to prevent damage to the alveolar bone.

- Habitual biting on *foreign objects* such as toothpicks, hairpins, pencils, and pipe-stems can irritate the gums and tooth ligaments by putting too much pressure on them. Repeatedly jabbing sharp objects like toothpicks between the teeth can irritate the gums directly. Even interdental stimulators should be used gently so as not to abrade the gums.
- Overzealous *brushing,* especially with stiff, pointed bristles, can damage both the gums and the adjacent parts of the teeth.
- *Malocclusion*— a "bad bite" from misaligned teeth—can contribute to periodontal disease in several ways. First, crowded, malposed teeth can become hard-to-clean "plaque traps." Second, malocclusion cause unbalanced chewing pressures, irritating the periodontium, just as biting on foreign objects does. Some severe malocclusions, such as *open bite* and *long face syndrome,* make closing the lips difficult, and exposure to air dries and irritates the gums.

  Malocclusion can be remedied by restorative dentistry, orthodontics, or orthognathic surgery (see Chapters 13, 16, and 15).
- *Clenching* and *grinding (bruxing)* are habits that wear down the teeth, and damage the gums and ligaments through excessive pressure. They are also thought to contribute to temporomandibular disorders.
- Poorly installed or badly maintained *orthodontic appliances* may press into the gums or permit the buildup of plaque and calculus. Conscientious home care is essential during orthodontic treatment, and fixed appliances (braces) must be removed periodically so the teeth can be thoroughly cleaned.
- Poorly constructed or ill-fitting *dental restorations,* such as fillings, crowns, and partial dentures, can irritate the gums, either directly or by harboring plaque and calculus that are not easily reached.
- Harmful habits such as *thumb-sucking, tongue-thrusting,* and *mouth breathing* (see page 94) can irritate and inflame gums, as well as malpose teeth. Habitual mouth breathers tend to have dry and chapped gums, which can sometimes be protected by coating them with petroleum jelly.
- *Tobacco* in any form—smoked or chewed—is extremely harmful to the soft tissues of the mouth. Tobacco not only increases the risk of periodontal disease but also greatly intensifies inflammation; its use often renders treatment ineffective.
- Strong *acids* in the mouth can irritate the gums as well as endanger the enamel of the teeth. Those who habitually suck on lemons run this risk. So do those who are afflicted with the eating disorder *bulimia,* which is characterized by alternately bingeing on food and vomiting. Sucking on aspirin to relieve sores in the mouth is especially dangerous. Aspirin is a strong acid that can easily burn soft tissues (see page 263).

HORMONAL CHANGES

Attacks of gingivitis often occur at particular stages of life, and are believed to be at least partly caused by hormonal changes. Adolescents often experience such attacks just after puberty (see page 101). So do pregnant women (see page 83). Some older people suffer from a gradual degeneration of the gums. The condition is particularly common among women after menopause, but there is no evidence that it results specifically from decreases in estrogen levels.

NUTRITIONAL DEFICIENCIES

Severe deficiencies of protein, and of such vitamins as the B complex and C, can cause gum inflammation, among other symptoms. In our society, such deficiencies are relatively uncommon. It is generally agreed that the health of the gums, and the health of the body as a whole, is helped by a balanced and nutritious diet.

MEDICATIONS

Certain medications may cause inflammation or swelling of the gums as side effects. The most notorious drug is *Dilantin (phenytoin)*, which is commonly used to control epilepsy (see page 229). Others include certain birth-control pills, and medications for hypertension and heart disease such as *propranalol (Inderol)*. Sometimes the inflammation can be treated by reducing the dosage or by switching to a substitute.

PREVENTION OF PERIODONTAL DISEASE

You are most likely to avoid chronic periodontal disease through a combination of regular professional treatment and conscientious home care. At home, essentially the same techniques serve to protect both the teeth and the gums.

Periodontal disease is especially likely to begin in areas between the teeth, so it is crucial to clean these areas thoroughly. With age, the gums often recede, exposing larger spaces between the roots of the teeth. To clean these spaces, you may find it helpful to use an interdental stimulator, a mechanical irrigator, or a small brush designed for the purpose.

Brushing your gums along with your teeth tends to make them firmer. There is no evidence, however, that such massage eliminates the risk of periodontal disease. Moreover, it is possible to overdo massage, and to damage the gums. If your gums are healthy, but brushing causes them to bleed,

you may be using too much pressure, or too stiff a toothbrush.

BASIC PERIODONTAL TREATMENT

Regular professional care is essential for the diagnosis and treatment of periodontal disease. As the disease progresses through its four stages, treatment becomes more complex.

STAGE ONE: GINGIVITIS

Simple gingivitis can usually be treated without much difficulty, if it is caught early. Each regular visit to your general dentist ought to include a periodontal examination. Plaque and calculus should be removed from each tooth, right down to the bottom of the sulcus, and the tooth surfaces polished. Routine professional treatment twice a year, accompanied by thorough home care, will be effective in most cases.

STAGE TWO: EARLY PERIODONTITIS

Treatment is similar to that for gingivitis but more thorough. Under local anesthesia, plaque and calculus are carefully scraped off, to the bottom of each pocket. In addition, inflamed and severely damaged tissue is removed with a spoon-shaped *curette* from the wall of the pocket. This *curettage* process gives the eroded gum a better chance to heal.

STAGE THREE: MODERATE PERIODONTITIS

Treatment continues to include scraping of each tooth surface and curettage of the damaged gum. The tooth root may be not only scraped but also *planed* to provide a smooth surface for the regenerating gum to attach to. In the most severe cases, periodontal surgery (see below) may become advisable.

STAGE FOUR: TOOTH MOBILITY AND LOSS

At this stage, scraping, curettage, and root planing are seldom enough to heal the gum. The treatment of choice becomes periodontal surgery, and even this may not save the affected tooth or teeth.

PERIODONTAL SURGERY: GINGIVECTOMY AND FLAP SURGERY

Periodontal surgery is similar to other forms of oral surgery, except that a periodontist rather than an oral surgeon usually performs it. It generally takes place under local anesthesia, and in as sterile a manner as the bacteria-laden mouth will allow. If many teeth are involved, the operation may be performed in two or more sessions. The surgery takes two main forms: *gingivectomy* and *flap surgery.*

Gingivectomy means literally "cutting away the gum." As periodontal pockets become deeper, the gum is more apt to become reinflamed, even after thorough scraping and curettage. Gingivectomy reduces the depth of the pockets by cutting off the upper part of the loose "cuff" of gum tissue. The remaining tissue is more likely to heal without reinfection, and the area will be easier to keep clean. Even if more of the root "shows" above the gum, the tooth is better off than it would be if it were surrounded by inflamed pockets.

Flap surgery is sometimes necessary to eliminate very deep pockets, especially those that have caused the bone to resorb. This more sophisticated, more versatile procedure has, in fact, largely replaced gingivectomy. The periodontist cuts loose the whole side of the pocket, and folds back the resulting "flap" to expose the pocket itself, plus the tooth root and the crest of the alveolar socket. All dam-

GINGIVECTOMY

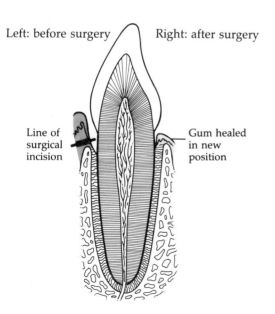

Left: before surgery   Right: after surgery

Line of surgical incision

Gum healed in new position

FLAP SURGERY

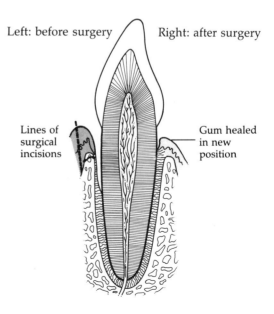

Left: before surgery   Right: after surgery

Lines of surgical incisions

Gum healed in new position

aged bone and soft tissue are removed, and the root is scraped clean and planed smooth.

If bone has been lost through resorption, the periodontist may attempt to rebuild it. Grafts of your own bone or of artificial bone may be used. Fragments of bone can be "harvested" from the jawbones or other parts of the body, and inserted into the eroded areas.

The periodontist then moves the flap back in place, and sutures it snugly against the tooth. In this closed, protected environment, inserted fragments should become bonded to the remaining alveolar bone by new bone growth—just as the ends of a broken bone "knit." New gum tissue, periodontal ligament, and cementum should also form, to connect the tooth firmly to its socket.

Sometimes a great deal of gum tissue has been lost from around the root of a tooth. As part of flap surgery, a *gingival graft* may be transferred to the area from healthy gum tissue elsewhere in your mouth. The graft will become integrated with the gum next to it, and the area from which it was taken will heal.

When gum surgery is completed, the periodontist applies a putty-like, medicated *periodontal pack* over your teeth and gums to protect the area from contamination, and to reduce swelling and pain. It hardens in a few minutes, and you will be able to chew fairly normally.

After surgery, an antibiotic, to protect further against infection, and a mild analgesic, to alleviate pain, may be prescribed. Ice is also effective in reducing swelling and soreness. A relatively soft diet will help prevent irritation. In about a week, when healing is well under way, the periodontal pack and any sutures are removed.

ROOT RESECTION

When bone resorption has occurred around a molar, one of its multiple roots may become exposed. The periodontist may then choose, while doing flap surgery, to cut off, or *resect*, the exposed root, since the remaining roots will support the tooth. New bone tissue will often form in the empty alveolar socket, just as it does after a tooth is completely extracted.

Sometimes not only the root, but part of the crown as well, will be resected. After the gum heals, the remaining parts of the tooth may have to be covered with an artificial crown.

In either case, whenever part of a root is cut away, root canal therapy must be performed to keep the remaining pulp from becoming infected.

FRENECTOMY

A procedure that sometimes accompanies gingivectomy or flap surgery (but is sometimes performed by itself) is *frenectomy*. A *frenum* (from a word meaning "sail") is a vertical membrane that extends from the gum to the lining of the mouth. Your mouth contains several of them—you can easily touch the two most prominent, by stretching the tip of your tongue over and beyond your center teeth in each jaw.

Normally the frena are attached to the gums well away from the teeth. Sometimes, however, they are too close, and lip movements tend to pull the gums away from the teeth. This process can make periodontal disease more severe. *Frenectomy* is a surgical procedure in which part of the frenum is cut away from the gum, so its attachment will be farther away from the teeth.

CHEMICAL THERAPY AS AN ALTERNATIVE TO SURGERY

Periodontal surgery is the most widely utilized treatment for serious (stages three and four) periodontal disease. In recent years, however, some practitioners have developed an alternate approach, using antiseptics.

First, pockets are cleaned out in the usual way, with scaling, curettage, and root planing. Then they are treated, both in the office and at home, with an antiseptic paste; its chief ingredients are salt, baking soda, and hydrogen peroxide. This treatment is designed to remove eroded tissue, reduce bacterial contamination, and prevent reinfection until healing can occur.

Most periodontists question the effectiveness of this procedure as a substitute for surgery. It was formerly believed to be useful in treating moderate periodontitis, but recent studies indicate that it is no more beneficial than ordinary care. Hydrogen peroxide, moreover, must be used with caution. It is a highly reactive chemical, and can easily irritate soft tissues such as gums and ligaments.

RESTORATIVE DENTISTRY

Sometimes, especially among older patients, neither conservative periodontal treatment nor periodontal surgery will succeed in stabilizing the teeth. Some form of *restorative dentistry* may be needed.

EQUILIBRATION

If your teeth are loose but sound, the procedure called *equilibration* is often used to help stabilize them. The term is based on a Latin word meaning "balance." The basic goal of equilibration is to ensure that the teeth in both jaws mesh together evenly, in what is known as a *balanced bite*. When the bite is properly balanced, chewing pressure is directed straight down each tooth to the root. Loose teeth are not so likely to "rock" in

their sockets, which would make them even looser.

The procedure consists of selectively grinding and smoothing any "high spots"—areas on individual teeth that stick up too far, or that meet those in the other jaw at the wrong angle. Only the hard, outer enamel is affected, so the process is painless and won't harm your teeth.

The dentist locates high spots by having you bite upon a sheet of special paper—rather like carbon paper—which leaves marks on the teeth wherever they contact the teeth in the other jaw. If extensive equilibration is required, the dentist may also take impressions of your jaws, from which models can be cast. These models can be used to "try out" the treatment before it is performed on your teeth.

Sometimes equilibration is carried out on only a few teeth. But periodontal patients may require *full-mouth* equilibration, which involves all or most of the teeth in both jaws, and essentially rebuilds the bite.

Equilibration is also commonly used in connection with other kinds of dental treatment, such as orthodontics and the treatment of temporomandibular disorders.

SPLINTS

If your teeth are loose but sound, your dentist or periodontist may bind them together for mutual support, using a *dental splint*. Splints are often used following periodontal surgery to stabilize the teeth while the supporting tissues heal. A temporary splint may be fashioned from stainless steel wire, woven around the teeth, and covered over with a layer of acrylic plastic. If more permanent support is needed, an *A-splint* may be imbedded in the teeth, to connect them with one another, and with more firmly anchored *abutments* (see page 130).

PROSTHETIC RESTORATIONS

When the teeth of periodontic patients become so loose or so otherwise damaged that they cannot be saved, it becomes necessary to replace them with prosthetic restorations. If only a few teeth need replacing, a fixed bridge may be inserted. If, however, the losses are substantial, a removable denture, either partial or complete, may be necessary (see page 133).

Implants (see Chapter 14) are increasingly being used as a foundation for bridges and dentures. Periodontists, because of their experience with gum and alveolar bone surgery, are among the specialists equipped to insert such devices.

SEEKING PERIODONTAL TREATMENT

Periodontics is a recognized dental specialty. It requires at least two years of advanced training in a certified graduate program, followed by board examinations. Most periodontists belong to the American Academy of Periodontology (see Appendix 281).

Many general dentists also provide periodontal care. Some even perform periodontal surgery, though others choose to refer advanced or severe cases to a specialist.

If your dentist or periodontist recommends a procedure as extensive as gingivectomy or flap surgery, you should consider obtaining at least one additional opinion (see page 14).

OTHER FORMS OF PERIODONTAL DISEASE

Chronic periodontal disease is the most common disorder of the periodontium. But there are also other disorders that produce gum inflammation as a primary or secondary symptom.

INFECTIONS

Several types of bacterial, viral, and fungal infections cause inflammation of the gums. Some afflict the gums alone; others, the soft tissues of the mouth in general.

Acute Necrotizing Ulcerative Gingivitis (ANUG)

This severe disorder, also called *Vincent's infection* and *trench mouth*, is an infection of the gum margins, especially those between the teeth. It appears suddenly and may recur periodically. It is not contagious but rather appears to result from a sudden, extreme overgrowth of normal mouth bacteria. Physical fatigue and psychological stress are thought to be precipitating factors, as are smoking and poor dental hygiene.

Inflammation can be severe and painful, with bleeding, ulceration of the gum tissue, and a foul taste and breath. It is sometimes accompanied by fever. Treatment includes careful cleaning of the teeth and gums, rinsing with salt water and mild antiseptics, and rest. Antibiotics are occasionally prescribed. If left untreated, the disorder can cause permanent damage to the tissues of the periodontium.

Herpetic Gingivostomatosis

Unlike acute necrotizing ulcerative gingivitis, this is a highly contagious infection, caused by the herpes simplex virus. It is most common among children—adults often develop an immunity to the virus. It can affect the lips and the entire lining of the mouth as well.

Pericoronitis

Sometimes the gum may become inflamed by an infection near a tooth that is partly erupted, or impacted. This condition is called *pericoronitis*, and it occurs most often over third molars, or "wisdom teeth" (see page 152).

Other Infections

Other infections that can involve the gums, such as candidiasis (oral thrush), tuberculosis, syphilis, and herpes simplex, are discussed in Chapter 19 (page 219).

SYSTEMIC DISEASES AND HEREDITARY CONDITIONS

A number of systemic disorders and hereditary conditions either produce gum inflammation, or make patients especially susceptible to it. They include diabetes, leukemia, Down syndrome, lupus erythematosis, allergies, and hypothyroidism (see Chapters 19 and 20).

DESQUAMATIVE GINGIVITIS AND PERIODONTOSIS

The causes of two other serious periodontal disorders are unknown. Fortunately, both are relatively rare.

Desquamative gingivitis is a painful inflammation in which the outer layers of the gums become soft and often peel off. Most sufferers are adult women. There may be a hormonal factor involved, since treatment with the female hormone estrogen is often effective. A predisposing factor may be allergy.

Periodontosis is a severe breakdown of certain, specific areas of alveolar bone. It usually appears during adolescence, and tends to attack the bone supporting the front teeth (incisors) and the first ("six-year") molars. The teeth loosen and shift outward, and spaces open up between them. Some researchers have suggested that the disorder originates when these teeth begin to develop—at about the time of birth. But no one knows what the basic cause might be. Unfortunately, the condition often fails to respond to treatment, and the affected teeth may be lost.

TEN

PEDIATRIC DENTISTRY: MEETING THE SPECIAL NEEDS OF INFANTS, CHILDREN, AND ADOLESCENTS

I t has always been important to take good care of young people's teeth, but it is especially important now. Since tooth decay and gum disease are no longer inevitable, proper care can ensure that today's children will have sound, healthy, natural teeth throughout their lives.

But reaching this goal requires a systematic, conscientious program of dental care, starting in the earliest years. And the dentist can't do it alone. Maintaining dental health requires the active participation of *both* parent and child.

PRENATAL DENTAL CARE: WHAT THE EXPECTANT MOTHER CAN DO

Dental care for children should start before birth. Generally speaking, healthy mothers produce healthy children, with healthy teeth. There are several factors worthy of attention.

NUTRITION

Good nutrition plays an essential role in maternal health. A pregnant woman's diet should be balanced among the basic food groups, it should have enough calories to assure a steady weight gain, and it should include adequate amounts of vitamins and minerals. Vitamins A, C, and D and the minerals calcium and phosphorus are especially important to the development and maintenance of bones and teeth.

Under normal circumstances, however, the mother's diet doesn't seem to have much *direct* effect on her child's teeth. Only severe nutritional deficiencies damage developing teeth. The most important benefit of good nutrition is to reduce the chance of premature birth and low birthweight, both of which are associated with many health problems, including dental abnormalities such as defective enamel (see page 251).

TOOTH DECAY AND GUM DISEASE

It is *not* true that the developing fetus "robs" the mother's teeth of calcium or that she is doomed to "loose one tooth per child." These are just myths. It *is* true, though, that pregnant women are more susceptible to tooth decay and gum disease, either of which can lead to tooth loss.

Increased susceptibility to tooth decay results mainly from changed eating habits. Many pregnant women crave frequent snacks, particularly of sweets. Such snacks produce more plaque and high levels of acid, which attacks the teeth. The best solution is to avoid between-meal snacks as much as possible, and to be especially careful to brush and floss at least once, and preferably twice, a day.

Higher levels of certain hormones in the blood cause the gums of pregnant women to become more sensitive to the irritants in plaque. Inflammation of the gums often results—a condition so common that it is known as *pregnancy gingivitis.* This is another reason to be conscientious about daily brushing and flossing, especially near the gums. A balanced, nutritious diet is also important to keep the gums healthy, as is an adequate daily intake of vitamins such as A, C, and D.

If gingivitis does occur during pregnancy, it should be treated as early as possible, while it is still relatively mild and doesn't require medications that might harm the fetus.

INFECTIONS

To protect the dental health of the developing fetus, the expectant mother should try to minimize the chance of catching any infectious disease—especially during the first three and last three months of pregnancy. Infections during pregnancy can result in serious birth defects, including damage to the developing teeth (see page 251).

Many infectious diseases are preventable.

Any woman planning to have a child should make sure she is immunized beforehand against such viral diseases as measles, mumps, and, most important of all, rubella (German measles). She should also be certain that she is not infected with any sexually transmitted disease (STDs), such as gonorrhea or syphilis.

The best protection against many infections is a properly functioning immune system—another reason for good nutrition and other measures to assure maternal health during pregnancy.

RADIATION AND MEDICATIONS

It is advisable for a woman to inform her dentist, and any other health professional treating her, that she is pregnant as soon as she knows it. In general, any but the most essential medical or dental treatment should be postponed if possible, especially during the first and last three months of pregnancy. X-Rays should be avoided, or at least performed with maximum protection of the abdomen. Also, medications should be kept to a minimum.

One medication that can directly affect developing teeth is the antibiotic *tetracycline,* in any of its several variations. If tetracycline is taken by the mother during the last two months of pregnancy, the child's primary teeth (baby teeth) may be discolored. Moreover, if tetracycline is given to the child, up to the age of eight, the *permanent* teeth may be discolored (see page 89). Most physicians now know enough to avoid tetracycline if an antibiotic is needed for an expectant mother or a young child.

DENTAL CARE DURING INFANCY AND EARLY CHILDHOOD

Ordinarily, a newborn has no visible teeth. The teeth are there, though. All twenty *pri-*

mary teeth (also known as *deciduous, milk,* or *baby* teeth) are at least partly formed. Over the first two to three years of life they will *erupt,* in sequence, through the gums. Then, starting about age six, the primary teeth will begin to drop out, or *exfoliate,* to be replaced and supplemented by the 32 *permanent* teeth (see illustrated chart of development, pages 96–99).

DENTAL DISORDERS OF THE NEWBORN

In addition to problems arising during pregnancy, certain disorders may affect the mouths and teeth of newborn children. Most of these are discussed in other chapters (see below). Here we will describe only a few, relatively common conditions.

Natal and Neonatal Teeth

Some newborns have one or more teeth that have already erupted *(natal* teeth); and some infants have teeth that erupt shortly after birth *(neonatal* teeth). Usually these teeth are poorly formed, and drop out in a few weeks. They pose a problem mainly when they do drop out: the expelled tooth may be *aspirated* (breathed in), causing the infant to choke. Such premature teeth should be examined promptly by a dentist, but should be removed only if they pose a danger, interfere with nursing, or irritate the tongue.

Bednar's Aphthae

A newborn baby's mouth is often cleaned out to assure unobstructed breathing. Sometimes in the wiping process the inside surfaces of the upper jaw are slightly injured, and whitish lesions may form. They heal in a few days and require no treatment.

White Cysts

Small pale sacs, or *cysts,* that contain a tough, fibrous protein called *keratin,* appear inside the mouths of many newborns. Depending on where in the mouth they appear, they are called *Epstein's pearls, Bohn's nodules,* or *dental lamina cysts.* They require no treatment and will go away within a few weeks.

Tongue-tie (Ankyloglossia)

Newborns have a small membrane that "ties" the tongue to the floor of the mouth, and prevents it from extending freely. This has a useful function: it helps position the tongue for nursing. Usually it disappears after a few days. Sometimes, though, it remains, growing thicker and stronger, impeding speech. In severe cases, surgery may be needed to correct it.

See Chapter 19, for developmental defects such as cleft lip or palate, imperfect tooth formation (amelogenesis imperfecta, dentinogenesis imperfecta), and tongue anomalies; for infections such as oral thrush, canker sores, and herpes infections; and for tumors, such as fibromas, hemangiomas, papillomas, and oral cancer. See also Chapter 20 for special medical conditions that affect dental treatment, such as diabetes, heart disease, hemophilia, asthma, and Down's syndrome.

HOME CARE: CLEANING THE MOUTH

You should begin a regular program to assure your child's dental health in infancy, even *before* the teeth begin to erupt. When your baby is about five months old, it is time to start cleaning his or her mouth. At least once a day, after a feeding, you should lightly wipe the mouth, gums, and tongue with a piece of moistened gauze or the corner of a washcloth. You may moisten the gauze or cloth with plain water or a fluoride rinse (see below). Delay the use of toothpaste until the child has enough muscle control to spit most of it out.

The main purpose of cleaning the gums before the teeth appear is to get the child used

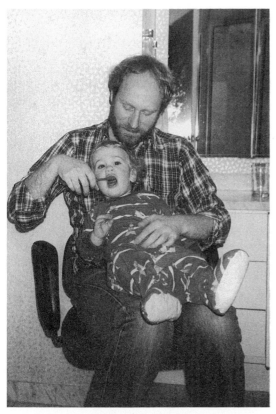

Position for brushing child's teeth
Photograph by Barry Dale

to the procedure, as a familiar and even pleasurable experience. Once the teeth erupt, daily cleaning will be needed to remove food residues and check the buildup of plaque. Since primary teeth have relatively thin enamel, decay proceeds rapidly once it starts.

During cleaning, the best position for the child is lying on your lap, with the head toward you. This position gives the clearest view of the whole mouth. You can use the same position later for brushing the child's teeth, until about age six.

TEETHING

The eruption of the primary teeth is popularly known as *teething*. Sometimes the process is preceded or accompanied by irritation of the gums, which become reddish or slightly swollen. Teething babies may become unusually fussy and wakeful, lose their appetite, or drool more than usual.

Teething babies may be made more comfortable by gently massaging the gums, or by providing a pacifier, teething ring, or hard food such as dry toast to chew on. Anesthetic, "numbing" salves for the gums are also available.

Occasionally, an *eruption cyst* may appear on the gums where a tooth is about to erupt. This is a soft, bluish, watery sac which is seen most often over emerging molars. The best thing to do about an eruption cyst is nothing. Eventually, it will rupture as the tooth pushes through. Trying to puncture or remove it can lead to infection.

When the incisors first erupt, the biting edges may contain three small bumps called *mamelons*. They are harmless, and ordinarily wear off with use.

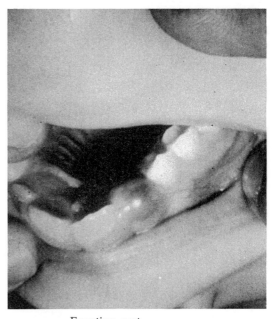

Eruption cyst
Photograph by Jeffrey Leeds

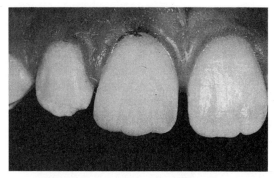

Mamelons on edges of upper incisors
Photograph by Kenneth Aschheim

At one time, teething was thought to be responsible for medical symptoms such as fever, diarrhea, and rash. It is now generally agreed, though, that teething produces no disorders by itself. If the baby suffers any such symptom, the cause is likely to lie elsewhere, and a pediatrician should be consulted.

FLUORIDES: THE GREAT TOOTH SAVERS

Teeth are protected from decay by the mineral content of their outer layer, the enamel. The principal minerals in enamel are calcium and phosphorus. For decades, it has been known that enamel can be strengthened by various fluorine compounds, or *fluorides.*

Fluorides help teeth resist decay in five ways:

- They strengthen the enamel of teeth as the teeth are being formed.
- They appear to help the developing teeth form shallower grooves on the biting surfaces. Shallow grooves tend to retain less decay-producing food debris and plaque than deep ones.
- They continue to reinforce the enamel in fully formed, erupted teeth.
- In saliva, they help minimize acid from decay-producing bacteria, and inhibit their proliferation.

- They also act with minerals in saliva to restore enamel during the earliest stages of decay.

There are two basic ways in which fluorides become incorporated into teeth:

- *Systemic ingestion.* Fluoride compounds are taken internally, and then travel through the bloodstream to the teeth. Ingested fluoride particularly helps developing, unerupted teeth.
- *Topical application.* Fluorides are applied directly to the surfaces of the erupted teeth.

For maximum prevention of decay, both ways are important.

The simplest, most reliable way of ingesting fluoride is by drinking fluoridated water. Fluoridation of the water supply is still politically controversial in some areas. Yet there is no scientific evidence that it has ever harmed anyone. There is overwhelming evidence, however, that it reduces tooth decay.

In areas where the water is fluoridated, no other form of systemic ingestion is ordinarily necessary. It is, in fact, possible to ingest too much fluoride, which can cause unsightly mottling of the enamel, called *fluorosis.* But fluorosis occurs almost exclusively in areas where the drinking water contains an overabundance of natural fluorides, not in water systems that are artificially fluoridated.

If your water supply is not fluoridated, you can use a fluoride supplement. Such a supplement may take the form of tablets or drops, and is sometimes mixed with vitamins. These can be added to water or formula. Your dentist or pediatrician should prescribe the exact dosage.

Since systemic ingestion is most effective before the teeth erupt, it should begin at birth and continue at least until the second permanent molars erupt, about age twelve. Topical applications should continue past that age, however.

There is no conclusive evidence that mothers can pass on systemic fluoride to their offspring, either through the placenta before birth or through breast milk afterward.

Once the teeth have erupted, topical fluoride application augments the protective action of systemic ingestion. Topical application should begin when the first teeth appear, and continue at least through puberty. You can start at home, by moistening a piece of gauze with a few drops of an over-the-counter fluoride rinse, and rubbing it gently over your child's teeth and gums. When the child is ready, you can substitute fluoride toothpaste, and continue the rinse as a daily mouthwash. Twice-yearly applications of "professional-strength" compounds should begin at the first regular visit to the dentist, around age two-and-a-half (see page 89).

With topical application, you can't get too much of a good thing. When you combine daily application at home with regular treatment by a dentist, you don't risk fluorosis, but you do obtain better protection against decay.

FEEDING CONSIDERATIONS

The health of children's teeth and gums is greatly affected both by *how* they are fed and by *what* they are fed.

Encouraging Healthy Oral Habits

Breast feeding has several advantages over bottle feeding. One of them is the development of healthy patterns of chewing, sucking, and swallowing.

Bottle nipples of traditional design are too large, extend too deeply into the mouth, and are pierced too generously to give an infant's jaws and tongue the kind of exercise they need. Such nipples encourage bad habits like

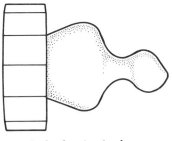

Orthodontic nipple

tongue-thrusting—in which the tongue is thrust forward between the front teeth when the infant swallows (see page 95).

Some mothers can't breast feed. Fortunately, *orthodontic* nipples are now available. Their special shape and relatively small opening help the child to chew, suck, and swallow correctly.

Sucking and chewing are natural activities, and they are of benefit to developing teeth and jaws. They should be encouraged. Whether breast-fed or bottle-fed, the infant should be held upright, to help prevent choking and to give the mouth more exercise. Sucking on thumbs, fingers, or pacifiers is natural and usually harmless, unless it persists into later childhood (see below). Even before their first birthday, children should at least try out solid food such as dry toast (zweiback), which requires and encourages chewing.

Incidentally, pacifiers, teething rings, and any toys that children can put in their mouths should be large enough so they can't be swallowed, and made of a material that can be easily cleaned. If you give your child a pacifier, it should have an orthodontic nipple, and you shouldn't offer it too frequently.

A Healthy Diet

Good nutrition is essential to all aspects of

an infant's health, including the condition of the teeth and gums. Mother's milk and formula usually contain all needed nutrients. And once the infant is weaned to solid food, the diet should be balanced among the basic food groups, and he or she should receive adequate amounts of vitamins and minerals. Vitamins A, C, and D, and the minerals calcium and phosphorus are especially important to healthy teeth and gums.

Limiting Contact with Sugar

The great dietary enemy to sound teeth is sugar. The most harmful form is *sucrose*—the form in table sugar—but other sugars, such as *lactose* (milk sugar) and *fructose* (fruit sugar), can lead to decay as well. In the mouth, the bacteria that cause plaque, tooth decay, and gum disease feed on sugar.

It is virtually impossible to eliminate sugar entirely from the diet. Just about all foods contain it, including mother's milk and formula. Furthermore, carbohydrates in some form are essential to nutrition. But it is possible, and very important, to limit sugar intake.

Heavily and artificially sweetened drinks should be avoided for unweaned infants. Instead, provide unsweetened milk and natural fruit juices. You should also avoid artificially sweetened baby foods, and you should not add sugar to make them "taste better."

In general, children should not be allowed to become *accustomed* to sugar-containing foods as a reward, or as a regular part of their diet.

Nursing-Bottle Syndrome

It is important not only to limit a child's intake of sugar but also to limit the time the sugar remains in the mouth. In particular, a nursing bottle should not be allowed to remain in the mouth for an extended period of time.

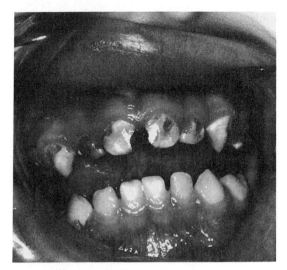

Nursing bottle syndrome
Photograph by Kenneth Aschheim

Even formula and unsweetened milk contain substantial amounts of sugar. When the bottle remains in the mouth for several hours such liquids "pool" there, increasing the food supply of bacteria. *Nursing-bottle syndrome* often results, with severe decay, first in the upper front teeth, and then in the back teeth of both jaws.

In general, a nursing bottle should *not* be used as a pacifier or an aid to sound sleep, if it contains anything but plain water. Furthermore, it is wise to wean a baby from bottle to cup as early in life as possible—usually at about one year.

Though this syndrome is most often the result of bottle feeding, it can occur in breast-fed babies, if they sleep all night with their mothers and are allowed to feed at will.

DANGERS OF INFECTION

Children's dental health depends to a large extent on their general health. There are certain infectious diseases, for instance, that directly affect the mouth, gums, and teeth. In addition, many other infections can indirectly affect teeth by altering the body's chemical balance while the teeth are developing. The result can be teeth with thin or uneven enamel, which increases their susceptibility to decay (see page 251).

Children should be protected against infection as much as possible. Their immune-system defenses should be kept strong through good nutrition and adequate sleep. They should also be immunized against infections—not only smallpox, diphtheria, whooping cough, and scarlet fever but also "less serious" diseases such as mumps, measles, and German measles. And if they do become ill, they should be treated promptly, to minimize the length and severity of the illness.

When your child first goes to the dentist (see below), it is advisable for you or your pediatrician to provide a record of past illnesses. You should also inform the dentist of any illnesses that occur between visits.

AVOIDING TETRACYCLINE

Tetracycline is a broad-spectrum antibiotic, offered in several formulations and under several names. It is widely used (and very useful) in treating infections. But one of its side effects is often severe, permanent discoloration of developing teeth. The danger to a child's primary teeth, when the mother takes tetracycline during pregnancy, has already been described (see page 83). Since the permanent teeth start developing soon after birth, this antibiotic should be avoided, if possible, up to about age eight.

Tetracycline staining, if it does occur, can be treated in later life through aesthetic dentistry (see Chapter 17).

THE CHILD'S FIRST VISIT TO THE DENTIST

Experts do not agree about when a child should first see a dentist. Many pediatric den-

tists would prefer to see both the child and the parents within the first year, in order to provide guidance for home care and to head off problems such as those described earlier. Others believe that a conscientious, well-informed pediatrician can provide this kind of supervision during infancy, referring the child to a dentist only if treatment is needed.

There is general agreement, however, that a child should visit a dentist by the time all or most of the primary teeth have erupted, at about two-and-a-half years of age. By this age, the child is psychologically ready for such a new experience.

It is unwise to postpone the first visit much past the age of three. In particular, the visit should not be postponed until some definite dental problem, requiring emergency treatment, appears. The child is likely to respond with fear and anger, and may develop a lasting aversion to dental treatment.

At the first visit, the dentist is likely to do the following:

- Familiarize the child with the dental office and dental procedures, in a gentle and reassuring manner.
- Review the child's medical and dental history.
- Thoroughly examine the mouth, gums, and teeth.
- Counsel both parent and child about diet, teeth cleaning, and fluorides, in a program to assure future dental health.

In addition, the dentist may begin professional fluoride treatment. A gel is applied topically to the teeth, after they are thoroughly cleaned. The treatment should be repeated at each regular visit, every six months, until adolescence or even later.

The dentist will also attempt to determine whether the enamel of the primary molars is unusually susceptible to decay; if it is, a *sealant* may be applied to the biting surfaces.

Sealants, however, are more commonly used on permanent molars (see page 101).

The Pediatric Dentist: A Pediatrician for the Mouth

Most parents understand the advantages of having a specialist in childhood care—a pediatrician—attend to their children's medical health. More and more parents are now recognizing the advantages of a specialist—a pediatric dentist—in attending to their children's dental health.

Pediatric dentistry is a recognized dental specialty, and pediatric dentists receive at least two years of specialized training in this field. As a result of their training and their experience, pediatric dentists are more likely to have a thorough, up-to-date knowledge of child development, specific dental disorders of childhood, and effective methods of treatment.

Just as important, pediatric dentists are drawn to the field because they like children, and enjoy treating them. They are likely to be skilled in building positive, trustful relationships with their young patients, and in guiding them to positive attitudes toward dental treatment and home care.

How to Find a Good Dentist for Your Child

Finding a pediatric dentist is similar to finding a practitioner in any of the other established specialties, and is discussed in Chapter 2.

In some areas, you may not be able to locate such a specialist. Or you may prefer to have your own dentist treat your children. In either case, make sure that treating children is a regular part of your general dentist's practice.

Dealing with Dental Fear

Many adults are afraid to go to the dentist, and some of them, because of painful past experience, have reason to be. But there is no reason for their children to share that fear. Dental treatment doesn't have to be painful, and should not be. Perhaps the most important goal of pediatric dentistry is to teach children that they need not fear or avoid dental treatment.

Dentists who treat children use a variety of methods to prevent and overcome fear.

- They make a special effort to provide an attractive, nonthreatening office environment.
- To build confidence and trust, they use techniques such as "Tell–Show–Do": Before starting a procedure, they first *tell* the child, in carefully selected, reassuring language, what they are going to do. Next they *show* the procedure, by an actual demonstration. Only then will they actually *do* what they have described and shown.
- To overcome fear, they use relaxation exercises and desensitization, as described on page 47.

Every once in a while, despite such reassurance, a child is so severely frightened, panicky, or defiant, that the dentist may have to employ stronger measures to overcome resistance to treatment, including gentle but firm restraint. Only in rare instances is it necessary to use a sedative to calm a child for treatment. But if sedation is necessary, an experienced pediatric dentist is best qualified to administer it effectively (see page 52).

In preventing dental fear, parents play a crucial role. You should try to avoid behavior likely to provoke fear, such as telling "dentist jokes" or reciting dental horror stories, and you should forcefully instruct older siblings not to do so. And *never* use the prospect of "a visit to the dentist" as a threat or punishment.

In preparation for the first visit to the dentist, the following guidelines are recommended:

- Inform the child about the visit, in truthful but positive terms. Describe the dentist as "a special doctor who takes care of your teeth."
- Don't represent the visit to the dentist as something extraordinary. Don't promise special rewards for good behavior.
- In talking about the visit, be general, rather than specific, about procedures. Leave explanation to the dentist, since a proper choice of words is crucial.
- Don't describe your own experiences at the dentist, or take the child along when you visit your own dentist. Adult treatment is different in many respects, and the child will get an inaccurate impression of what to expect.
- If the child asks specific questions, such as, "Will it hurt?" give answers such as: "I don't think so, but we'll talk it over with the doctor." Indeed, write down such questions, to be discussed with the dentist.
- Emphasize that the dentist is someone who can be trusted, and who is genuinely concerned about helping children be healthy.

You can also help to reassure your child during the dental visit, primarily by reinforcing the dentist's own efforts. For example, depending on the circumstances, the dentist may request that you be present during treatment, or completely out of the room. Sometimes the dentist will encourage you to be present, but not in the child's direct line of vision. Unless your child is very young—under two years—it is usually not necessary or desirable for you to hold him or her during treatment.

Dental fear is not inherited, it is learned. Most children learn it from parents who are themselves afraid. Conscious efforts not to transmit such fear often do not work. Children intuitively sense your fear, and pick it up. Very often, the best way for parents to head off dental fear in their children is to con-

front and overcome their *own* fear (see Chapter 6).

CARE OF THE PRIMARY TEETH

Primary teeth may be only temporary, but they are important. For at least four reasons, they deserve continuous care.

- *Function.* The child needs teeth, not only to chew food but also to facilitate speech and to achieve a proper facial contour.
- *Comfort.* Tooth decay can lead to painful toothache and gum disease, in children as well as adults.
- *Appearance.* In childhood, as in later life, healthy teeth significantly contribute to appearance, which, in turn, often affects self-confidence and self-esteem.
- *Succession.* Primary teeth also significantly affect the permanent teeth that succeed them. If primary teeth, especially primary molars, are lost prematurely, the permanent teeth are not guided into their proper positions, and are more likely to grow in crooked and misaligned. Moreover, infection from decayed or injured primary teeth can damage the permanent teeth developing under them.

CLEANING THE PRIMARY TEETH

Keeping the primary teeth clean and free of plaque is essential. But until about age 6, it is your responsibility—not your child's. A small child lacks both the physical coordination and the psychological determination to do the job properly.

The most effective position for examining and cleaning a child's mouth has been described earlier (page 84). For the first year or so, when the earliest primary teeth are coming in, you need only wipe the teeth, gums, and tongue with a piece of moistened gauze. Once six to eight primary teeth have erupted, switch to a toothbrush.

The toothbrush should be small enough to fit comfortably in the child's mouth; an adult brush is too big. The bristles should be soft, made of nylon, and rounded at the ends. The working surface should be flat.

An electric toothbrush does a good job, but not a significantly better one than an ordinary toothbrush. Some parents buy an electric toothbrush in the hope that the child will become better motivated to brush regularly. This strategy usually doesn't work—or at least not for long.

Toothpaste is not absolutely necessary, and shouldn't be used until the child is old enough not to swallow it. It is the scrubbing action of the brush that loosens food particles and breaks up plaque. The main benefits of toothpaste are its refreshing taste, which makes brushing more agreeable, and (even more important) its fluoride content.

When the child is ready for toothpaste,

start out by using a very small amount—a pea-sized blob—and make sure it is rinsed out afterward. Use a fluoride toothpaste, one that bears the "Accepted" seal of the American Dental Association. Fluoride toothpaste has only limited value in protecting the teeth, but it helps.

There is no single best way of brushing a child's teeth. We customarily recommend a simple "scrub-brush" technique, which is described below. Whatever method is used, it is important to brush all surfaces of all the teeth, together with the adjoining gums.

Slight bleeding of the gums after brushing is not necessarily something to worry about. But it probably does indicate that areas of the teeth near the gums are not being brushed sufficiently. Bleeding usually stops after a week or so of regular, thorough brushing.

Most dentists recommend brushing twice a day, after the first and last meals. To prevent the buildup of plaque, it is essential to clean the teeth thoroughly at least once every 24 hours.

BRUSHING CHILDREN'S TEETH: THE "SCRUB-BRUSH" METHOD

1. Establish a systematic, habitual order for brushing, so that no teeth will be missed. Such an order might be: all the upper teeth, outside and inside, and then all the lower teeth. Or the order might be one quarter of the mouth, outside and inside, at a time.

2. Brush no more than two teeth at a time, and then move on to the next pair.

3. Place the brush horizontally against the teeth and adjoining gum. Brush with short, scrubbing strokes back and forth. Be gentle—it takes very little pressure to break up plaque, and hard

brushing can damage the teeth and gums.

4. Exception: It may be easier to brush the insides of the center teeth, the incisors, by holding the brush vertically, and brushing up and down.

5. Don't miss any surface of the teeth. Brush the tops of the molars after the insides and outsides. The molars and the insides of the lower incisors are most often neglected.

6. After brushing, rinse the mouth thoroughly, and use a fluoride mouthwash.

After brushing, a fluoride mouthwash should be used, but only if the child spits it out consistently. Fluoride mouthwash, like fluoride toothpaste, offers some protection against decay, but not as much as ingested fluoride or topical fluoride applied by a dentist.

Do not use any mouthwash, or any toothpaste, in the expectation that it will "kill germs." It is not possible—or desirable—to kill all microorganisms in the mouth. Brushing the teeth simply cuts down the amount of food debris and bacteria enough to help prevent tooth decay. And except for fluoride, no ingredient in any mouthwash or toothpaste has been proven effective in preventing decay.

Using dental floss is less important for primary teeth than for permanent teeth. Primary teeth have naturally large spaces between them, compared to the narrow spaces between permanent teeth. Until the age of six or seven, it is usually possible to clean all surfaces of the teeth just by thorough brushing.

Plaque is not visible to the naked eye. You can use disclosing solutions or tablets (see page 32) with older children to demonstrate any plaque that remains after brushing.

Children cannot be expected to do a complete job of brushing on their own until they are about six years old. But they should certainly be encouraged to start much earlier. The best way for you to encourage your child is to set a good example. You might allow the child to watch you brushing your own teeth, and then imitate the procedure. It sometimes helps to give a child an extra, personal toothbrush to practice with.

LIMITING SUGAR

Sugar is the main enemy of sound teeth, and children should eat as little of it as possible. The problem is, of course, that children *like* sugar (and so do parents). Completely eliminating it from the diet is virtually impossible.

However, you can *limit* your child's sugar consumption if you are firm, and set a good example. The amount of sugar intake is less important than the length of time it spends on the teeth. For this reason, several overlapping strategies are advised:

- Limit the number of times sugar is eaten during the day. Do not include sugar in every meal. Even more important, avoid sweet snacks between meals, or at least limit them to one special treat a day.
- If possible, substitute nonsweet foods for snacks, such as popcorn, nuts, pretzels, or raw vegetables—or even fresh fruit, which contains relatively little sugar. Firm, fresh fruit and raw vegetables also encourage vigorous chewing, which stimulates and cleanses the teeth and gums.
- Avoid or limit sweet foods that "stick around" in the mouth. Such long-lingering sweets include hard or chewy candy, cookies and pastries (and even white bread), presweetened cereals, dried fruits such as raisins and fruit roll, chewing gum (other than sugarless gum), jams and jellies, and sweetened drinks (other than plain fruit juice). "Fruit" drinks, by the way, often contain little fruit juice; the rest is largely sugar water.

Theoretically, it should be possible to prevent decay by brushing *immediately* (within 20 minutes) after *every* meal or snack. For most people, such a regimen is simply impractical. Furthermore, that much brushing could actually damage the teeth and gums.

PROTECTING AGAINST ACCIDENTAL INJURY

Next to decay, the chief cause of damaged or lost primary teeth is accidents. Accidental blows can chip teeth, knock them out, or even break a jaw.

We will discuss this subject in greater detail on page 101. To protect a small child, the most important measure you can take is to install a restraint system in your car (they are compulsory in many states) and to use it faithfully. Protective seats and seat belts save lives—and teeth!

PROFESSIONAL CARE OF PRIMARY TEETH

Following the first visit, a child should visit the dentist every six months. Regular visits enable the dentist to make sure the teeth are in good condition—free of cavities, and growing properly—and to treat problems before they become serious. Regular visits also help control dental fear.

During these visits, the dentist will take X-rays of the child's teeth and jaws. Modern equipment and techniques make these procedures safe, and they are essential tools in assuring dental health. They reveal conditions of the primary teeth, such as small areas of decay, that might be missed in examination or that cannot be seen any other way. Even more important, they show how the *permanent* teeth are developing in the jaws, which is crucial information for the prevention and early treatment of orthodontic problems (see page 178).

Following examination, any lingering plaque, tartar, or stains will be removed from the child's teeth. The dentist will also continue topical applications of fluoride.

Any cavities should be promptly filled. If a tooth is badly decayed or damaged, covering it with a stainless-steel crown is usually preferable to extracting it. The fact that the primary teeth aren't permanent is no reason to leave them untreated. The last ones won't be shed until about age twelve.

If a child does lose a primary tooth—particularly a primary molar—through decay or injury, the pediatric dentist or an orthodontist may have to insert a *space maintainer* to keep the adjacent teeth from drifting into the gap (see page 175).

INTERVENTION AGAINST HARMFUL HABITS

In the years just before the permanent teeth begin to appear, the dentist will probably recommend intervention against certain oral habits that can harm a child's teeth and jaws, if allowed to persist.

Thumb-Sucking

For infants, sucking the thumb or fingers is natural and healthy. Older children often continue the habit for psychological comfort. It is relatively harmless unless it persists as the permanent teeth come in. Then it can misalign the front teeth and deform the jawbones, causing or aggravating a *malocclusion* (see page 170).

To break the habit, gentle persuasion usually works best. Advise your child that the habit is harmful and that getting rid of it is part of growing up. The child often sucks the thumb unknowingly, and simple, repeated reminders—"You're sucking your thumb"—can be enough to motivate the child to stop. The example of siblings and peers can also be helpful.

Avoid negative, judgmental pressure, or ridicule. Praise and rewards will often work; threats and punishments seldom do. Under emotional stress, children often regress, and tend to suck their thumbs even more.

If your child sucks a thumb while sleeping, you can use a physical "reminder" such as a glove or a mitten, or an elastic bandage around the elbow so it will be harder to bend the forearm toward the mouth.

In extreme cases, a pediatric dentist or an orthodontist can fabricate a special habit-control appliance that will keep the child from finding comfort in thumb-sucking (see page 174).

Tongue-Thrusting

More damaging, and harder to eliminate, is the habit of thrusting the tongue against or between the front teeth when swallowing. It is thought to have its origins in feeding from a bottle without an orthodontic nipple (see page 87). The repeated pressure of the tongue can lead to a serious form of malocclusion called an *open bite,* in which the front teeth fail to meet when the jaws are closed (see page 169).

Breaking this habit will often require professional intervention. The child may have to practice certain exercises to retrain the muscles. Or, again, a habit-control appliance may be fabricated to retrain the tongue and prevent it from moving too far forward.

Biting Habits

Teeth are designed for chewing food. When they habitually are used to bite on other things—like fingernails, lips, cheek linings, or pencils—they can eventually be forced out of place, causing malocclusion. As with thumb-sucking, the best treatment is usually reminder and persuasion.

Grinding the Teeth (Bruxism)

Many children habitually grind their teeth, while awake or asleep or both. The habit usually goes away by itself and does no harm. Only if it persists into adolescence does it deserve attention. Adults who clench and grind their teeth can do serious harm not only to the teeth but also to the temporomandibular joints (see page 204).

CARE OF PERMANENT TEETH

Starting at about age six, a child's primary teeth begin to loosen and fall out (exfoliate). The loosening is the result of the natural resorption of the roots. After a few weeks, the permanent teeth begin to erupt into the spaces left vacant. For the standard pattern of succession, see the chart on pages 96–99.

Variations of six months, or even a year, from the usual schedule of exfoliation and eruption are not uncommon. You don't have to worry about such variations unless loss and replacement of the primary teeth occur in the wrong order, or there is insufficient space in the jaw for the permanent teeth. Monitoring succession is an important part of dental checkups during these years of *mixed dentition* (see page 179).

The structure of permanent teeth differs slightly from that of primary teeth. Hence, their color differs slightly; it is yellowish, rather than milky white. Most permanent teeth are also considerably larger than primary teeth, and more closely spaced. One of the most common orthodontic problems is teeth that are too tightly crowded together, for lack of enough space in the jaws to accommodate them (see page 166).

There is ordinarily no need to pull out loose primary teeth—they will fall out eventually. Nevertheless, loose teeth can irritate the gums, and children often become impatient to be rid of them, and to receive a reward from the tooth fairy. When a tooth is extremely loose, it can usually be removed by gripping it firmly between thumb and forefinger, and pulling sharply and quickly. If the tooth doesn't come out readily, try being patient for another few days. If the child's anxiety level is especially high, the dentist can remove the tooth, using a topical anesthetic to assure that there will be no pain.

After a primary tooth comes out, the gum

ERUPTION OF THE TEETH

All the ages listed in this chart are approximate; there is a very wide normal range. In general, girls' teeth develop earlier than those of boys, and the lower teeth erupt before the upper ones. The sequence of eruption, as shown here, is far more important than the precise time when it occurs.

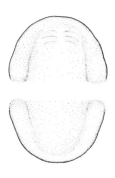

At birth, no teeth are visible. But all the primary teeth are at least partially formed, and the development of the permanent teeth, deep in the jaws, has already begun.

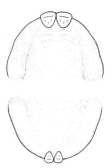

Starting as early as six months, the four *central incisors* erupt. They usually appear two at a time, and in the lower jaw before the upper.

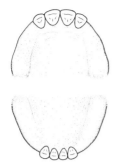

After the central incisors are in, starting at about seven or eight months, the four *lateral incisors* erupt next to them. The primary teeth are bluish white in color.

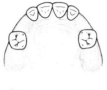

At about twelve months, the *primary first molars* erupt, leaving temporary spaces between them and the lateral incisors.

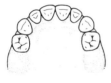

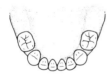

At about sixteen months, the primary *canines,* or *cuspids,* appear in the spaces between the lateral incisors and first molars. Usually there is a slight gap in front of the canines in the upper jaw and behind those in the lower jaw.

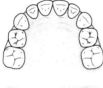

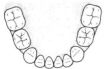

At about two years, the *second primary molars* erupt, completing the set of primary teeth. By age three, they are fully erupted, with completely formed roots.

Continued on next page

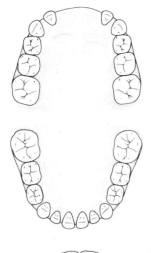

Starting about age four, the jaws grow significantly, and gaps appear between the primary teeth. About age six, the period of *mixed dentition* begins. The *permanent first molars,* or *six-year molars,* erupt, behind the primary second molars. Meanwhile, the roots of the primary teeth, starting with the incisors, start to *resorb,* causing the teeth to loosen and fall out (*exfoliate*).

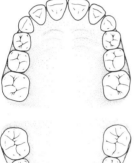

At age seven to eight, the primary incisors are replaced by permanent ones. The permanent teeth are noticeably darker in color, and also larger and more closely spaced, especially in the lower jaw. There may still be spaces between the upper incisors (sometimes called the "ugly duckling" look). About the same time, the jaws undergo another growth spurt.

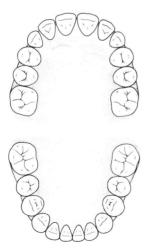

The permanent lower canines replace the primary ones at about age ten—noticeably earlier than the succession in the upper jaw. Soon after the lower canines appear, the primary molars begin to give way to permanent *premolars,* or *bicuspids.* The first premolars erupt about a year before the second ones. Unlike most permanent teeth, the second premolars are smaller than their primary predecessors, and after they erupt, the permanent first molars shift forward to fill the extra space.

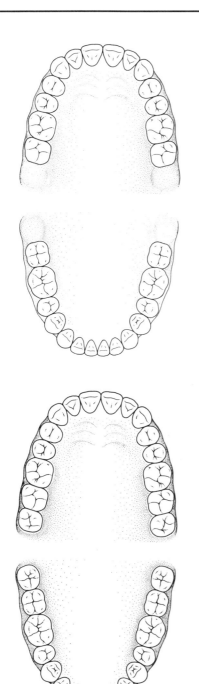

By age thirteen or so, the permanent upper canines have replaced their primary predecessors. As they erupt, they usually force the upper incisors together, closing the spaces between them. Meanwhile, the permanent *second molars*, the *twelve-year molars*, come in behind the first ones.

The last teeth to erupt are the *third molars*, or *wisdom teeth*, starting at about age eighteen. It is not unusual for a person to lack some or all of these four teeth. They also have a tendency to be *impacted* within the jaw, so they cannot erupt properly and may have to be extracted.

may bleed. Pressing a piece of gauze over the area should stop the bleeding quickly. Sometimes a child swallows a shed tooth. It is small and smooth enough to pass through the digestive system as harmlessly as a cherry pit.

By the time the permanent teeth begin to come in, the child should be ready to assume more responsibility for their care. This includes daily brushing and flossing, and the use of disclosing dyes at least once a week (see page 28). The new molars are especially susceptible to decay, and their surfaces must be regularly and thoroughly cleaned of plaque.

Avoiding frequent and prolonged contact with sugar continues to play a crucial role in preventing tooth decay (see page 93). It is important for older children to understand clearly the effects of sugar on their teeth, so they themselves will be motivated to limit its intake.

Small children usually don't suffer from gum disease. But when the permanent teeth come in, gum inflammation (gingivitis) may occur. The most common cause is the buildup of plaque at the junction of tooth and gum, the result of insufficient brushing. The first symptoms are swelling, tenderness, and bleeding. Sometimes the condition can be corrected at home, with vigorous brushing along the gumlines. But if it persists more than a week, you should take the child to the dentist for a periodontal examination.

CONTINUING PROFESSIONAL CARE

Regular, semiannual visits to the dentist become more important than ever as the permanent teeth come in. The dentist will begin to give the child the same basic treatment as an adult receives. Topical applications of fluoride will continue, since young, recently erupted teeth are especially susceptible to decay. The dentist will also watch out for any

orthodontic problems that may arise as the permanent teeth erupt.

In addition, the dentist may apply a *sealant* to the biting surfaces of the permanent back teeth—the molars and premolars. This is a plastic coating that seals out decay-producing plaque. It can be applied easily and painlessly, and lasts two or three years before it needs renewing. A sealant is especially effective in protecting the creviced biting surfaces of the molars, which are difficult to keep free of debris and plaque.

If decay does occur, it is important to fill cavities promptly. If cavities are treated when they are still relatively small, they can often be filled with tooth-colored composites rather than silver amalgam. Such small fillings usually don't require any anesthesia, and sealants will stick to them, to help protect against further decay.

DAMAGE FROM INJURY

Accidents are a very common cause of damage to children's teeth. The front teeth are especially susceptible to being broken or knocked out. Lost teeth not only mar appearance but may also cause speech and orthodontic problems (see page 171).

The best "cure" is prevention. From an early age, children should receive safety training to avoid injury, and should wear protective gear when taking part in active sports.

A broken tooth can sometimes be mended, if the tooth fragment can be found. Otherwise, it can often be recontoured or otherwise restored (see page 186). In any event, a child with a broken tooth should be taken promptly to the dentist.

Permanent teeth that are knocked out can often be successfully reinserted. If a tooth does get knocked out, carry out the following steps *right away.*

SAFETY PRECAUTIONS TO PROTECT YOUR TEETH

- *At the swimming pool.* Use the ladder to climb out. Don't try to haul yourself up onto the side. Don't run alongside the pool. Don't push anyone in.
- *On a swing.* Remain seated until the swing has stopped. Don't jump off a moving swing, or walk under it.
- *On a bike.* Be especially careful in rainy weather. Wet pavements and wet leaves can be very slippery. Never ride in icy weather.
- *In a car.* Be prepared for sudden stops. Always wear a seat belt—even if you're sitting in the back, or the trip is short.
- *When someone is drinking.* Don't hit, push, or throw anything at someone who is drinking from a container or a drinking fountain.
- *When walking, running, or playing.* Watch where you're going. Look out for trees, stumps, curbs, or other obstacles you might trip over. Don't trip or upset a playmate.
- *When using skates or a skateboard.* Keep your skateboard under control. Don't push or trip another skater or try to "hitch a ride."
- *Climbing a tree.* Don't try to climb a wet tree. The footing is too slippery.
- *Sports equipment.* Wear a properly fitted helmet and mouth guard when playing sports like football, ice hockey, and lacrosse. Always wear a mouth guard for boxing and for rough games of basketball. For baseball, if you are catching pitched balls, always wear a catcher's mask.

- Hold the tooth by the crown (not by the root), and if necessary rinse it clean of dirt or blood under running cold water.
- If possible, reinsert the tooth. If that isn't feasible, keep the tooth damp by putting it in a container of milk or even under the child's tongue..
- Take the child to a dentist *immediately;* the probability that reimplantation will be successful drops sharply after 30 minutes.

Unfortunately, treatment of a broken, loose, or reimplanted tooth isn't always successful. After a while, the root may start to resorb, and the tooth will then be lost. Or the tooth pulp may be damaged, causing the tooth to discolor or the pulp to die (see page 116 and page 184).

DENTAL CARE DURING ADOLESCENCE

The permanent molars continue to erupt during adolescence. The third molars, or "wisdom teeth," may not appear before adulthood (see illustrated chart of development, pages 96–99). Sometimes these teeth do not erupt in their proper locations: They may become *impacted* against the adjoining molars, or tightly bound *(ankylosed)* to the underlying bone. In such instances they may have to be surgically extracted (see page 151). An even more common problem is that these back molars are hard to clean, and are thus especially susceptible to plaque buildup and to decay.

Gum inflammation (gingivitis) is not uncommon during adolescence. It is usually mild, but may occasionally become severe enough to endanger the teeth. The causes of adolescent gingivitis are not completely known. Some researchers think it results from hormonal changes at puberty. Others believe that improper diet and poor control of plaque are mainly responsible.

Behavioral habits do cause many adolescent dental problems. Fast-growing adolescents have big appetites, and often snack. Their snacks are likely to be high in sugar. Furthermore, teenagers commonly become lax about cleaning their teeth regularly and thoroughly, and about visiting the dentist. As a result, their teeth become more susceptible to decay, and gingivitis is more likely to occur.

Teenagers may also begin experimenting with tobacco—smoked or chewed—which can damage their teeth and gums.

Persuading adolescents to take good care of their teeth may seem an uphill struggle. As in earlier years, the best thing parents can do may simply be to set a good example. Nagging, or the recital of unpleasant consequences, isn't likely to work. One tactic that may be effective is appealing to the teenager's desire to be physically attractive. A bright, clean smile does make a difference.

ELEVEN

GERODONTICS: DENTAL HEALTH IN LATER LIFE

It is no secret that people live longer than they used to, or that the number of older people in our population is rising. In 1970, about 10 percent of the population was 65 or older. By the year 2000, the ratio will approach 20 percent.

Modern medicine concentrates not only upon helping people survive into old age, but also upon assuring them a good quality of life once they get there. Its aim is not so much adding years to life, as adding life to years. More and more attention is being paid to preventing disorders through healthy habits, and the early treatment of minor disorders before they become major problems.

Modern dentistry shares these goals, especially in its emphasis on preventive care and early intervention. Some of the dental problems of the elderly are directly related to the aging process; others are caused, indirectly, by disorders common in old age. But many of them can be alleviated, if not prevented, through steady, ongoing home care and regular professional treatment.

The total loss of teeth in old age is no longer inevitable. Modern knowledge and techniques greatly increase your chances of retaining your natural teeth for your lifetime. Longer life expectancy, moreover, makes taking care of your dental health a most worthwhile investment. But conscientious dental care, at home and in the dentist's office, is crucial.

Geriatric dentistry is not a recognized dental specialty—at least not yet. But dentists are increasingly aware that dental treatment of older people poses special problems and requires somewhat different solutions. Professional organizations such as the American Society for Geriatric Dentistry (see Appendix) give dentists opportunities to share their research and clinical experience. Such organizations, as well as local dental societies, can help older people find qualified practitioners in this field.

THE AGING PROCESS

As the body ages, fundamental cellular changes gradually reduce some of its functional capacities. Some of the mass of the muscles, for example, is lost, so strength diminishes. Reflexes slow, prolonging reaction times, and food is metabolized at a lower rate. The heart may become less able to pump blood, and the lungs to breathe air.

The body also tends to become more susceptible to illness. The immune system becomes weaker, and less able to resist "opportunistic" infections. "Wear-and-tear" disorders, such as osteoarthritis of the joints, are more common. The bones may become more porous and brittle, to pose a greater threat of fractures. And recovery from illness or injury tends to be slower and less complete.

Physical limitations may be accompanied by psychological problems. Only a relatively small minority of older people, such as those suffering from Alzheimer's disease, become mentally disabled or incompetent. More common are occasional lapses in short-term memory, and a slowing down of mental processes.

Most common of all are problems of self-image and attitude toward life. Some find the losses and disabilities of aging—diminished strength and function, diminished health, and diminished control over their lives—difficult to accept. Chronic depression is not unusual, as well as a low sense of self-worth.

These psychological burdens are not only painful in themselves, they can also have a negative effect on physical health. Some older people react by fiercely defending their independence and denying the existence of any disability. Others become resigned to ill health, concluding that "nobody cares," or, "nothing will help." Denial or resignation can lead to harmful neglect of health and to delay in seeking care until minor disorders become severe.

CHANGES IN THE MOUTH

As people age, certain natural changes take place in the teeth, gums, jawbones, and other tissues of the mouth. Some of these changes are harmless. Others, though, threaten dental health, and require intervention.

DARKENING OF THE TEETH

Over the years, the enamel of the crowns tends to become more transparent, revealing more of the dentin underneath. Moreover, the dentin itself darkens. If the teeth are neglected, this natural darkening may be compounded by stains from food or tobacco.

NARROWING OF THE PULP

With time, additional dentin forms inside the teeth, and the pulp space becomes narrower. Sometimes the pulp may disappear.

As the pulp is reduced, or disappears, the teeth tend to become less sensitive. Also, once they are no longer nourished by the blood vessels of the pulp, they become drier and more brittle. They are more likely to fracture, either under chewing pressure or during attempts at dental restoration.

WORN TEETH

Through long use, the teeth are likely to become worn and to lose some of their substance. There are three main forms of wear: *attrition*, *abrasion*, and *erosion*.

Attrition

Decades of chewing wear down the biting surfaces of the teeth. Sometimes the enamel is completely worn away, exposing the inner dentin. This process hastens the recession of the pulp, and is itself hastened by the destructive habit of grinding the teeth (bruxism). In severe instances, the face may lose some of its *vertical dimension*—the distance separating the nose from the chin.

Abrasion

This type of wear occurs just below the enamel of the tooth crown, in the weaker cementum that covers the roots. It is more prevalent on tooth roots that are partly exposed by receding gums (see below), and is thought to be caused mainly by overly forceful brushing.

Erosion

Acids in the mouth, even if they are not strong enough to cause decay, may etch away parts of the tooth surfaces. Erosion is likelier to occur if the mouth is dry (see below). It is also associated with habitually sucking on acid foods, such as lemons and lemon drops.

RECESSION OF THE GUMS

In many older people, the gums become thinner and less dense. They retreat from the crowns, particularly on the outer sides, exposing some of the cementum covering the

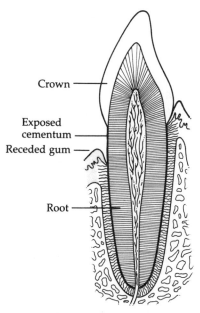

Recession of gum

roots. Gum recession contributes to both abrasion and decay of these exposed surfaces.

WRINKLING OF THE SKIN

When the skin ages, the cells contain less water, and the tissues contain less fat. A typical result is the "purse-string effect" of wrinkles radiating from the lips.

If tooth wear or loss reduces the vertical dimension of the face, particularly deep wrinkles may appear at the outer corners, or angles, of the mouth. Successive wetting and drying within these deep creases may cause them to become inflamed, a condition called *angular cheilitis*. This condition is also associated with vitamin deficiencies, particularly a deficiency of vitamin B_2, and may be accompanied by infections such as *candidiasis* (see page 257).

BONE RESORPTION

Many older people have lost most or all of their natural teeth. When individual teeth are lost, the alveolar bone around them may partly regenerate. But when several teeth are lost, the alveolar bone loses its function and is likely to dissolve, or *resorb*. The lower jaw, or mandible, tends to resorb more swiftly than the upper jaw, or maxilla. Bone loss may be hastened by *osteoporosis*, a condition in which bone density and strength are reduced (see page 276).

MOUTH DRYNESS (XEROSTOMIA)

For a variety of reasons, the salivary glands may generate less saliva. Mouth dryness, or *xerostomia*, appears to result, in part, from the natural aging process. But there can be other causes as well, including diseases such as diabetes and Sjögren's syndrome, and the side effects of radiation treatment and certain

Labels in figure: Crown, Exposed cementum, Receded gum, Root

medications (see page 272, and table, pages 231–233). Smoking and excessive drinking also contribute.

CHANGES IN THE TONGUE

The veins on the underside of the tongue may become more prominent, and the upper surface may become more deeply furrowed. More significant, though, are changes in the tongue that alter the sense of taste.

From about age 45, there is a progressive loss of taste buds. Particularly affected are those that register sweet and salty tastes. This loss is compounded and complicated by the atrophy of the sense of smell, by mouth dryness (to be tasted, substances must be wet), by upper dentures that cover the palate, and by certain diseases and medications (see page 269, and table, pages 231–233). As a result, the sensation of taste may become diminished, distorted, or both.

COMMON DENTAL PROBLEMS

The changes in the mouth that occur with aging are likely to cause—or at least contribute to—dental problems such as tooth decay and periodontal disease.

TOOTH DECAY

After childhood, the teeth usually become less susceptible to decay, and remain so through most of adulthood. But with advancing age, a certain kind of tooth decay, *cervical caries*, becomes more common.

The main reason is gum recession. The shrinking gum tissue exposes the upper parts—the necks—of the roots. The cementum covering them is far less resistant than enamel to the acids generated by bacteria. Thus decay in the exposed necks—cervical caries—becomes more prevalent.

This decay may be accelerated by mouth dryness. The reduced saliva flow may not flush food particles from the teeth, and it may not be as effective in *buffering*, or neutralizing, the acids produced by bacteria.

Other factors contribute to decay. The diet of older people often tends to be relatively soft, sticky, and high in sugars, which enriches the food supply for the bacteria that form plaque. Older people may also lose the manual dexterity needed to brush and floss their teeth efficiently, especially if they suffer from arthritis, Parkinson's disease, or the effects of stroke.

Because of the narrowing of the pulp, the nerves in the teeth are less likely to be sensitive, and so decay is less likely to produce the warning symptom of pain. Cervical decay may eventually undermine the whole crown of the tooth, causing it to break off.

PERIODONTAL DISEASE

The likelihood of periodontal disease also increases with age. Major contributing factors are bacterial plaque and calculus, mouth dryness, and reduced resistance to infection. Inflammation of the gums also accompanies common diseases of advancing age, such as diabetes (see page 270).

Periodontal disease accelerates the resorption of the alveolar bone, and leads to the loosening and loss of teeth. Scrupulous home care and regular professional treatment are crucial in later years to keep the often insidious progress to this disorder in check.

TOOTH LOSS AND MALOCCLUSION

Because the teeth of older people are more brittle, and more susceptible to decay and periodontal disease, they are more likely to be lost. If not promptly replaced by such prosthodontic devices as bridges and dentures, the

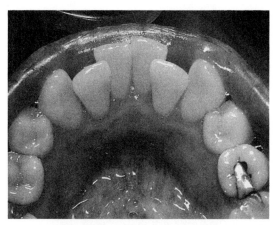

Crowding of lower front teeth
Photograph by Gordon Gaynor

losses may lead to malocclusion, or "bad bite."

If many of the teeth are lost, the bite may lack so much of its vertical dimension that it "collapses." Furthermore, teeth next to open spaces may drift and tip into them, or the opposing teeth in the other jaw may grow out too far, or *overerupt* (see page 131). Malocclusion can make chewing very difficult and inefficient.

In old age, one form of tooth misalignment is very common. Chewing pressure causes all the teeth to move gradually forward. The front teeth—particularly those in the lower jaw—may become crowded and overlapping. Keeping these teeth cleaned and flossed becomes more difficult. Otherwise, the problem is likely to be more aesthetic than functional. It can sometimes be at least partly corrected by selectively *recontouring* the teeth (see page 190).

BAD BREATH

A common source of social embarrassment for older people is bad breath *(halitosis)*. It is especially prevalent among wearers of dentures. There are several potential causes, in-cluding tooth decay, periodontal disease, mouth dryness, systemic disease, smoking, and the side effects of medication. But the most common cause—insufficient home care—should be remediable.

BURNING TONGUE

Many older people, most of them women, suffer a persistent soreness or burning sensation in the tongue, called *glossitis*. Occasionally the burning occurs in the rest of the mouth as well. The causes seem to be multiple, and are not completely understood. They are thought to include the following:

- An imbalance of the female hormone estrogen. The disorder occurs mostly in women after menopause, when the natural production of estrogen is reduced.
- Mouth dryness, or xerostomia (see page 105).
- Vitamin and mineral deficiencies, especially of vitamin B_{12}, folic acid, and iron (see page 268).
- Other medical disorders such as diabetes and stroke.
- Psychological stress, bereavement, and depression.

Treatment concentrates upon these presumed causes. Older women may be given supplemental estrogen. Artificial saliva (see page 110) or other aids may be used to relieve mouth dryness. Diet changes and supplements may help correct deficiencies. Counseling and medications may be used to alleviate stress or depression. Sometimes the symptoms may be relieved by rinsing the mouth with a mixture of an antihistamine such as Benadryl, a topical anesthetic such as Xylocaine, and the coating agent kaopectate. Unfortunately, the condition sometimes doesn't respond to any form of treatment.

DENTURE PROBLEMS

Tooth loss makes it necessary for many older people to wear removable prosthodontic appliances—partial or complete dentures. Over time, these can cause or contribute to a variety of problems.

Poor Fit

As the gums shrink, and the bones of the jaws resorb with age, dentures—particularly complete dentures—may no longer fit. They become increasingly uncomfortable, and are more likely to shift about in the mouth. And since a film of saliva helps keep complete dentures in place, mouth dryness makes the problem worse.

Ill-fitting dentures hinder efficient chewing and clear speech. They may also cause or intensify mouth sores. In severe cases, the discomfort becomes so great that the dentures can't be tolerated.

Particularly painful is the condition that results when the bone of the lower jaw, the mandible, resorbs to such an extent that the *mental* nerves that pass through it on each side lose their bony protection. The pressure of a lower denture is transmitted through the thinned bone to the nerves, and the resulting pain makes chewing virtually impossible.

Mouth Sores and Infections

Dentures, especially if they don't fit properly or are never removed from the mouth, often cause sores of the gums, palate, and tongue. In older people, tissues are irritated easily and heal slowly. Among the most common mouth lesions are *pressure sores, denture stomatitis,* and overgrown tissue on the palate or tongue *(papillary hyperplasia)* or on the gums *(epulis fissuratum)* (see page 141).

Dentures that are not removed regularly and cleaned carefully provide a moist, dark, warm environment ideal for the growth of fungi and bacteria. The most common form of infection is *candidiasis,* or *oral thrush* (see page 257).

Other Denture Problems

Some people with new dentures complain that the plates have a bad taste. Usually the dentures themselves are not to blame. Altered taste sensations tend to be common in later years. Moreover, a complete upper denture covers the palate, which registers some taste sensations. When the palate is covered, these sensations are changed or lost.

Dentures must often be removed during medical treatment—particularly hospitalization. Under these circumstances, it is easy to lose them. They should be permanently marked for identification, with the wearer's name and Social Security number. Some states now require such a built-in record.

With time, dentures may not only lose their fit but also wear down. These artificial teeth may become so worn that the vertical dimension of the bite is reduced. Worn or ill-fitting dentures can be repaired by *relining, rebasing,* or replacement of the prosthetic teeth (see page 141). A whole new denture may be necessary. However, for older wearers, whose mouths have become accustomed to their old dentures, repair is usually far preferable.

Nutritional Deficiencies

For at least two reasons—natural changes and behavioral changes—older people are likely to suffer from nutritional deficiencies that contribute to dental disorders, or otherwise affect dental health adversely.

Aging can alter the digestive system. The body is less able to derive nourishment from food. In particular, it becomes less able to absorb vitamins and minerals. Older people are also likelier to suffer from such digestive disorders as constipation and irritable bowel.

Nutritional deficiencies also stem from harmful changes in diet that may occur when taste sensations fade or alter, the energy for food preparation wanes, and interest in eating generally diminishes. Chewing difficulties from the loss of teeth further contribute to the problem. Complete dentures, for example, cannot withstand the same chewing pressures as natural teeth.

As a result, older people tend to depend more upon prepared, soft, convenience foods—which are too often high in fat, sugar, salt, and cholesterol and relatively low in protein, vitamins, minerals, and fiber. They also tend to eat and drink fewer dairy products, thus depriving their bodies of needed calcium.

Nutritional deficiencies have an adverse effect on dental health both directly and indirectly. Lack of the B vitamin riboflavin, for example, is associated with the fungal infection candidiasis. Calcium deficiency is thought to play a role in osteoporosis, which hastens bone resorption (see page 276). Deficiencies in vitamin B_{12}, folic acid, and iron lead to various forms of anemia, of which a sore, burning tongue is a common symptom (see pages 268–269). A diet rich in sugars and fats contributes to the risk of diabetes, which can cause mouth dryness and gum inflammation, and of heart disease, which complicates dental treatment in several ways.

MEDICAL DISORDERS AND COMPLICATIONS

The aging body has less resistance to disease and heals more slowly and less completely. Moreover, each disorder further stresses the body, making it even more vulnerable.

Certain disorders of the mouth and teeth are especially prevalent among older people. Some of these have already been described: they include angular cheilitis, cervical decay,

mouth dryness, burning tongue, and the fungal infection candidiasis. These and other medical conditions that produce symptoms in the mouth are discussed in greater detail in Chapter 19. Among the most significant are the following:

- Diabetes.
- Hemangioma.
- Oral cancer.
- Paget's disease.
- Pemphigus and bullous pemphigoid.
- Sjögren's syndrome.
- Trigeminal neuralgia.

Some medical disorders, even if they do not produce oral symptoms, can affect how the dentist treats the patient. They are discussed in Chapter 20. For older people, the following are among the most important:

- Adrenal insufficiency, such as occurs in Addison's disease.
- Diabetes.
- Heart and blood vessel diseases.
- Inflammatory joint diseases, such as rheumatoid arthritis and osteoarthritis.
- Liver disorders, such as cirrhosis.
- Lung diseases, such as emphysema.
- Mental impairment, such as occurs in Alzheimer's disease.
- Motor nerve disorders, such as Parkinson's disease and stroke.
- White blood cell disorders, such as leukemia.

GUIDELINES FOR DENTAL HEALTH IN LATER YEARS

Despite the limitations and impediments of aging, maintaining dental health in later life is both possible and worthwhile. What is required is a program of home and professional care, and the determination to carry it out.

HOME CARE OF THE TEETH, GUMS, AND MOUTH

Daily brushing, flossing, and using interdental stimulators continue to be the best ways of assuring the health of your teeth and gums throughout your life. It cannot be stressed too much how desirable it is to retain as many teeth as possible. Even if some teeth are lost, those remaining can provide support for fixed bridges or removable dentures.

For a variety of reasons, such as arthritis, Parkinson's disease, stroke, and a natural decrease in strength, older people may find it difficult to use a standard toothbrush. Often the main difficulty is that the handle is too small to be held firmly and controlled precisely.

Sometimes just making the handle larger can remedy this problem. A rectangle of foam rubber can be wrapped around the handle and taped in place. Or a short length of cast-off garden hose or a flexible bicycle handgrip can be slipped over the handle. A tennis ball with holes punched through the sides can also serve as a handle extension. Finally, you may find that an electric toothbrush provides both a larger handle and more brushing control.

Similarly, if you have trouble holding dental floss between your fingers, you can use a floss holder (see page 31). And the handle of an interdental stimulator, like the handle of a toothbrush, can be built up to make it easier to grip.

A mechanical irrigator, such as a Water Pik, can be very useful in flushing food particles from between teeth or from under fixed bridges. But it is not a substitute for thorough brushing and flossing, since it does not remove plaque.

Moreover, an oral irrigator must be used with caution. If the gums have been damaged by periodontal disease, the jet of water may drive infectious organisms deeper into the pockets, and the infection may spread by way of the bloodstream to other parts of the body. Such infections are especially dangerous to people with heart valve disease or artificial joints (see page 219).

In later years, fluoride becomes even more valuable in fighting tooth decay, especially cervical decay. Topically applied fluoride is absorbed by the cementum of the roots even more effectively than by the enamel of the crowns. Continue to use one of the brands of fluoride toothpaste approved by the American Dental Association. You may supplement it with a fluoride mouthwash or a fluoride compound prescribed by your dentist.

As you get older, it becomes more advisable to brush your tongue when you brush your teeth. Its furrowed, uneven upper surface tends to harbor both the bacteria that cause tooth decay and the fungus *Candida albicans* that causes candidiasis. Brushing the tongue also refreshes the mouth and fights bad breath caused by mouth dryness.

A tendency toward forgetfulness is not unusual in later years. To avoid neglecting regular home care, it may be helpful to use reminders such as a daily checklist or a small sign posted on your bathroom mirror. It is also wise to mark your calendar in advance when an appointment with your dentist becomes due.

REMEDIES FOR MOUTH DRYNESS

Excessive mouth dryness is not only unpleasant in itself; it also contributes to tooth decay and periodontal disease and makes the retention of dentures more difficult. There is no simple, long-lasting remedy. Sometimes the condition can be alleviated by treating underlying conditions that cause it or by adjusting the dosage of medications that contribute to it (see page 231).

Certain medications, called *sialogogues*, tend to stimulate the flow of saliva. But they are not very reliable, and often have undesirable side effects. A simpler method of stimulation is to suck on lemon-flavored hard candies. You must be sure, though, that these contain only artificial sweeteners—sugar will just lead to decay, especially in a mouth that is customarily dry.

You may also be able to relieve mouth dryness by taking frequent sips of water. Some people find it helpful to rinse the mouth periodically with a mouthwash such as Glycothymoline, or with a 10 percent mixture of glycerin in water. Or an artificial saliva may be used. There are several brands available; these include Xerolube, Salivart, Saleze, and Saliacid, which are packaged in squeeze bottles, pump bottles, or the like. Glycothymoline, glycerin solution, and artificial salivas lubricate soft tissues somewhat better than plain water and are especially helpful to denture wearers. One caution: Some artificial salivas contain sodium and should be avoided if you are on a low-sodium or a sodium-free diet.

DIET

A balanced, nutritious diet is very important in preventing dental problems as well as in maintaining general health.

You may have difficulties in chewing, especially if you wear dentures. Nonetheless your diet should include such foods as fresh vegetables and fruits. Cutting chewy or crunchy foods into small pieces, or cooking them slightly, can make them easier to chew. A denture wearer, for example, might not be able to eat a whole raw apple, but would have little or no difficulty chewing thin apple slices, stewed apple, or applesauce.

Older bodies need extra calcium, to maintain bone strength and density. The best source is milk, about two cups a day, unless you are allergic to it or are lactose intolerant. If you are allergic to cow's milk, you may be able to tolerate goat's milk. And if you are lactose intolerant, you can take lactase orally, in order to digest the lactose, or milk sugar.

Ordinarily a nutritious diet will supply you with all the vitamins and minerals you need. But medical conditions may limit your diet, or may place special demands on your system. In such situations, vitamin or mineral supplements, prescribed by your physician, may be advisable.

REGULAR PROFESSIONAL CARE

Some people tend to forego regular dental treatment during what they regard as their "last" years. This is a mistake. Regular professional attention is, if anything, even more important than before, to prevent problems such as decay and periodontal disease and to keep minor disorders from becoming severe. You should continue to visit the dentist for preventive treatment at least every six months—more often if your dentist recommends it.

During these regular visits, the dentist may resume topical applications of fluoride to strengthen root surfaces exposed by receding gums. And if cavities do occur in these areas, the teeth can often be restored with inconspicuous, tooth-colored composite fillings.

Teeth loosened by periodontal disease can often be preserved with *splints*. Attaching unstable teeth to those that are still well anchored can add years to their useful life. The most simple forms are wire *ligatures*—lengths of wire woven around and between the teeth, which are then covered with a layer of composite to prevent irritation of soft tissues. Even stronger and longer lasting support can be provided with *A-splints* (see page 130).

Even if you have lost all your teeth and wear complete dentures, you shouldn't assume that regular professional attention is no longer necessary or helpful. Your mouth will continue to change, and periodic adjustments will be needed to keep your dentures fitting properly. Moreover, your dentures will become worn, and may eventually need repair or even replacement.

Discomfort from dentures is not inevitable if they are fitted properly and cleaned conscientiously. If your mouth does become irritated by pressure sores or denture stomatitis, or if an infection such as candidiasis develops, your dentist can prescribe remedies ranging from antiseptic rinses to antibiotics.

At least once a year, as part of your dental examination, your mouth should be examined for oral cancer. Dentists are trained to spot any suspicious growths at an early stage. When caught early, oral cancer is usually curable. Neglected, it can devastate your health and threaten your life (see page 260).

Every time you visit the dentist, be sure to up-date your medical history, and include any new symptoms, disorders, medications, hospitalizations, or operations. You should also encourage communication between your dentist and your physician—many conditions require a team effort.

Some older people have trouble simply getting to the dentist's office: they cannot drive, or they cannot walk, or they can do neither. If you have this problem, and if you do not have friends or family to take you to the dentist, inquire whether your community or local medical center either provides a transportation service for you or has mobile vans that can bring treatment facilities to you.

Many dental offices provide access to the handicapped—wheelchair ramps, automatic or easily opened doors, elevators, and the like. Also available, though not as widely as it should be, is special equipment for treating disabled patients. There are, for example, special mechanized bases for wheelchairs.

Without having to get up, a patient in a wheelchair can be placed on such a base, and maneuvered into position for treatment, as if the wheelchair were a dental chair. Even simpler is a headrest that can be clamped to the back of a wheelchair, allowing it to be used for at least routine dental treatment.

DENTAL CARE IN A NURSING HOME

Nursing homes often provide only minimal dental care. If you have the responsibility for a patient in a nursing home, you should try to see that the patient receives regular dental attention. If the patient is incapable of cleaning his or her teeth, the task should be performed by a member of the staff. And the patient should have a professional examination at least once a year. If absolutely necessary, you should arrange to have the patient taken to the dentist.

THE IMPORTANCE OF ATTITUDE

A major impediment to dental health in later years is a psychological barrier. Many older people become apathetic and depressed, and tend to neglect their health in general and their dental health in particular. Or dental care is dismissed as "less important" than other medical concerns. But taking care of your teeth and mouth at home, and obtaining regular professional treatment, can contribute significantly to your comfort, your general health, and your quality of life. To a large extent, your dental health depends on your own choices and determination.

The dentin is normally covered and protected by the enamel on the crown, or the cementum on the root. But if the dentin loses part of that protection, exposing its microscopic tubules to such irritations as heat, cold, or acid, the odontoblast cells may become at least mildly irritated. The tooth is then said to be hypersensitive.

Hypersensitivity is very common. By itself, the irritation usually causes no lasting damage to the pulp. In later life, as the pulp becomes narrower, sensitivity is likely to diminish and disappear. But before that it can cause a great deal of discomfort. Eating ice cream, for example, or even brushing can provoke a sharp short pain in an affected tooth.

Hypersensitivity can generally be alleviated without difficulty. Two approaches can be used: sealing the exposed tubule openings and reducing the ability of the affected nerves to transmit pain.

Your dentist seals tubules by applying such chemicals as strontium chloride or stannous fluoride, which cause additional calcium to solidify in the openings. Alternatively, the dentist can cover over the openings with the bonding agents and composite materials used for fillings and other restorations.

Many people find relief just by brushing regularly with a standard fluoride toothpaste. A special '"desensitizing" toothpaste containing strontium chloride can also be used. Another type of desensitizing toothpaste contains potassium chloride, which appears to block the transmission of pain through the nerves. Both types require several applications before they take effect. You may have to try both of them to determine which one works best for you.

Hypersensitivity occurs most often near the gumline, where a receding gum has exposed the relatively thin cementum. Here a flexible gum stimulator can be helpful, with or without desensitizing toothpaste, to burnish the exposed surface of the dentin.

ODONTOBLAST TUBULES ON SURFACE OF DENTIN

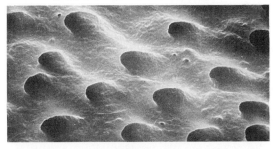

Open

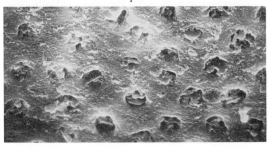

Chemically sealed
Photomicrographs by Block Drug Company

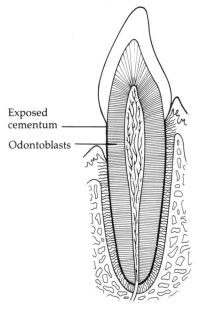

Exposed cementum

Odontoblasts

Hypersensitivity

If sensitivity is severe, the dentist may make you a flexible plastic plate—rather like an athletic mouthguard—that fits over one or both dental arches. It is coated inside with desensitizing chemicals and should be worn for several hours at a time (usually at night). Dentists use the same technique to apply fluorides to teeth that are especially susceptible to decay.

Sometimes, despite repeated efforts to alleviate it, hypersensitivity is severe and persistent. As a last resort, the dentist may perform root canal therapy to eliminate the problem.

PULP INFLAMMATION (PULPITIS)

If the dentin is extensively exposed or lost, damage to the odontoblasts can be severe, and the nerves may become inflamed, a condition called *pulpitis*. A bacterial infection may result, either through the damaged dentin or through the root.

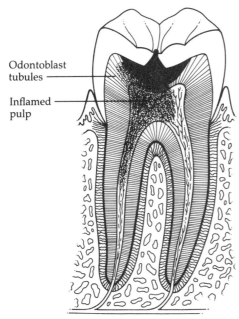

Odontoblast tubules

Inflamed pulp

Pulp inflammation (pulpitis)

The most common symptom of pulpitis is increased sensitivity to specific stimuli, but pulpitis feels somewhat different from the sensitivity of exposed dentin. Rather than a short, sharp, "stabbing" pain, pulpitis tends to cause a lasting, throbbing ache.

Dentists categorize pulpitis as either reversible or irreversible. Reversible pulpitis eventually heals with only conservative treatment, such as removing decay and inserting fillings, or periodontal scaling. Irreversible pulpitis, however, usually requires root canal therapy to keep the condition from growing worse.

To determine whether pulpitis is reversible or irreversible, your dentist is likely to ask you certain questions and perform some simple tests:

- Do you have a history of pain? Have you suffered attacks of pain in the past, or is this the first? If this is the first attack, the pulpitis is more likely to be reversible. If it is the latest in a series of attacks over weeks or months, the pulpitis may be irreversible.
- During the current attack, is your pain steady or intermittent? And do you find relief from mild analgesics like aspirin or Tylenol? If the pain comes and goes, and can be relieved with low doses of analgesics, the pulpitis is more likely to be reversible. If the pain is steady and persistent, if it gets worse when you lie down, or if analgesics give little or no relief, the pulpitis is more likely to be irreversible.
- Is the tooth sensitive to cold and sweets, but *not* to heat or pressure? This is evidence that the pulpitis is still reversible. If, however, the tooth is sensitive to heat, and *relieved* by cold, it is likely to be irreversible.
- Is the tooth sensitive to pressure or tapping? Does chewing provoke pain? Does gentle pressure on the gum near the

PART III

ADVANCED PROFESSIONAL CARE

TWELVE

ENDODONTICS: INSIDE THE TEETH

At the center of each of your teeth is a structure of soft tissue known as the *pulp*. It occupies a pulp chamber inside the crown, and extends to each root apex through a slender root canal. Its elements include the following:

- *Blood vessels*, which carry oxygen and nourishment to the tooth and remove carbon dioxide. The blood cells help to maintain and rebuild the tooth, and to protect it from damage and infection.
- *Odontoblasts*, specialized cells that make up the outer lining of the pulp. They have fine, threadlike extensions that radiate outward from the pulp through narrow channels, or *tubules*, in the dentin. Their chief function is to form new dentin from minerals and other substances conveyed by the blood.
- *Sensory nerves*, which respond to stimuli such as hot and cold, pressure, electricity, and acidity. They may respond to these stimuli directly, but more often they respond indirectly, when the odontoblasts are stimulated.

- Fibrous *connective tissue*, which supports the pulp. With age, the fibrous tissue makes up an increasingly large proportion of the pulp.

Ordinarily, odontoblasts are shielded from the environment outside the tooth by the enamel and the cementum. But if this shield is thin or damaged, the odontoblast tubules may be exposed to irritating stimuli, and may then communicate the irritation to the nerves. The nerves respond by registering pain, which may range from mild sensitivity to severe discomfort.

When the teeth first erupt in childhood, the pulp is relatively large and close to the outer surface. As a result, children's teeth tend to be more sensitive than the teeth of adults. Later in life, additional dentin forms inside the tooth, making the pulp chamber smaller and the root canals narrower. The teeth of older people thus become relatively insensitive. Eventually, the chamber and canals may fill in almost entirely, so that very little pulp remains.

At any time, the enamel and cementum of

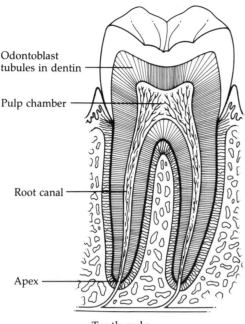

Odontoblast
tubules in dentin

Pulp chamber

Root canal

Apex

Tooth pulp

a tooth may become damaged, exposing the dentin, or even the pulp itself, to "insult." As a result, the pulp may become sensitive or inflamed, or it may even die. The sources of damage include the following:

- Severe tooth decay, penetrating deep into the dentin, if not actually reaching the pulp (see page 61). This is the most common cause of pulp damage.
- Trauma to the tooth or its supporting alveolar bone, from an accident or blow. The tooth may be fractured—cracked or broken. Or it may be *avulsed*—completely dislodged from the jaw. But even if the tooth is not visibly damaged, the shock of trauma is often enough to injure the pulp.
- Severe wear of the tooth surfaces, through attrition, abrasion, or erosion.
- Advanced periodontal disease, in which the pulp is infected through the sides or the end of the root.

- Tooth *reduction*, the process of grinding down the tooth enamel and dentin. Your dentist may have to reduce a tooth substantially, either for a deep filling or for the insertion of an artificial crown or fixed bridge. The friction of such a procedure can produce heat, which, in turn, inflames the pulp. Also, the materials used to take impressions, to fill a cavity, or to fasten a restoration in place may irritate or damage the pulp.

The specialty in which pulp damage and pulp death are treated is called *endodontics*, a term derived from words meaning "inside the teeth." The most prevalent form of endodontic treatment is the removal and replacement of the pulp, a process called *root canal therapy*.

Endodontic treatment is performed by general dentists, as well as by endodontic specialists. General dentists are more likely to refer to endodontists those patients whose conditions are relatively complex or whose treatment holds greater risks of complications (see page 125). If you need to find a specialist on your own, you can follow the procedures described in Chapter 2. Many endodontists belong to the American Association of Endodontists, which can supply you with a list of its members in your area (see Appendix).

DEGREES OF PULP INJURY

The degree to which the tooth pulp may be injured varies widely, from mild irritation to nerve death.

HYPERSENSITIVITY

The mildest response of the pulp is simple *hypersensitivity*. It results from the exposure of tooth dentin.

tooth reveal swelling or sensitivity? All these symptoms suggest that the pulpitis is not only irreversible but has spread from the root to the *periapical* tissues beyond.

Often the pain will be generalized, and your dentist must perform tests to identify the specific tooth affected. One such test is to run a mild electrical current through a tooth. If it produces a tingling sensation, the pulp is still vital. If no reaction is produced, the pulp may have been so badly damaged that it is dead.

A more precise test is to inject a little local anesthetic next to a suspected tooth. If the anesthetic produces prompt relief from pain, that tooth is probably the one affected.

Another possible symptom of pulp damage is darkening of a particular tooth. Such darkening may be caused by leakage of blood from damaged pulp into the surrounding dentin. (Blood contains iron, which stains the tooth brown or gray.) Your dentist can sometimes remove this stain during root canal therapy, but it may require special treatment, such as bleaching, afterward (see page 124).

NERVE DEATH AND PERIAPICAL ABSCESS

Pulpitis, especially if it is caused by tooth decay, usually works its way from the pulp chamber through the root canal to the root apex. Bacterial infection, which gravely damages the pulp, often occurs. By the time the infection reaches the root apex, the nerve is dead.

The tooth itself may become insensitive, but pain in the *periapical* area beyond the root often continues, or even becomes worse. At this stage, root canal therapy is usually essential, to keep the infection from spreading farther into the surrounding tissues. The only other alternative is extracting the tooth.

Inflammation and infection of the pulp

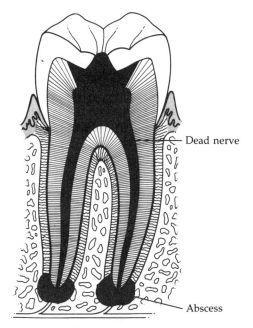

Nerve death and periapical abscess

may cause the adjacent bone to erode, forming a pus-filled *abscess*. The accumulating pus may exert pressure on the already inflamed periapical nerves, causing severe pain—a classic "toothache." The pressure of the pus may also force the tooth slightly out of its socket, so that it meets the opposing teeth prematurely when you chew, and the pain is intensified.

At this stage, you may suffer from swelling of the soft tissues of your face *(cellulitis)*, accompanied by fever and other symptoms of spreading infection. Generalized, *systemic* infection is fairly rare, but even in this age of antibiotics it can be very dangerous. When cellulitis appears, your need for root canal therapy is likely to be urgent. Usually the tooth will still be salvageable, but sometimes the only course of action is extraction.

An abscess is usually visible on an X-ray. It may also reveal itself by a *fistula*—a channel that forms in the bone, allowing the pus to drain out through the gum. To establish the precise location of an abscess, your dentist will sometimes pass a length of material opaque to X-rays through the fistula and back to its source.

But you will not always feel pain with pulp inflammation or periapical infection. Occasionally, these processes can occur without any symptoms you are aware of, until your dentist discovers the problem during an examination. That's one reason that regular professional care is so important.

PULP CAPPING AND PULPOTOMY

Although the standard remedy for pulp inflammation and nerve death is root canal therapy, more conservative techniques are sometimes used. If damage to the pulp is very slight, very recent, and therefore reversible, your dentist may attempt to save it by *pulp capping*. If the damage is irreversible, your dentist may nonetheless prefer to delay root canal therapy by performing a transitional procedure called *pulpotomy*.

Dentists generally use pulp capping (see page 67) for teeth that are deeply decayed—that is, the decay comes close to, or even reaches, the pulp. Pulp capping is often performed on recently erupted teeth of children or adolescents, before their roots have completely developed. If the pulp can be kept alive, even temporarily, the roots are more likely to form normally.

Sometimes the capping procedure effectively isolates the pulp, and it returns to normal. Often, however, the procedure is only a temporary solution. The pulp eventually becomes inflamed or dies, and root canal therapy is necessary.

Moreover, root canal therapy may be more difficult to perform following a pulp-capping failure. The calcium hydroxide used in pulp capping stimulates the formation of additional dentin inside the tooth, including the

root canal or canals. The extra dentin may close off a canal so that the dentist cannot penetrate it.

If there is evidence that the pulp is irreversibly damaged but not yet dead, the dentist may choose to remove it *only* from the pulp chamber, leaving the pulp in the canal or canals undisturbed. This procedure is known as *pulpotomy* (literally "cutting the pulp"). Once the pulp chamber is cleaned out, the dentist packs it with a material like zinc oxide and eugenol, and seals it with a temporary filling.

Like pulp capping, pulpotomy is often performed on incompletely formed teeth of children or adolescents, to give the roots a chance to develop fully. It is sometimes used for damaged primary teeth, to keep them from being lost prematurely. In adults, pulpotomy is usually an emergency procedure, to bring relief from pain until root canal therapy can be performed.

Pulpotomy thus is a temporary expedient. Sooner or later, complete root canal therapy will be needed. Otherwise the pulp is likely to become infected, eventually causing a painful abscess and the risk of losing the tooth.

ROOT CANAL THERAPY

The symptom most likely to make canal therapy necessary is pain, when the pulp is irreversibly damaged. The only alternative is extracting the tooth.

Even before you go to the office for treatment, your dentist may prescribe an analgesic to relieve the pain. You may also find it helpful to apply a cold pack to the part of your face over the affected tooth.

Two things you should *not* do. First, don't apply a *hot* compress—if the inflammation is accompanied by infection, heat can make it spread. Second, don't try the folk remedy of placing an aspirin tablet in the painful area. It may provide temporary relief, but it will burn the soft tissues of the gums and cheek.

Before the development of modern anesthetics and analgesics, patients faced root canal therapy with justifiable dread. There is still some discomfort connected with the procedure, but current techniques have greatly reduced it. Moreover, the discomfort is far less severe than the pain of pulp inflammation or an abscess. Most important, root canal therapy can save teeth that otherwise would have to be extracted.

At your first visit, the affected tooth may be obvious. Otherwise the dentist will probably perform some diagnostic tests and studies, such as those described earlier. These are likely to include a fairly extensive series of X-rays, taken from different angles, to locate the pulp, and to evaluate damage to the tooth and the alveolar bone. Other possible causes of pain, such as sinusitis or neuralgia, must be ruled out.

Root canal therapy has three steps:

- Removal of the pulp from the chamber and each canal, a process called *pulpectomy*.
- Cleaning, shaping, and smoothing the chamber and canal surfaces.
- Drying out the empty cavity, and filling it with an inert material.

In rare instances, these steps may all be carried out in a single office visit. More often, though, two, three, or more visits are required.

PULPECTOMY

Before removal, or *debridement*, of the pulp begins, your dentist will administer an anesthetic—generally an injected local anesthetic—and will isolate the tooth, usually with a rubber dam (see page 63). The dentist

ROOT CANAL THERAPY

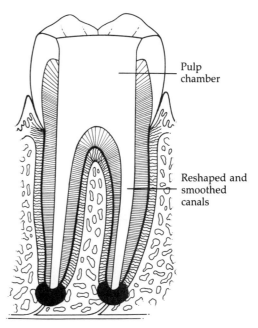

Pulp chamber

Reshaped and smoothed canals

Pulpectomy

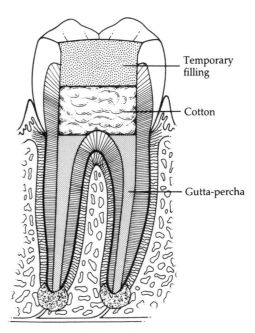

Temporary filling

Cotton

Gutta-percha

Pulp replacement

may grind away a little of the enamel on the biting surface to reduce the amount of pressure upon it from the opposing teeth. An access channel is then drilled through the enamel and dentin into the pulp chamber.

The pulp chamber is usually large enough so the pulp can be removed with the power handpiece. But the canals are so fine, and often so irregularly shaped, that they must be debrided with small hand instruments, described collectively as *endodontic files*.

It is important to remove the pulp tissue as thoroughly as possible—any that remains is likely to become a source of infection. Even if the pulp in only one canal of a multirooted tooth is damaged, the pulp in all the other canals must be removed as well.

Throughout the procedure, your dentist will periodically irrigate the area with antiseptic solutions, which usually contain sodium hypochlorite or hydrogen peroxide (the same active ingredients as in household bleaches). Irrigation helps dissolve and carry away pulp material; it also helps destroy any bacteria in the area.

Pulpectomy is usually completed in one visit. At the conclusion of the visit, and of every successive visit until treatment is completed, your dentist will dry the pulp chamber, insert pellets of cotton into it, and then cover it with a temporary filling or a crown.

One of the immediate goals of treatment is to relieve pain. Pulp inflammation can sometimes be alleviated just by opening the chamber and affected canals. A periapical abscess, similarly, may be relieved by releasing the accumulated pressure of pus and gas.

Nonetheless, once the anesthetic has worn off, you are likely to experience discomfort for a few days, until the tissues around each root apex calm down. Again, your dentist may prescribe a mild analgesic to relieve the pain. If there is evidence of bacterial infection, antibiotics may be prescribed as well.

CLEANING, SHAPING, AND SMOOTHING

Once the pulp has been removed, the chamber and each canal must be prepared to receive the inert material that will replace the pulp. Using files and antiseptics, your dentist continues to clean the area of any remaining pulp tissue. Very fine files are used to smooth and shape the walls of each canal. The ideal shape would be a completely straight channel, tapering gently toward the apex, but the natural irregularity of tooth roots and their canals usually makes this goal difficult to achieve.

After completing this process, your dentist may delay the next stage until a later visit, so that the surrounding tissues can recover from irritation. Cotton pellets are again placed in the chamber, and sealed with a temporary filling or crown.

FILLING

Once the pulp is removed, the chamber and canals must not be left empty. The final step is filling them with an inert material. The one almost all dentists use is a natural, flexible resin called *gutta-percha*.

Gutta-percha is manufactured in slender, tapered "points." Your dentist dries the pulp chamber and each canal as thoroughly as possible, and then inserts the points, lightly coated with cement, one at a time. The points are pressed, or *condensed*, against the walls until the whole cavity is fully packed, and X-rays are taken to confirm that the insertion is complete and snug, right down to the apex of each root. The dentist then seals the access channel with a filling, which may be temporary or permanent.

The treated tooth retains much of its strength, and should be serviceable for a number of years. Nevertheless, it no longer has a pulp, and its blood supply is much reduced, so it is likely to become brittle and more susceptible to fracture. The natural crown must often be replaced with an artificial one, once root canal therapy is completed. And if the tooth needs even more strengthening, a *post* can be inserted.

POST INSERTION

During or after root canal therapy, your dentist may determine that the root needs additional reinforcement, or that too little of the natural crown remains to support an artificial crown.

Under these circumstances, a metal *post* may be inserted into the treated tooth.

First, your dentist drills a tapered hole for the post into the gutta-percha packing. The hole must extend deep into the root canal, but not so deep that it pierces the sealed apex.

The post may take either of two forms. The first is a metal pin or screw, inserted into the hole, and cemented in place. The dentist then builds up the top of the pin with silver amalgam or composite resin, to make a *core* for an artificial crown.

The second form is a combined, single-unit *post and core,* cast in a dental laboratory from an impression of the hole. Like the built-up post, the cast post-and-core is cemented into the hole to support the artificial crown.

APEXIFICATION

In certain instances, dentists perform a special kind of root canal therapy called *apexification.* It is most commonly used on children's permanent teeth, when they have first erupted but still have incompletely formed roots. Ordinarily, a root canal narrows to a very fine passage at the apex, and this passage can be sealed off with gutta-percha. But if the root is not completely formed, or if it has been damaged, the canal may "flare" open at the apex, making it impossible to be sealed with gutta-percha.

If the pulp isn't too badly damaged, the dentist may simply perform a pulpotomy (see page 121), which leaves the canal undisturbed while the root completes its development. But if the pulp in the canal is severely damaged or dead, the dentist must perform a pulpectomy, right down to the flared apex. The canal is then cleaned, dried, and temporarily filled with calcium hydroxide paste, instead of gutta-percha.

Calcium hydroxide stimulates the formation of additional dentin around the canal. The new dentin *apexifies* the tooth; it builds up the apex. Once the canal has sufficiently narrowed, it can be filled with gutta-percha.

Apexification doesn't always work. If it does not, the apex may have to be removed and sealed off by the surgical procedure of *apicoectomy* (see page 125).

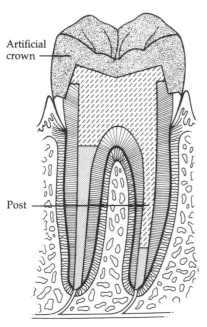

Artificial crown

Post

Cast post and core

TOOTH WITH FLARED ROOT

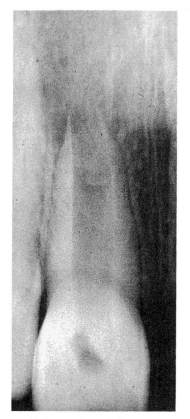

Before root canal therapy

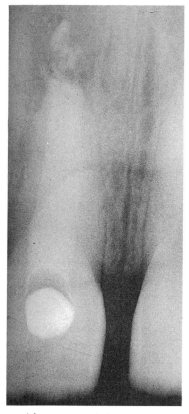

After root canal therapy
Radiographs by Morton Brenner

BLEACHING

As described earlier, a tooth with damaged pulp may become discolored, usually from the iron in the blood that leaks into the tubules of the surrounding dentin. Often the staining results from trauma to the tooth, and it may be the first sign that the pulp has been damaged. More rarely, it appears after root canal therapy.

A treated tooth may have to be stabilized with an artificial crown, which will also cover up any discoloration. But if the natural enamel remains, the iron stain can often be removed by *internal bleaching.*

Your dentist first completes basic root canal therapy as usual, and allows time for the tissues to recover from irritation, usually a few days. Then the pulp chamber is re-entered and emptied. Your dentist introduces a strong solution of hydrogen peroxide, and applies heat from a warm instrument or a light beam to hasten the bleaching process. More than one bleaching treatment may be necessary to achieve satisfactory results.

Between office visits, you may be treated

with a *walking bleach.* Your dentist inserts cotton saturated with a relatively mild bleach (sodium perborate) in the partly emptied pulp chamber, and covers it with a temporary filling. You then "walk around" while the contained bleach gradually lightens the tooth.

Once a satisfactory degree of lightening is achieved, your dentist will insert a filling to seal up the pulp chamber and access channel. Bleaching, however, doesn't always remove iron stains. If a stain has existed for a long time—more than six months or so—bleaching is less likely to remove it. Other techniques, such as composite bonding or veneering (see Chapter 17) may then be used to hide the discoloration.

RISKS AND COMPLICATIONS OF ROOT CANAL THERAPY

The success rate of root canal therapy is high, over 90 percent. Nevertheless, it is not always effective, and complications may develop later.

Some teeth just can't be treated properly. The canals may be too narrow or too obstructed or too sharply angled to be debrided. Sometimes these problems can be remedied by surgical removal of the root apex, the procedure called *apicoectomy* (see below). In some instances, however, the only solution is extraction.

Sometimes roots contain, instead of a single canal leading to each apex, additional canals or side branches that cannot be reached with instruments. If these additional canals are close to the root apex, they may be removed by apicoectomy. But occasionally the whole tooth must be removed.

Despite your dentist's best efforts, things may go wrong during treatment. For example, a complete, perfect pulpectomy is very difficult. Cleaning out and sterilizing the narrowest part of the canal near the apex is es-

pecially challenging. And even a tiny bit of pulp left in a canal can cause bacteria to pass through the apex to infect the periodontium beyond. If this occurs, root canal therapy may have to be repeated. If the problem persists, the apex may have to be removed, or the tooth may have to be extracted.

Endodontic files are fine and fragile. Inside a canal, the end can easily become separated from the shank, especially if the canal is narrow or sharply angled, and it is usually impossible to remove the separated piece. Sometimes the dentist can pack gutta-percha around it, but apicoectomy may have to be performed, to seal off the apex directly.

Sometimes files perforate the sides of roots or accidentally penetrate the apex, and thus widen the opening. Or some of the gutta-percha may be forced through the apex. All these accidents reduce the chances for successful healing.

During either the shaping or filling process, a tooth may fracture, leaving a crack that cannot be sealed. Bacteria can seep through the crack to cause a continuing infection. In such an instance, the tooth must be extracted.

Finally, the infection around the roots of teeth, or damage from trauma, can cause the roots or the surrounding bone to dissolve, or *resorb.* Root canal therapy will often halt this process. Occasionally, however, resorption will occur even after repeated treatments. Inserting a post (see above) or surgically removing the infected apex may stabilize a tooth enough to save it. But sometimes the tooth will have so little support that it will be lost.

APICOECTOMY

When root canal therapy cannot successfully seal off a root apex, the surgical procedure

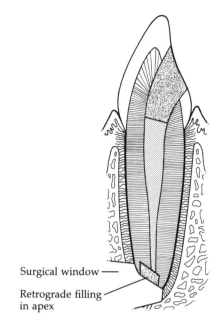

Surgical window ———

Retrograde filling
in apex

Apicoectomy

called apicoectomy may be used as a supplementary procedure. Apicoectomy may be performed as part of root canal therapy, or separately. Many dentists choose to refer such cases to an oral surgeon.

To reach the apex, the surgeon cuts a "window" through the gum and bone. Any infected tissue around the root is removed. If necessary, the apex itself is cut back to sound tissue. The canal is then sealed with a *retrograde filling*, usually of silver amalgam. When a tooth has more than one root, the whole defective root may be removed, a procedure called *root resection*.

T H I R T E E N

PROSTHODONTICS: MAJOR REPAIRS AND REPLACEMENTS

For any of several reasons, your teeth may suffer extensive damage. The teeth themselves may be severely decayed, discolored, or fractured, or they may become loose in their sockets because of periodontal disease. The damage may prevent them from functioning properly or may cause them to be lost entirely. Such conditions may require *prosthodontic* treatment. The term comes from Greek words meaning "replacement of teeth," but prosthodontic techniques are used to repair teeth as well as replace them. Prosthodontics has three main purposes:

- *Restoration of function.* Loose teeth may be supported, damaged teeth may be repaired, and missing teeth may be replaced to make normal chewing possible and to improve the *occlusion*, or bite.
- *Prevention of further damage.* Loose teeth can be stabilized to prevent them from loosening further. Damaged teeth can be repaired to halt further decay or fracturing. Lost teeth can be replaced to prevent the remaining teeth from tipping, drifting, or growing where they don't belong.

- *Improvement in appearance.* Damaged, discolored, or missing teeth are often unsightly, if not disfiguring. Appropriate restorations can make the mouth look more "like new."

Prosthodontics is one of the recognized dental specialties. Prosthodontic treatment, however, is often provided by general dentists.

Most prosthodontic restorations fall within a few basic categories.

- Damaged but salvageable teeth can be repaired with *onlays* or *artificial crowns.*
- Loose teeth can be stabilized with *splints.*
- Missing individual teeth, or a few missing teeth, are often replaced with *fixed bridges.*
- More than a few missing teeth may need to be replaced with *removable dentures,* either *partial* or *complete.*

Prosthodontic dentistry often involves several teeth at a time, and it may be necessary to use more than one type of treatment. A complete treatment plan, including detailed diagnosis, a description of the type of treatment to be used, and a thorough analysis of likely outcomes, is particularly important. If extensive treatment is recommended, a second opinion may be advisable.

ONLAYS

Onlays are essentially large fillings. The term *onlay* is used when a substantial portion of the tooth crown needs to be replaced, and at least one protruding cusp is involved.

Onlays are used to restore teeth severely damaged either by decay or wear. Since they are often subjected to heavy chewing pressures, they must be made of very durable material. In most instances, this means gold or some other cast metal that can withstand chewing pressures without shattering or deforming (see page 65). Porcelain is sometimes used. It has the advantage of matching the tooth in color, but it tends to be brittle and

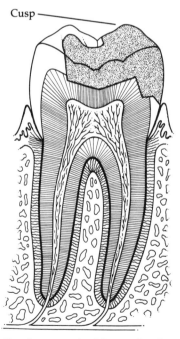

Cusp

Tooth restored with metal onlay

may become "leaky" around the edges (see page 65).

The use of metal onlays is generally limited to the back teeth, where they are not so visible. They are fabricated, inserted, and cemented in place just like cast metal fillings.

ARTIFICIAL CROWNS

If one or more of your front teeth are substantially damaged, or if the back teeth are in too poor a condition for onlays, they may be restored with artificial crowns, sometimes called *caps*. Teeth that have been treated by root canal therapy must almost always be restored in this way.

An artificial crown replaces the enamel and some of the dentin of the natural crown of the tooth. Any of several materials may be used.

- Gold or other cast metal is often used for crowns on less-visible molars. Metal is stable, durable, and long-lasting.
- On the more visible front teeth and premolars, crowns are often made with a core of gold or other metal and covered partly or entirely with a tooth-colored material—acrylic plastic or porcelain. Modern acrylic is fairly durable and easy to work with. Porcelain is even stronger and looks more like natural tooth enamel. Porcelain, however, is so hard that it can cause significant wear on the opposing teeth.
- Occasionally, all-porcelain *jacket crowns* are used. They can be made to match teeth closely but tend to be brittle. Some new porcelain formulations have been developed under such brand names as Cerestore and Dicor, which appear to be more resistant to shattering. They have been available for too short a time, however, for their long-range reliability to be judged.

If one of your teeth requires an artificial crown, the dentist will start by preparing the tooth. The dentist administers an anesthetic, usually an injected local, and removes the enamel and some of the dentin of the natural crown to a level slightly below the gumline. What remains is a peg-like core of dentin. If the nerve of the tooth is dead or exposed, root-canal therapy will be required, and the root should also be reinforced with a *post* (see page 123).

The dentist then takes impressions of both jaws (see page 24). The impression of the prepared tooth must be extremely accurate, and it must extend under the gumline even farther than the level of preparation. Usually, the dentist packs a length of chemically treated *retraction cord* around the neck of the tooth before taking the impression, to push back the gum, and to prevent contamination from saliva or blood.

The impression of the opposing jaw is called a *counter impression*. The dentist also takes a third impression, of the biting surfaces of the teeth of both jaws together, to record the relationship between them. This impression is known as a *bite*. In a dental laboratory, models will be cast of the two jaws, and mounted together in the relationship registered by the bite.

If a tooth-colored material is to be used for the crown, the dentist provides the laboratory with a specific selection from a *shade guide*—a set of color samples—so that the crown will match the adjacent teeth as closely as possible. Meanwhile, the dentist will cement a temporary crown over the prepared tooth, to protect the exposed dentin between visits.

At the laboratory, the crown is carefully fabricated on the model of the prepared tooth, to meet following criteria:

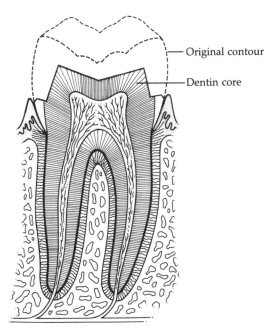

Tooth prepared for artificial crown

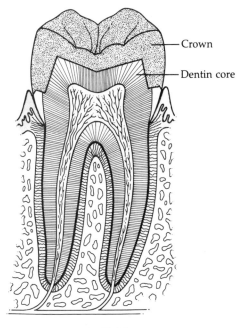

Artificial crown

- It must fit the prepared tooth precisely, forming a tight seal over the reduced dentin, and a smooth, unbroken contour with the surface of the root.
- If it is to be tooth-colored, it must match the color selected from the shade guide.
- It must harmonize with the adjacent teeth in size and shape, and must fit between them snugly, forming definite *proximal contacts* on each side.
- It must meet the opposing teeth so that the bite is correct.

When the crown is returned by the laboratory, the dentist performs a *try-in*, slipping it over the prepared tooth to evaluate its appearance, comfort, and function. It is not unusual for the crown then to be returned to the laboratory for reshaping, recoloring, or polishing.

In rare instances, the crown may be so unsatisfactory that additional impressions must be taken, and a new crown fabricated. But often a crown is judged to be satisfactory at the first or second try-in. It is then cemented in place, either temporarily or permanently.

Temporary cement gives you an opportunity to wear the crown for several days to evaluate it, and to have it removed for further adjustment if needed. But only an all-metal or metal-core crown can be temporarily cemented; an all-porcelain jacket crown is too brittle to be safely removed once it is inserted. To make removal easier, a metal-based crown

is usually constructed with a small knob or button projecting on the tongue side. Just before permanently cementing the crown, the dentist may grind off the removal button.

Sometimes the nerve of a tooth may die after a crown is permanently cemented. It is still possible to save the tooth with root-canal therapy, either by drilling a hole through the restoration, or by performing an *apicoectomy*—surgery through the gum and bone to reach the apex of the root (see page 125).

Crowns are customarily used to restore individual teeth, but when adjacent crowned teeth are loose, as from periodontal disease, the crowns can sometimes be soldered together to form a stabilizing *splint*.

SPLINTS

Teeth may become loose, or *mobile*, from a variety of causes. By far the most prevalent is advanced periodontal disease, which erodes the supporting bone. If teeth are not too mobile, and otherwise sound, they may be stabilized with a splint, which binds them to firm adjacent teeth and to each other, and thus distributes the pressures of chewing among them.

A widely used form is the *A-splint*. It may connect a single mobile tooth to a single firm *abutment* tooth, or it may connect a group of mobile teeth to abutments on either side.

To create an A-splint, the dentist cuts continuous channels into the involved teeth—the top surfaces of back teeth or the sides of front teeth. Lengths of wire, or even nylon filament (rather like fishline) are laid into these channels. The dentist then fills the channels with a stabilizing material—often the same kind of tooth-colored composite used to fill cavities to hold the wire or filament in place and to bind the teeth together.

A-splints are relatively inconspicuous and can be inserted quickly and easily during a

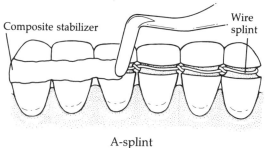

Composite stabilizer — Wire splint

A-splint

From: Dale, B. G., and Aschheim, K. W., Esthetic Dentistry: A Clinical Approach to Techniques and Materials. © 1991, Lea and Febiger

single office visit. Another, more elaborate form of restoration that may serve as a splint is the *Maryland bridge* (see page 132). Aside from its greater cost, it has one major disadvantage. One or more of the splinted teeth may come loose, and it is then difficult, if not impossible, to refasten them to the bridge.

For a good appearance and lasting reliability, neither A-splints nor Maryland bridges can match splints of full artificial crowns, soldered together to form a single, fixed unit.

THE NEED TO REPLACE LOST TEETH

When teeth are lost, they should be promptly replaced. There are a few exceptions to this rule, such as the third molars, or "wisdom teeth." But the rule applies to virtually all other teeth, for several reasons.

For most people, the most important reason is probably appearance. Gaps left by missing teeth are unsightly. And when many teeth are lost, the mouth is likely to look caved in and collapsed. Deep creases may form at the outer corners of the mouth, which often leads to an inflammation called *angular cheilitis* (see pages 265–266).

Even more important are disorders of function that result when teeth are lost. Missing teeth obviously affect your ability to chew efficiently; and they also tend to throw your bite off balance, causing *malocclusion,* or "bad bite." Then damage to the remaining teeth, such as fracturing, becomes more likely. So does periodontal disease. Malocclusion is also believed to be one of the possible causes of temporomandibular disorders.

Perhaps most serious of all are misalignments of the remaining teeth. These teeth don't just stay in their sockets. If deprived of the support and restraint of the teeth next to them, they may move. Back teeth, in particular, tend to rotate, tip over, or shift into the empty gaps. Moreover, when teeth fail to

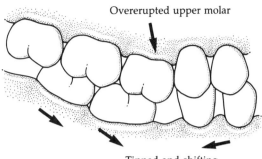

Overerupted upper molar

Tipped and shifting lower teeth

Tipping, shifting, and overeruption following loss of lower first molar

meet resistance from matching teeth in the other jaw, they may grow out too far, or *overerupt.* All these misalignments make malocclusion even more severe.

FIXED BRIDGES

If only a few of your teeth are missing—usually no more than four adjacent front teeth, or two side teeth, they may be replaced by a *fixed* restoration called a *bridge.* A dental bridge, like a highway bridge, ordinarily has two elements. It is supported by *abutments,* sound teeth on either side of the empty gap. The span, or *pontic* (from a Latin word meaning "bridge"), is a metal framework attached to the abutments at each end, with one or more artificial teeth attached to it.

For stability and durability, there should be at least as many sound, firmly fixed abutment teeth as there are teeth to be replaced. Moreover, these abutments must usually have artificial crowns, even if they are healthy in themselves.

Sometimes an entire dental arch is restored with a single fixed bridge. Crowns are placed on *all* the sound teeth in the jaw, not just those next to the pontics. This is known informally as a "roundhouse."

On a properly made bridge, the artificial

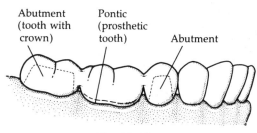

Abutment (tooth with crown)

Pontic (prosthetic tooth)

Abutment

Fixed bridge

teeth and abutment crowns should not only match your natural teeth in shape and color, they should also look as if they are growing out of the gums. In fact, though, the pontic should barely touch the gums. Putting unnecessary pressure on the gums and underlying bone can damage them. Furthermore, there should be enough space beneath the pontic so dental floss can be passed along the underside, to keep the restoration clean.

THE MARYLAND BRIDGE

To avoid having to remove all the enamel of healthy abutment teeth, dentists at the University of Maryland have in recent years developed an alternative, the *Maryland Bridge.* Here, the abutments are not complete crowns but simply metal onlays, bonded to the inside (lingual) surfaces of front teeth and the biting surfaces of molars.

The main advantage of a Maryland bridge

is that the natural teeth are largely undisturbed. It is also likely to be less expensive than a standard bridge. The main disadvantage is that the Maryland bridge is more likely to come loose from the abutment teeth. For long-term reliability, a standard bridge is preferable.

CANTILEVER BRIDGE

Ordinarily a bridge is composed of abutments with a pontic between them. Under certain circumstances, however, the pontic may be supported at one end only. This is known as a *cantilever* bridge.

A cantilever bridge is most commonly used in two situations:

- If a lateral incisor is missing, it may be replaced with a cantilever bridge anchored to the adjacent canine, which makes a relatively strong, well-anchored abutment.
- If all three adjacent molars are missing, the first molar may be replaced with a cantilever bridge. The bridge must be supported by at least *two* abutment teeth—the adjacent premolars—that have connected crowns. Moreover, the cantilever extension should extend no farther than the single molar, so its benefits are more aesthetic than functional.

Cantilever bridges are by no means as stable as bridges supported at both ends. They

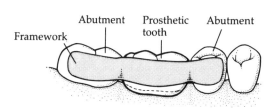

Framework

Abutment

Prosthetic tooth

Abutment

Maryland bridge (view from within)

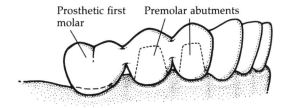

Prosthetic first molar

Premolar abutments

Cantilever bridge

are more likely to come loose themselves, or to loosen the abutment teeth, causing periodontal damage. Often they are fabricated to meet the opposing teeth only lightly, to minimize chewing pressures upon them.

REMOVABLE PARTIAL DENTURES

If several of your teeth are missing, or if the adjacent teeth are not strong enough to serve as abutments, some form of *removable* restoration may be used. If some serviceable teeth are still present, the appliance is likely to be a *partial denture*. A partial denture usually costs less than a fixed bridge.

Partial dentures have three basic elements:

- A *framework* that fits against the gums and other soft tissues of the mouth.
- Attachments, such as *clasps* and *rests*, which connect the framework to remaining natural teeth.

- Artificial, or *prosthetic*, teeth, mounted on the framework.

Unlike fixed bridges, partial dentures are not entirely supported by adjacent teeth; rather, some of their support is from the gums and jawbones upon which their frameworks rest. The framework of a partial denture is made of a light, strong, noncorroding metal—most often, a chrome–cobalt alloy. It is cast to conform closely to the tissues underneath. The thin film of saliva that is inevitably trapped under the framework helps it stick to the gums.

In the upper jaw, the denture framework may extend across the palate to the other side of the jaw, or it may be shaped like a horseshoe, leaving much of the palate uncovered. A denture for the lower jaw must leave room for the tongue, so its framework is usually horseshoe-shaped.

Some partial dentures still in use don't have this kind of extended framework. Instead, they are simply fastened by clasps to

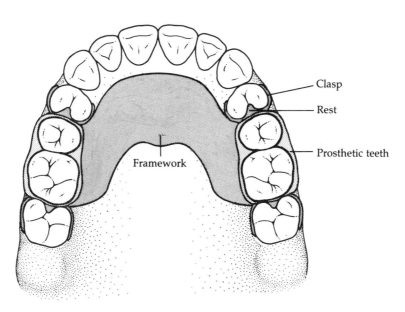

Partial denture with rests

adjacent teeth. This form is often called a *Nesbit*. Many dentists would rather not use Nesbits because they are not as well-anchored as standard partial dentures, and because they might even be swallowed if they come loose in the mouth. The greater bulk of a standard framework may strike patients as awkward and intrusive, but it is at once safe and more stable.

Another small partial denture still in general use is known popularly as a *flipper*. It consists of one or more artificial teeth mounted on a small plastic framework. The flipper is used as a temporary replacement for missing teeth (usually upper front teeth), and it serves only an aesthetic purpose. It can also "flip" readily out of the mouth—hence, the name.

PROSTHETIC TEETH

Artificial, or *prosthetic,* teeth are either acrylic plastic or baked porcelain. Either material can be shaped and colored to harmonize with your natural teeth. The best prosthetic teeth are said to be *fully characterized;* they have slight irregularities in shape and alignment, and subtle gradations in color, just as natural teeth do.

Porcelain teeth are stronger, and more resistant to wear and staining, than acrylic teeth. But modern acrylic is quite strong and easy to keep clean. Acrylic teeth have one significant functional advantage. Plastic is more resilient than porcelain, and doesn't transmit as much chewing pressure to the underlying gum and bone tissues. It is also less susceptible to fracture.

PARTIAL DENTURE ATTACHMENTS

A partial denture, even if not fully supported by your natural teeth, is attached to them whenever possible, to help prevent loosening

or shifting. The type of attachment will depend on whether the denture is *tooth borne, tooth-and-tissue borne,* or *tissue borne:*

- A *tooth-borne* denture is used when the toothless *(edentulous)* area is bounded on either side by fairly firm natural teeth, to which the denture framework can be connected. Thus, a tooth-borne denture derives much of its support, and sometimes almost all of it, from the natural teeth.
- A *tooth-and-tissue-borne* denture is used when the edentulous area is not bounded on both sides by natural teeth, or when the natural teeth are somewhat mobile. It derives some of its support from the teeth, but as much or more support from the gum and bone tissues.
- An entirely *tissue-borne* denture must be used when few natural teeth remain, and those that do tend to be mobile. Such a denture must derive virtually all of its support from the gum and bone tissues.

The frameworks of tooth-borne and tooth-and-tissue-borne dentures are usually attached by metal clasps, which slip around

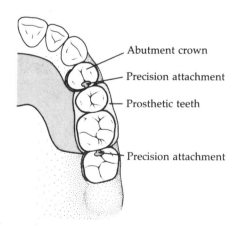

Partial denture with precision attachments

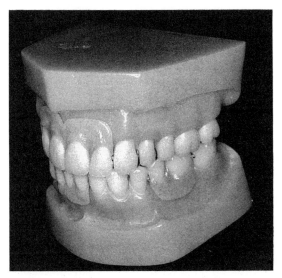

Model of partial dentures with outside clasps
Photograph by Dr. Jerome Goodman

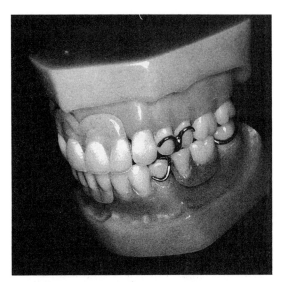

Model of partial dentures with precision attachments
Photograph by Dr. Jerome Goodman

sound natural teeth. But such a partial denture may instead be stabilized by *internal attachments,* sometimes called *precision attachments.*

Internal attachments require special preparation of adjacent natural teeth. Either inlays or crowns are used, and these have dovetail-shaped, vertical slots cut into them. Matching dovetail keys, extending from the framework, slip into the slots, and hold the denture firmly in place. Such internal attachments are very stable, and they eliminate the need for visible clasps. However, they must be fabricated and inserted with great exactness (see below).

When a partial denture must be entirely tissue borne, the framework is often made of acrylic plastic rather than metal. Such a framework is called a *base,* which is similar to the base of a *full* denture. The clasps place little or no pressure on the remaining teeth, and the denture will usually have no *rests* (see below). A tissue-borne partial denture is often considered a *transitional* denture, which may eventually have to be replaced with a full denture.

RESTS

It is advisable to reduce the pressure that partial dentures place on soft gum tissues as much as possible. Tooth-borne and tooth-and-tissue-borne dentures are therefore equipped with rests. These are small metal tabs that protrude from the denture framework, and fit shallow notches cut into your natural teeth. When you chew, some of the pressure is transferred through the rests to your natural teeth, rather than entirely to the gums.

FABRICATION AND INSERTION

The fabrication and insertion of a partial denture requires several visits to the dentist, and a sequence of many separate steps.

1. First, your natural teeth must be in the best possible condition. At the very least, they must be cleaned of all plaque and calculus, and any tooth

decay or periodontal disease must be treated.

2. Tooth loss may have caused some of your adjacent teeth to shift toward the edentulous space, or may have caused opposing teeth to overerupt. Such malposed teeth may have to be selectively ground, or *recontoured*. Sometimes the teeth may be moved into their proper positions by orthodontics.

3. Any of your teeth that cannot be salvaged must be extracted, and the sockets allowed to heal.

4. Extraneous mouth tissues that might interfere with the denture may have to be surgically removed. For instance, some people have a *torus*, or bulge of extra bone, either in the roof of the mouth, or inside the lower jaw (see page 279). Such a torus may keep the denture framework from fitting properly. For the same reason, extraneous growths of soft tissue, such as *epulis* (see page 141), may also have to be removed.

5. Sometimes the alveolar bone of the empty sockets becomes severely enough resorbed that the remaining bone ridge will not provide sufficient support for the denture framework. As a preparatory step, the bone may be surgically reshaped, or even built up with grafts of natural or artificial bone (see pages 111 and 157).

6. Impressions are taken of both your jaws, from which study models are cast. The dentist will use these models to prepare a comprehensive plan of treatment.

7. At the next visit, after reviewing the treatment plan with you, the dentist prepares notches for rests in your natural teeth, and takes final impressions of your jaws. The metal alloy framework of the denture is then fabricated in a dental laboratory upon models cast from these impressions.

8. The next visit is a trial fitting, or *try-in*, of the framework in your mouth. Additional visits may be needed if more than a minor adjustment is required. The biting relationships of your natural teeth are measured and recorded, and the colors, sizes, and materials of the prosthetic teeth are selected. The laboratory then prepares a *setup* of the denture, temporarily attaching the artificial teeth to the framework with pink wax.

9. A try-in of the waxed setup is performed at the next visit. It is evaluated by both you and the dentist for fit, appearance, and chewing accuracy. Again, additional visits may be required before the restoration is judged satisfactory. At the laboratory, the wax is then removed, and the artificial teeth are permanently attached to the framework.

10. At the final visit, the completed restoration is inserted. Follow-ups are usually necessary to assure proper fit, and to take care of any irritation that may develop as you wear your denture.

The process is somewhat more complex if your denture is to have precision attachments. First, the natural teeth that will be next to the denture are fitted with inlays or crowns with vertical slots. Then, *two* sets of impressions are made, one in the usual rubber-like material, the other in a more rigid material, such as plaster. The plaster provides a more accurate model of your teeth and jaws, which the precise fit of the framework "keys" makes necessary.

FULL DENTURES

Often, despite all efforts, all the teeth in a jaw are lost. The cause is most likely to be ad-

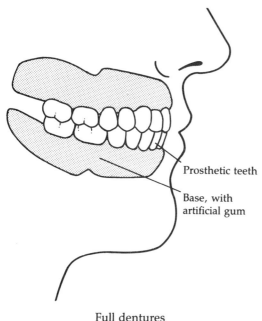

Prosthetic teeth

Base, with
artificial gum

Full dentures

vanced periodontal disease, but decay and injury also contribute.

For both functional and aesthetic reasons, it is wise to replace the missing teeth with a *full denture*. The framework of a full denture, called the *base*, covers more of your jaw than that of a partial denture. It is ordinarily made of pink acrylic plastic and covers the whole dental ridge. The base of an upper denture covers your palate as well; that of a lower denture must be horseshoe-shaped to leave room for your tongue.

A full denture is not supported by natural teeth, but only by the underlying gum and bone tissues of the dental ridge. The base is made to conform closely to the ridge, and is held in place mainly by a thin film of saliva.

An upper denture is also partly held in place by the vacuum created when the base is seated over the gums and palate, and its edges form a seal with the surrounding soft tissues of your mouth. A lower denture will rely less upon vacuum and more upon pressure from your cheek muscles and tongue to help maintain its position.

A full denture is far less stable than a partial denture, and a lower denture, with its limited base, is less stable than an upper denture. Moreover, a full denture can stand only very limited chewing pressure—much less than natural teeth, or even a tooth-supported partial denture. For this reason, many people find a denture on just one jaw harder to manage than matching dentures on both jaws. A single denture on the lower jaw is especially likely to be unstable and uncomfortable.

BONE RESORPTION

Making a denture fit firmly and comfortably over the edentulous ridge may be difficult. And even if the denture fits well when it is first inserted, it is likely to become loose in time. The principal reason is shrinkage, or *resorption*, of the bone in the ridge. When all the teeth are lost, the alveolar bone tissue that formerly supported them has no function. It then gradually resorbs, sometimes to the level of the underlying *basal* bone.

Moreover, the alveolar bone doesn't resorb uniformly, especially if the individual teeth were lost at different times. The eroded ridge may be bumpy and uneven, making the denture both less stable and less comfortable. A bony ridge that resorbs to a thin, sharp edge under the gum is particularly uncomfortable.

Resorption of the lower jaw may proceed so far that it approaches one or both of the *mental nerves*, which pass through channels in the bone, and then emerge to the outer surface on each side. As the bone resorbs under a lower denture, more and more pressure will be transferred through the denture base to the exposed nerves. The resulting pain is likely to make chewing all but unbearable.

The dentures may actually contribute to bone resorption. The pressure of the dentures sometimes irritates the tissues enough to hasten the process.

It is sometimes possible to smooth an uneven ridge surgically, or to build up a severely resorbed ridge with grafts of natural or artificial bone (see page 157). But resorption is likely to continue. As a result, dentures may have to be periodically *relined* (see page 142), or even completely replaced. One of the principal aims of prosthodontics is to prevent bone resorption or to slow it down as much as possible, particularly through the use of *immediate dentures, overdentures,* or *implants.*

IMMEDIATE DENTURES

Traditionally, if you needed a full denture, any remaining teeth you might have had were removed and the sockets allowed to heal before the denture was inserted. Meanwhile you were left toothless—possibly for months. To avoid this problem, many dentists now provide *immediate dentures*—so called because they can be inserted immediately after the last teeth are removed.

Two main stages are involved. First, your remaining back teeth (molars and premolars) are removed and the sockets are given time to heal. The more visible front teeth are allowed to remain temporarily. Impressions are taken of your jaws, and models cast from them, just as they would be for partial dentures. But the remaining front teeth are cut off the model and the plaster is recontoured to approximate the eventual shape of your dental ridge. The denture is fabricated on this altered model.

In the second stage, your remaining front teeth are extracted, and the edentulous ridge is surgically reshaped, if necessary. As soon as this process is completed, the denture is inserted. The sockets are allowed to heal under the denture base.

The obvious advantage is appearance; you never have to go toothless. But there is another benefit as well. Covered and protected by the base, the front sockets actually tend to heal faster and with less discomfort.

The disadvantages are that the process is more complex, requires more time and skill, and is more costly. When the denture is first constructed, its base will conform only approximately to the front of your dental ridge. To be safe, the laboratory will often make the base thicker than necessary, and the dentist will have to grind it down substantially to make it fit. Moreover, at least some bone resorption is inevitable after your front teeth are removed, so the denture must be refitted a few months after it is inserted. Sometimes a whole new denture must be constructed.

OVERDENTURES

It was once customary, before inserting a full denture, to remove all the remaining teeth in the jaw. No longer. Now dentists often try to save sound individual teeth, no matter how few there are, and to use them to support *overdentures.*

Actually, only the roots of the teeth are used. The crowns are ground down to the gumline, and root canal therapy is performed on the exposed pulps. The denture is then fabricated and inserted over the roots and gums.

There are at least three major advantages to this procedure:

• The tooth roots provide better support for the denture, and last longer. Not only do they themselves tend not to resorb, their presence also slows down or even prevents the resorption of alveolar bone.
• The sensation of biting is much closer to that with natural teeth. Chewing with overdentures feels more comfortable and more stable than chewing with conventional dentures.
• The roots can be used as anchors for mechanical devices that connect with the denture and improve its stability. For ex-

ample, posts or bars may be attached to the roots, and the denture attached to them with spring clips. Or magnets may be built into the denture, which are attracted to steel "keepers" attached to the roots.

The only disadvantage to an overdenture is that it is difficult to keep clean. The tooth roots under the denture are very susceptible to decay and periodontal disease.

LIVING WITH DENTURES

Partial and full dentures can be visually very convincing. They may be virtually indistinguishable from your natural teeth, especially when the prosthetic teeth are "fully characterized." But dentures don't really feel or function like natural teeth, and they require special care to keep them in working order.

THE PERIOD OF ADJUSTMENT

When a new denture is inserted in your mouth, especially if you have never worn one before, your mouth will take some time to adjust to it. Dentures are hard, rigid objects placed upon soft, flexible tissues. At least initially, they are likely to cause discomfort and other problems.

It is unlikely that any denture will fit perfectly when it is first inserted. The teeth supporting a partial denture may feel sore, and friction may produce sore spots on the soft tissues under either full or partial dentures. You may have to make several visits to the dentist before the fit is satisfactory.

For mouth soreness, a soothing rinse of a teaspoon of salt in a glass (eight ounces) of warm water is likely to be most effective. If you must limit your intake of sodium, you can substitute epsom salts (magnesium sulfate) for sodium chloride. It is generally un-

wise to use other medications, such as topical anesthetics, unless they are prescribed by your dentist.

If a denture causes persistent discomfort, take it out to give the soft tissues a rest, and see your dentist as soon as possible to check the fit. But *replace* the denture for at least an hour before the visit, to help pinpoint the source of the irritation. The dentist will mark the inflamed area with an indelible pencil or a pressure indicator paste, and will reinsert the denture to transfer the mark to the corresponding surface on the base. The "high spot" can then be reduced to ease the contact.

When a denture is first inserted, your mouth may react to it as if it were something to eat, and may flood it with extra saliva. Some saliva is necessary for proper retention of the denture, but excessive flow loosens it. Patients sometimes comment that their new denture feels like a boat floating in the mouth. The only solution is patience. The salivary glands usually get used to the denture in a few days and reduce their output.

The new denture will feel bulky in your mouth. Your tongue may feel that there is too little room for it, and normal speech may be difficult. Again, the lips and tongue are likely to adjust to the denture within a few days, with a little patience and practice.

Dentures—especially upper dentures that cover the palate—do reduce the sensitivity of the mouth. Sensitivity to heat, in particular, will diminish. This can be dangerous, for you may not realize how hot a food or drink is. You should be aware of the problem, and should be especially wary of hot liquids, such as coffee and soup, or a pizza right out of the oven.

LEARNING TO EAT WITH DENTURES

Dentures are nowhere near as strong or stable as natural teeth. To some extent, first-time denture wearers must learn to eat all over again.

Ordinarily, the chewing process has three steps. First, "bite-size" pieces of food are cut off by your front teeth. Then, they are ground into small particles by your back teeth, and lubricated with saliva. Then the chewed particles are formed into a ball by your tongue, and swallowed.

Adjustment to dentures requires relearning these steps in reverse order. First, you must learn to shape food with your tongue, and swallow it. A soft diet will be necessary until you fully master this skill.

Then, you must learn to grind food with your back teeth. At this stage, your food should be cut into relatively small pieces, which need only to be chewed fine before they are swallowed.

Finally, you must learn how to use your false front teeth to bite off fragments of food too large to be eaten whole. This is the most difficult and challenging step, and should not be undertaken until the other steps are mastered. Try not to bite "straight on" with the incisors, but rather, obliquely, in the area of the cuspids. Also, if possible, push the food (such as a sandwich) *against* your front teeth, so as not to dislodge the dentures.

You may have to accept some permanent limitations upon what you can eat. Full dentures, and tissue-borne partial dentures, simply cannot bear the same chewing pressures as natural teeth. Full dentures, in fact, can withstand only one tenth the chewing pressure of natural teeth. Crunchy foods, such as nuts, whole raw apples and carrots, and corn on the cob, may have to be foregone.

CARE OF DENTURES, AND THE MOUTH

A denture must be kept "like new." You should at least rinse it of food particles after every meal, and thoroughly clean it at least once a day. Plaque and calculus will form on it (as on all dental restorations) even more readily than on natural teeth. Liquid cleaners alone won't prevent plaque buildup—only thorough brushing will. Once calculus has formed, only professional cleaning can safely remove it.

Ordinary toothpaste, however, may be too abrasive for a denture. You should clean a denture with soap and lukewarm water, or with a commercial denture cleaner. In selecting a cleaner, look for the American Dental Association seal of acceptance.

Many wearers of full dentures prefer the feeling of stability commercial denture adhesives provide. Some may actually need such adhesives. Their salivary glands may not generate enough saliva to hold dentures in place or the saliva consistency may be too thin and watery or the dental ridges may have resorbed too far to keep dentures in place. If you do use an adhesive, it should be scrubbed off completely when the denture is cleaned, to prevent contamination.

Any remaining teeth, as well as the trimmed roots under overdentures, must be carefully brushed every day. Even if your mouth is completely edentulous, you should gently but regularly brush your gums, or at least rub them with a gauze pad.

Except under very special circumstances, neither partial nor full dentures should remain permanently in your mouth. The tissues of the mouth need periodic rest. Many dentists advise removing dentures at night, while you sleep.

Most dentures are made at least partly of acrylic plastic. This material, like wood, absorbs water, and repeated wetting and drying is likely to cause your denture to warp. Therefore, when you remove a denture from your mouth, you should keep it moist. Most wearers submerge their dentures in water, but this isn't essential. When traveling, for instance, you may prefer simply to place the denture in a plastic bag, along with moist gauze pads. For protection from breakage, though, you should enclose it in a rigid container as well.

Your mouth is alive; a denture is not. Once teeth are lost, changes in the bone and soft tissues are inevitable. If you wear a denture, you should continue to visit the dentist regularly, not only for adjustment of fit and removal of calculus but also to have your mouth checked. In particular, you should be examined at least once a year for evidence of oral cancer. If a denture becomes loose or uncomfortable over time, over-the-counter linings and pads should *not* be substituted for professional care.

DENTURE DISCOMFORT

A denture that doesn't fit properly or that is not cleaned thoroughly or removed periodically is likely to irritate the gums and other soft tissues of your mouth. Such irritation may produce chronic inflammation, or the growth of excess tissue. It may also help bring on mouth infections. Common results of irritation include the following:

- *Pressure sores* are common among wearers of new or ill-fitting dentures. They are formed by pressure and friction of the hard denture upon the soft tissues. Sometimes they are temporary, and disappear spontaneously. Often, though, they are a sign that the denture should be adjusted to relieve pressure in these areas.
- If denture sores are neglected, excess soft tissue, called *epulis fissuratum,* may grow, in reaction to the continued irritation. These growths are usually painless and harmless. But it is usually wise to have them removed surgically, and have them checked by biopsy to make sure that no malignant cells are present. And they must generally be removed if a denture is to be repaired or replaced.

- *Denture stomatitis,* sometimes called *denture sore mouth,* is a more generalized inflammation of the soft tissues under and around a denture. It is especially prevalent on the roof of the mouth, the palate. The tissues become reddish and painful, and sometimes swell. The condition appears to be caused not only by mechanical irritation but also by contamination from bacteria and funguses. It tends to occur when the denture is not kept clean, or is not removed often enough from the mouth. The best remedy is good oral hygiene.
- Denture stomatitis is sometimes accompanied by enlargements of the soft tissue called *papillary hyperplasias* (see page 260). They occur most often on the palate. Sometimes, like epulis, they interfere with the fit of the denture and must be surgically removed.
- Soft-tissue *infections* are also likely to result from poor hygiene, as well as from irritation. The most common is the fungus infection *candidiasis,* or *oral thrush* (see page 257).

Discomfort from a denture is not inevitable, if you care for it conscientiously and have it regularly checked. If your mouth does become irritated by pressure sores or stomatitis, or develops infections such as candidiasis, your dentist can prescribe remedies ranging from antiseptic rinses to antibiotics.

DAMAGED OR WORN DENTURES

A denture may become damaged, bent, or broken. You shouldn't attempt to make repairs yourself, but should take the damaged denture, or its parts, to your dentist. In particular, you shouldn't try to glue the broken elements of an acrylic denture base back together. The glue can ruin the plastic.

There is no such thing as a completely permanent restoration of any kind. A denture, in particular, is subject to wear. A worn or ill-fitting denture is repaired in three main ways.

- *Relining.* New material, conforming to the present shape of the dental ridge, is added to the underside of the base.
- *Rebasing.* A new base is made on a model of the ridge, and the artificial teeth from the old denture are attached to it.
- *Replacement of teeth.* Worn artificial teeth are replaced with new ones, mounted to the existing base.

It is not unusual, after five to ten years of use, for complete replacement to be required.

THE COST OF PROSTHODONTICS

Restorative dentistry requires highly sophisticated techniques, and extensive professional time. Hence, it is a relatively expensive kind of treatment. The more complex the procedure, the greater the cost. Partial dentures with precision attachments, for example, are especially costly.

Dental insurance will usually cover part of the cost—but only if the treatment restores dental function. Treatment that is primarily cosmetic will probably not be covered (see page 238).

You can sometimes obtain good treatment at lower cost through a dental school or medical center clinic (see page 242). But you should be cautious of heavily advertised commercial clinics that promise prosthodontic treatment at cut rates. There is no substitute for quality. Treatment that is not carefully planned or skillfully executed can do more harm than good. An ill-fitting denture, for example, can permanently damage your mouth.

If you are considering advanced prosthodontic treatment, you should be fully aware of the costs and should consider the alternatives. Do not hesitate to get other opinions on treatment, and even other cost estimates. But at the same time, be aware of the advantages of timely, high-quality treatment. For instance, crowns, bridges, and partial dentures not only improve your appearance and chewing efficiency but also protect your remaining teeth, and may prevent their eventual loss. The expense of prosthodontic treatment, though considerable, is likely to be a worthwhile long-term investment.

FOURTEEN

IMPLANTS: A FIRMER FOUNDATION

Prosthetic devices, such as bridges and dentures, are often remarkably effective replacements for natural teeth, in both appearance and function. But even though they are successful for a majority of patients, they don't work for everyone.

A complete upper denture, for example, covers the roof of the mouth, and alters the position and sensation of the tongue. Some people find that this seriously interferes with normal eating and speech. And dentures, both upper and lower, may not fit securely. Lower dentures tend to be particularly unstable, which significantly limits the range of foods that can be chewed.

Another example is a partial denture that replaces all the teeth on one side of a jaw. It is sometimes difficult to establish an even, stable bite with such a prosthesis, or to attach it securely to the abutment teeth. Moreover, some people find that the bulky partial denture feels intrusive and annoying, compared with the natural teeth on the other side.

Another problem, particularly with a full denture, is that it may loosen after a while. Once the natural teeth have been removed,

the ridge of alveolar bone that once held them in place begins to shrink, or *resorb*. And as it resorbs, it provides less and less support for the denture over it. In fact, chewing pressure, exerted on the bone through the denture, speeds up the resorption process. As a result, the denture becomes looser and looser, and eventually has to be refitted or remade.

Even worse, resorption sometimes leaves the bone ridge thin and sharp. When a denture is placed over such a ridge, the pressure of chewing is concentrated on the gum directly over the sharp edge. The gum becomes so irritated and painful that the denture can't be used.

Finally, some people simply can't wear dentures. Their jaw ridges are too damaged—by an accident, disease, surgery, or a genetic defect—to support any conventional prosthesis.

For all these reasons, there have been efforts, going back about half a century, to make prosthetic teeth more stable and longlasting. Specifically, efforts have been made to insert, or *implant*, anchors that would connect such teeth to the underlying bone as securely as natural teeth are connected by their roots. The field of *implantology* is now one of the most active in dental research, with many advances in recent years.

SUBPERIOSTEAL IMPLANTS

Among the earliest forms to be developed were subperiosteal implants. They are no longer common but are still used under certain circumstances. They are called *subperiosteal* because they are inserted under the *periosteum*, a membrane that lies under the gum, next to the bone.

To create and insert a subperiosteal implant, the gum and periosteum are surgically cut open in the area where teeth are missing. An impression is taken of the bony ridge, and the soft tissue is then sutured back together. A cast is made from the impression, and a metal framework is then constructed over the cast, so it will fit snugly against the ridge. In a second operation, the gum is opened up again, and the framework is inserted.

The framework may be directly fastened to the bone, or it may simply rest upon it. Either way, fibrous tissue forms around the metal, holding it in place. The framework has abutment posts that protrude through the overlying gum, and removable dentures or fixed bridges can be attached to these abutments.

At every stage of this process, great care must be taken to avoid bacterial contamination—a difficult task in the bacteria-rich environment of the mouth. If the tissues around the implant become infected, the implant will fail, and must immediately be removed.

Otherwise, subperiosteal implants are initially more stable than ordinary dentures, but eventually they too can become loose, and may have to be removed or replaced. The problem, again, is bone resorption. The pressures of chewing, transmitted through a subperiosteal implant, cause the bone to resorb, thus depriving the implant of support. And the looser the implant becomes, the more the process is accelerated. Subperiosteal implants in the lower jaw usually last no longer than ten years at best. Those in the upper jaw, where the bone is softer and more porous, usually last no more than five years.

ENDOSSEOUS IMPLANTS: CYLINDERS AND BLADES

To get around problems such as infection and bone resorption, a second type of implant was developed. Such implants are called *endosseous* because they are placed inside the bone. They take two basic forms: wedge-shaped blades, which are inserted into cut slots, and cylinders, often threaded like screws, which are inserted into drilled holes. Like subperiosteal implants, blades and cylinders have abutment posts to which bridges or dentures can be attached.

At first, endosseous implants weren't much better than early subperiosteal implants. The procedures used to install them were largely to blame.

Cylinder implants, for example, required that holes be drilled into the bone. But the drills rotated too fast, producing so much heat from friction that the surrounding bone became "cooked," and did not provide a stable socket for the implant.

It was customary, furthermore, to install bridges or dentures right after implant surgery. Thus, implants were immediately "loaded" with the intense pressures of chewing. The bone around the implants was not allowed to heal fully, and the implants never became completely stable.

Finally, contamination during surgery remained a problem. The bone tissue around the implant often became infected and inflamed, which hastened its breakdown and resorption. In severe cases, so much bone was lost that the implants couldn't be replaced, and conventional prostheses could no longer be inserted either.

THE TITANIUM REVOLUTION

In the early 1960s, a Swedish scientist, Per-Ingmar Branemark (pronounced *Broh*-neh-mark), made a discovery that led to a major breakthrough. Professor Branemark was conducting basic research on the healing of bone, which required the surgical insertion of a metal appliance into the bones of experimental animals. He discovered, accidentally, that appliances made of the metal titanium became so firmly attached to bone that they couldn't be removed. They appeared to be *osseointegrated* ("integrated with the bone").

Branemark quickly recognized the implications of osseointegration in dental implantology. Implants had previously been made of inert metals, such as a chrome–cobalt alloy, which body tissues would tolerate reasonably well. But these materials seldom became osseointegrated. Instead, they became surrounded with a capsule of softer and less stable fibrous tissue.

Titanium, however, allowed bone tissue to grow right against it, forming an increasingly tight bond. Thus, titanium implants could be expected to become more firmly attached, rather than looser, over time. Branemark himself collaborated in developing a commercial system of titanium implants, and several other producers have followed. A wide variety of products is now available; they are all made of titanium or titanium alloy, and employ much the same technology.

Branemark made two other important discoveries during his research. One was that the bone being cut or drilled to receive an implant must not become heated by friction. "Cooked" bone will not integrate with an implant. The other discovery was that osseointegration takes time—usually several months. During this time, the implant must not be "loaded," or it will fail.

Some practitioners still favor subperiosteal implants and endosseal blade implants. The use of titanium certainly helps make these more stable and long-lasting. But the nature of the metal makes it particularly suitable for cylinder implants, especially those that are threaded to screw into the bone. Endosseal cylinder implants are increasingly becoming the first choice of implantologists.

Endosseal cylinder implants require very careful installation, involving two stages of surgery. The implants themselves are customarily inserted by an oral surgeon or a periodontist, or by a general dentist with extensive training and experience in this field. Prosthetic devices attached to the implants— bridges or dentures—may be prepared and inserted by a prosthodontist, or by a general dentist experienced in prosthetics. This team effort requires the close collaboration of all the members from the planning stage on.

Implantology is still a relatively new field, and it may require some effort to locate qualified practitioners (see Chapter 2 and Appendix).

IMPLANT SURGERY

Here, step by step, is how surgery for cylinder implants proceeds.

You are likely to come to the implantologist with a history of unsatisfactory restorative dentistry—unstable or broken bridgework, or ill-fitting and uncomfortable dentures. The first visit is diagnostic. In addition to taking a detailed medical history, and conducting a regional examination of your head and neck, the implantologist will take impressions of both your jaws, in order to cast study models.

You may also be referred to a radiologist, for a series of X-rays. These are likely to include *panoramic* views (often called *Panorexes*) of the complete jaws, *tomograms* that focus on one thin "slice" of an area at a time, and *cephalometric* X-rays that record the structural relationships of the bones of the face. *Computerized tomography* may also be used, for the highly detailed views it provides of bone and soft tissue.

If, after a careful evaluation, you are accepted for implantation, and if you have had no recent extractions (which may require a healing period of several months), the first surgery can be scheduled promptly. To minimize infection, you will probably be put on a short course of antibiotics.

This surgery can be performed in a dental office, but the operating environment must be comparable to that of a hospital. As mentioned earlier, contamination of the implant site must be avoided. If the bone, or soft tissue, becomes infected, the implant is likely to fail.

Anesthesia is similar to that used in other forms of oral surgery (see page 151). General anesthesia is usually unnecessary. The operation may take from one to three hours, depending on the complexity of the surgery, and may be divided into two or more sessions.

The implantologist begins by making an incision through the gum in the area where implants are to be inserted. The soft tissue is pulled back to expose the underlying ridge of bone. If the ridge has a sharp edge, the implantologist may reduce it slightly to provide a broader, smoother surface.

The implantologist then drills holes into the bone to receive the implants. The number of these will vary, depending on the kind of prosthesis to be used and the amount of bone available. The thickness of available bone will also determine the depth of each hole—

SURGICAL INSERTION OF IMPLANT

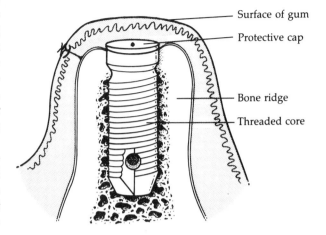

Insertion of core

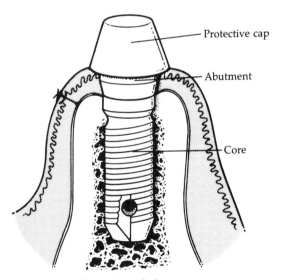

Insertion of abutment

usually between seven and eighteen millimeters.

At first, a small pilot hole is drilled, and then this hole is gradually enlarged, using drill bits of larger diameters. Special, slowly rotating drills are used, together with constant, cooling irrigation, to counteract heat from friction.

Cylinder implants vary somewhat in design. They are usually at least partially threaded. Each one is screwed slowly into place, until its top is about level with the bone surface. A temporary protective cap is then placed over it, and the gum tissue is sutured back in place, to heal. Buried under the gum, the implants must remain undisturbed and secure from contamination for anywhere from four to twelve months.

Postoperative care is similar to that following other surgery (see page 163). For two or three days, you may have some soreness, mainly from the cutting of the gum. Bruising of the lips and gums may occur, but "frank" bleeding is rare. Also, the lips may become chapped from the prolonged stretching of the mouth.

You can use ice to minimize pain and swelling, and you may be prescribed a mild painkiller such as Tylenol. Only rarely is a stronger analgesic, such as codeine or meperidene (Demerol), needed. Antibiotics will continue to be used to prevent infection. Also, you will have to follow a soft diet for several weeks.

Ten days to two weeks after the operation, your gums will be healed enough to remove the stitches. Until that time, it is advisable not to wear either a denture or a bridge. If you do have a denture, it can then be put into temporary use, after it has been cushioned with a soft relining material. Or a temporary bridge may be constructed, and attached to natural abutment teeth. But it is important to place little or no pressure on the gum over the implants.

At intervals in the following months,

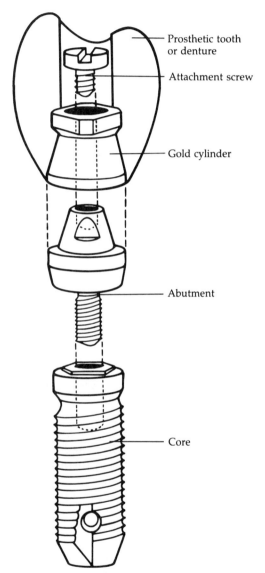

Prosthetic tooth or denture

Attachment screw

Gold cylinder

Abutment

Core

Complete endosseous cylinder implant

X-rays will be taken to see whether the bone is becoming dense and firm around the implants. The time for implant integration can vary greatly—usually three to six months in the lower jaw, and four to eight months in the less dense upper jaw. Only after the implantologist is satisfied that substantial integration has occurred will the second stage of the procedure begin.

This stage starts with a second operation. It is simpler than the first, and takes less time—usually under an hour. A small incision is made through the gum over each implanted anchor, to expose it. The temporary covers are removed, and, in their place, titanium abutment cylinders are inserted.

These abutments protrude slightly above the gum, and will eventually support the prosthetic denture or bridge. Meanwhile, they are covered with plastic healing caps. If necessary, the gum is sutured around them, but sometimes the abutments fit into the incisions so snugly that no suturing is needed. If sutures are used, they can usually be removed within a week.

RISKS AND COMPLICATIONS OF SURGERY

There are some possible complications to implant surgery that you should be aware of before consenting to the procedure.

Despite all precautions, the implant area may become infected and inflamed. There are several ways that infection-causing bacteria can invade the site—the mouth simply cannot be made completely sterile. One form of infection results when implants are placed in an upper jaw that has lost much of its bone. Drilling for an implant can penetrate the ridge completely, so the hole passes into one of the sinuses above. The implant cannot always be protected from contamination there.

If infection does occur, antibiotics may limit the damage. But sometimes the inflammation is severe enough to prevent osseointe-

gration, and the implant fails.

Implants may fail for other reasons. As mentioned earlier, osseointegration won't occur if the bone has become overheated in the drilling process. Also, in cases in which a lot of bone has already been resorbed, there may not be enough bone left to hold the implant securely. And the implant may fail if the hole drilled for it is too big or not perfectly round, or if the implant "strips" the threads in the bone as it is inserted.

If an implant does fail, it can be removed, and a new effort made in a different location. Or the bone may be allowed to grow back to fill the hole, and a second attempt may be made in the same location.

The wound of the first surgery may not heal properly. This usually occurs when a denture is worn too soon, or when the denture was not correctly relined with cushioning material. But it can also be the result of radiation treatment or systemic disease (such as diabetes) that has compromised the body's ability to heal. Or previous surgery in the area may have disrupted the blood supply. Nerves pass through both the upper and lower jaws, and these nerves must be carefully avoided when the implants are inserted. If any nerve is irritated or injured, tingling or numbness in the lower lip and chin or beside the nose may result. In rare instances, the numbness may persist.

INSTALLING THE PROSTHESIS

Once the implantologist has implanted the anchors and abutments, a general dentist may take over the responsibility for constructing and inserting the bridge or denture.

First, a new impression is taken of your jaw. In the process, the protective caps are removed from the abutments, and in their place are put *impression copings,* cylinders that are about the same diameter as the abutments. When the impression is taken, the impression copings are transferred to it. They then become guides for the precise placement of the prosthesis relative to the abutments.

The bridge or denture is constructed on a cast from the impression, in much the same fashion as a conventional bridge or denture. Its metal framework contains cylinders in the positions dictated by the impression copings, so they will be directly over the abutments. Screws or posts, passing through these cylinders, will fasten them to the tops of the abutments.

Artificial teeth may be built directly onto this metal framework. When fastened in place, the resulting bridge or denture will be securely fixed, and can be removed only by the dentist, for periodic cleaning and maintenance.

As an alternative, the metal framework may be a separate unit, and an *overdenture* is made to clip over it. You can easily remove the overdenture yourself, and clean it as you would a conventional denture.

A denture fastened to implants does not require a base, or an artificial gum, to make it stay in the mouth. An artificial gum may be constructed for the outer side of the denture, simply to hide the joint between the denture and the natural gum.

Neither does a bridge have to be attached to natural teeth. The implanted anchors, which are tightly bonded to the surrounding bone, are sufficiently strong to support it.

A bridge anchored by implants is, in fact, sometimes attached to natural teeth—to give *them* support, rather than to be supported by them. The firmly fixed bridge may help stabilize teeth loosened, say, by periodontal disease. Some practitioners, however, prefer not to connect implanted bridges or dentures to natural teeth under any circumstances.

If the denture or bridge is fastened directly to its abutments, the heads of the screws or posts are customarily covered over with tooth-colored plastic. Periodically the dentist will remove this plastic, and unscrew the

prosthesis for examination and cleaning. Incidentally, cleaning requires special care. The abutments, in particular, may be scratched during cleaning, which can lead to bacterial invasion.

RISKS AND COMPLICATIONS

Complications in the prosthodontic stage of treatment tend to be less severe and easier to remedy than complications of surgery. The most serious potential problem is that the implants may not be placed in the right location or inserted at the correct angle to give good, even support to the denture or bridge. As a result of such *uneven loading*, the connecting screws or posts, or the prosthesis itself, may break under the repeated pressure of chewing.

Some implants are now available with abutments that can be set at an angle, providing more leeway in the placement and attachment of the prosthesis. If necessary, one or more of the implants can be replaced in a better location. Close collaboration between the surgical implantologist and the prosthetic dentist is the best way to avoid such problems.

Titanium cylinder implants have a low rate of failure. But even if one of them does fail, the result of such a failure is usually not serious. It can be compared with the loss of a single tooth, which can be rather easily replaced. By contrast, the failure of a blade implant or a subperiosteal implant can be compared with the simultaneous loss of several teeth. Replacement is at best difficult, and severe, permanent damage may result.

ADVANTAGES OF TITANIUM CYLINDER IMPLANTS

Perhaps the most important benefit of titanium cylinder implants is that they appear to minimize the problem of bone resorption. During the first year following implantation, the crest of the bone ridge recedes slightly— about one millimeter. After that, its resorption is minimal—about one tenth of a millimeter each year. And the bone surrounding the implant seems to grow denser and stronger with time. Hence, this kind of implantation seems to offer the best prospect for a lasting replacement of natural teeth.

Moreover, implanted bridges and dentures are stable and comfortable—they feel and function like natural teeth. There is virtually nothing, from raw apples to caramels, that cannot be chewed.

THE COST OF IMPLANTS

For most people, the big drawback to implants is cost. Implantation is one of the most expensive procedures in restorative dentistry, and it can cost several times more than traditional restorations. The reason is obvious: the process requires extensive surgery, as well as the precise fabrication and installation of the implants and prosthetic devices. Dental insurance may pay for implantation, but policies vary, and the procedure is sometimes excluded from coverage (see page 238).

As a result, implant patients tend to be those for whom traditional methods have failed. They may find that they have to choose between implants that work and ordinary restorations that don't. Faced with this choice, more and more people are finding that implants are well worth the expense.

FIFTEEN

ORAL AND MAXILLOFACIAL SURGERY

The formal title of the surgical specialty in dentistry is *oral and maxillofacial surgery*. The oral and maxillofacial surgeon operates upon the mouth and teeth (oral surgery) and also upon the jaws and other bones of the face (maxillofacial surgery). For simplicity, we will use here the more traditional terms *oral surgery* and *oral surgeon*.

Oral surgery is in many respects similar to other medical surgery, except that it is performed upon very specific parts of the body. Oral surgeons receive their basic training in dental school. They then obtain their specialized surgical training during four years of hospital residency. Unlike most other dental specialists, oral surgeons are likely to do as much of their work in hospitals as they do in their offices.

Should you have need of an oral surgeon, you will almost certainly be referred by your regular dentist, or possibly your physician. If you should need to find a qualified practitioner on your own, you can use the process outlined in Chapter 2. Most oral surgeons belong to the American Association of Oral and Maxillofacial Surgeons (see Appendix).

TOOTH EXTRACTION

The most common form of treatment provided by oral surgeons is the extraction of teeth. Although many general dentists extract teeth, some prefer to send their patients to an oral surgeon, especially if the problem is severe or complex, such as impacted teeth. The oral surgeon's office is well enough equipped so that most extractions can be performed there, rather than in a hospital operating room.

TEETH THAT REQUIRE EXTRACTION

The philosophy of modern dentistry is to save teeth whenever possible, and to extract them only when necessary. The advantages of natural teeth over artificial teeth are so many and so great that dentists will make substantial efforts to salvage them through restoration, endodontic treatment, periodontic treatment, and orthodontics. For the same reason, dentists place heavy emphasis on preventive care, both at home and in the dental office.

Preventive care is by far the best way to save teeth.

Nevertheless, certain conditions can be remedied only by extraction. The following are among the most common:

- *Decayed* teeth, in which the decay has proceeded deep into the root, or has completely penetrated the root, causing an abscess underneath. Sometimes these conditions can be remedied with endodontic treatment. But in severe cases the teeth cannot be restored, and must be removed, if only to prevent widespread infection.
- *Periodontal disease* so advanced that the eroded alveolar bone and periodontal ligaments no longer support the teeth. The teeth simply "float" in what's left of their sockets.
- Teeth severely damaged by *trauma* from accident or violence. The teeth may have been shattered to their roots, or may be at the sites of jaw fractures. Also, the roots of teeth loosened by trauma may eventually dissolve *(resorb)* so they are no longer stable.
- *Overretained primary* teeth, which hinder the eruption of the adult teeth in the proper order and cause orthodontic problems (see pages 171 and 179).
- *Impacted* teeth, which cannot erupt properly because they are jammed against adjacent teeth. The teeth most likely to be affected are the third molars ("wisdom teeth"), the canines, and the first premolars.
- Severely *malposed* teeth that cannot be brought into position by orthodontics. These include *supernumerary* (extra) teeth and *ectopic* teeth (teeth that erupt outside the dental arch).
- Teeth located near sites of *diseases* of the mouth and jaws, such as cysts, oral cancer, or osteomyelitis (see pages 228 and 276–278).

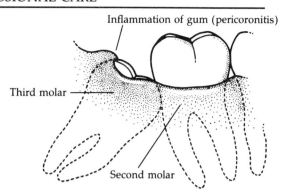

Impacted third molar, partly erupted through gum

THIRD MOLARS: A SPECIAL CASE

For several reasons, the third molars may fail to erupt properly. The basic reason is usually the lack of room in the dental arch—a side effect of human evolution. This crowding may cause the emerging third molars to tip or rotate in the jaws, and to become impacted against the second molars. Such malposed teeth may erupt only partly through the gum, and are thus susceptible to decay and a gum infection called *pericoronitis*.

In addition, many people naturally lack one or more of these molars. The opposing molars may then grow out too far, or *overerupt*. Moreover, since they have no chewing function, the opposing molars may become traps for food particles, making them susceptible to decay and infection.

When such problems exist, the usual solution is extraction. The third molars are not very visible, nor are they required for chewing. But sometimes they just fail to erupt, without causing (at least initially) any other difficulties. They are described as "sleeping" in the bone. Should they be extracted? There are two schools of thought.

Because extraction of teeth completely enclosed by bone is a difficult surgical process, and carries some inevitable risks (see page 155), some dentists advocate leaving "sleeping" molars alone until and unless they begin to cause trouble.

Other dentists believe that unerupted third molars should be removed before they have a chance to cause trouble—and even before they are fully formed. They advocate extraction whenever X-rays plainly show that the teeth won't erupt—usually between the ages of 18 and 21. Young, healthy patients are more likely to recover from surgery quickly and without complications, and the teeth are much easier to remove before their roots are completely grown.

These dentists also argue that "sleeping" third molars are likely to cause trouble eventually, and that the trouble is likely to be serious. If, for example, they are impacted against the adjacent second molars, they may cause those teeth to decay, or their roots to resorb. Or hollow cysts may form in the bone near the unerupted molars, and threaten the stability of other teeth. In rare instances, tumors called *ameloblastomas* (see page 279) may grow in the adjacent bone.

The decision to leave or extract unerupted third molars will also be strongly affected by individual circumstances. If an X-ray examination shows that you have this condition, you should discuss the options fully with your dentist. A second or even a third opinion may be advisable.

SIMPLE EXTRACTIONS

Most erupted teeth can be removed by a process of simple extraction. First, an anesthetic is injected locally to desensitize the area of the tooth. The dentist then loosens the tooth in its socket, gently rocking it back and forth with hand instruments. The instruments commonly used are *forceps* (essentially pliers) and *elevators* (short levers). They stretch the semirigid alveolar bone of the tooth socket and stretch and break apart the fibers of the periodontal ligament that holds the tooth in place. Once the tooth is loosened, it can be removed in one piece.

The dentist cleans the socket of debris. Any inflamed tissue, tumor, or cyst in the socket is removed. If the alveolar bone has been considerably displaced, it is pressed back into position.

You will experience some bleeding in the socket, and possibly some swelling as well. If the blood flow is heavy or persistent, the dentist may press gauze pads over the area or apply chemical clotting agents. Normally, though, the blood coagulates to form a clot within an hour or so, and this clot must remain undisturbed while healing takes place (see page 154).

COMPLEX EXTRACTIONS

More complicated procedures are required for teeth that cannot simply be loosened and extracted in one piece. These include severely malposed teeth and teeth that have failed to erupt. Impacted teeth may be especially difficult to remove.

These extractions may be performed under local anesthesia, but some dentists (and some patients) prefer the unconsciousness of general anesthesia. If the tooth is partly or completely unerupted, it may be necessary to cut through gums and bone to gain access. Then the tooth itself can be cut into pieces (*sectioned*) for removal.

Bleeding and swelling of the disturbed soft tissues are likely to be more severe than after a simple extraction. To help control the bleeding and to avoid contamination, the dentist may suture the soft tissue over the wound. As in simple extractions, the blood clot in the empty socket must be left undisturbed.

RECOVERY FOLLOWING EXTRACTIONS

A careful dentist endeavors to use the minimum force necessary to extract teeth, and to disturb the gums and jaws as little as possible. Nevertheless, extraction inevitably "insults" the tissues, and is likely to cause some measure of postoperative discomfort. This will be most severe during the first days following treatment but usually peaks four to six hours after the operation.

Pain relievers (analgesics) will be prescribed; their strength will be determined by the extent of the procedure. A simple extraction generally requires only a mild analgesic such as acetaminophen (Tylenol), whereas the extraction of an impacted wisdom tooth may need a more potent formulation with a narcotic such as codeine.

Keeping your head elevated, even when lying down, can be helpful in controlling bleeding and swelling after the operation. Ice packs may also be used for this purpose. You should apply the packs gently to the face, in the approximate area of the extraction, for periods of no more than twenty minutes or so in any hour. Cold helps constrict the blood vessels, and has a numbing effect as well.

You may also be given antibiotics to prevent infection. Many dentists don't find this precaution necessary, at least for simple extractions.

Bleeding after an extraction is normal, but a clot usually forms within an hour or so. If the socket continues to ooze blood, pressing a gauze pad over the area for twenty minutes or so will usually bring relief. You can often hold the pad in place simply by biting down on it. An alternative is a moist tea bag—the tannic acid in tea helps clots to form.

If the wound doesn't simply ooze blood, but bleeds "frankly," pressure will usually control the flow. But such bleeding suggests a serious complication, and you should seek professional help immediately.

The clot *must* remain undisturbed for at least 24 hours. Don't brush it or chew on it or even rinse it with a mouthwash. After that, you may find it soothing to rinse it with a mild salt solution or a commercial antiseptic mouthwash. After two days, enough healing should have taken place so that the tissues can withstand normal chewing.

The reason why the clot must be undisturbed until partial healing has occurred is that it forms the basis for regeneration of the bone and soft tissue. In the first week or two following the extraction, the gums heal over. Meanwhile, connective tissue invades the clot and, over a period from about six weeks to four months, is replaced by bone. Eventually, at least part of the empty socket is filled in with new bone.

The socket doesn't fill in completely, however. Once a tooth is removed, the alveolar bone that once supported it no longer has a function. During and after the healing process, some of it inevitably dissolves, or *resorbs*. Thus, the level of the regenerated bone is never as high as it was before the extraction, and is likely to resorb further over time.

RISKS AND COMPLICATIONS

There are slight risks in any procedure that requires anesthesia (see page 54). In general, local anesthesia has fewer potential problems than general anesthesia.

When a tooth is extracted from the upper jaw, there is a slight chance that the root may be long enough to penetrate one of the sinuses above. Should this happen, the dentist must seal off the opening, sometimes by suturing the gums together over the wound.

Most extractions heal without complications in about six to eight weeks. In rare instances, the wound may become infected, and must be treated with antibiotics. Sometimes the extraction will slightly damage a nearby nerve, causing temporary numbness in part of the lips or tongue.

One of the most unpleasant potential complications of extraction is *osteitis*, or *dry socket*.

The causes of this perplexing condition are not completely known. The blood clot in the socket fails to become organized into new connective tissue and bone, and the existing bone is exposed to air and saliva. The symptoms are a foul taste, a foul smell, and considerable pain.

Dry socket usually requires three or four daily treatments by the dentist. The wound is carefully washed out, or *irrigated*. It is then covered with a gauze dressing saturated with antiseptics and other medications. Sometimes an antibiotic must be prescribed to deal with bacterial contamination of the unprotected bone. After these treatments, the socket usually heals, but at a slower rate than normal.

DENTAL EMERGENCIES

Oral surgeons are often called upon to treat dental emergencies such as *avulsed* (knocked out) teeth, jaw dislocations, jaw fractures, and facial lacerations (cuts and other wounds).

REIMPLANTATION OF AVULSED TEETH

Teeth that have been knocked out of their sockets can sometimes be successfully reimplanted—if the treatment is prompt (see page 100). Reimplantation is more likely to be successful with children than adults. Sometimes, however, the pulp will die, so that root canal therapy is necessary. And sometimes the root will dissolve, or resorb, after being reimplanted, and the tooth is eventually lost.

A reimplanted tooth can become stable only if it is held firmly in place while the *periodontium* around it heals. After placing the tooth back in its socket, the surgeon may install a temporary splint of wire to support the tooth between its neighbors.

REDUCTION OF JAW DISLOCATIONS

Sometimes your lower jaw (mandible) may become partly or completely dislocated at the temporomandibular joints. The causes range from trauma to simply opening the mouth too widely. Often the jawbone will slip back into position by itself. But sometimes the *condyles* at the ends of the mandible may pass over the *eminences* on the cranium, and stick there. Also, your jaw muscles may go into spasm, hindering free movement.

Usually the dislocation can be reduced by simple manipulation. The back ends of your lower jaw are pulled downward, while the chin is pushed backward and upward. In severe cases, medication or even an anesthetic may be needed to relax the muscles.

In rare instances, the ligaments of the joints have become stretched, so that dislocation recurs. The problem can be remedied surgically, either by reducing the bulge of the eminences or by shortening the ligaments. This is major oral surgery, which must be performed in a hospital.

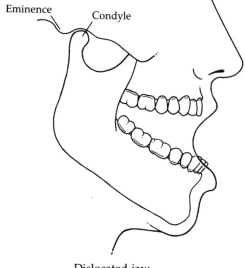

Eminence   Condyle

Dislocated jaw

REDUCTION AND FIXATION OF FRACTURES

As a result of accident or violence, one or both of your jawbones may be broken (fractured). Fractures of the lower jaw are more common than fractures of the upper jaw (maxilla). Fractures of the maxilla may be more serious, however, because other bones of the skull may be involved and because the upper jaw is so close to the brain.

There are three areas on each side of the mandible that are most likely to be fractured. One of them is the angle where the horizontal arch meets the vertical ramus. The second is the slender vertical extension of the ramus, just under the condyle. The third is anywhere in the horizontal arch under the teeth, but usually *between* teeth.

Bone fractures will heal themselves, if the broken ends are brought into close proximity—a process called *reduction*. New bone tissue will gradually form in the reduced gap. But the broken parts must be stabilized—one must be held immobile in relation to the other. Jaw fractures are usually kept stable by *intermaxillary fixation*. The broken jaw is bound to the unbroken one, and the natural meshing of the teeth helps keep the fractured parts in the proper position until they heal.

Intermaxillary fixation is most often accomplished with wire. Wires are woven around

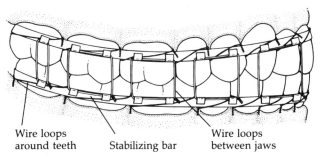

Wire loops around teeth　　　Stabilizing bar　　　Wire loops between jaws

Intermaxillary fixation

some or all the teeth in each of your jaws, forming a splint that helps support the teeth. Usually the splint is reinforced by a heavier wire or bar, extending around the outside of the arch.

The jaws are then connected to each other by short elastic bands or wire loops, with only a little play between them. Sometimes a splint of plastic is molded upon the biting surfaces of the teeth, which helps immobilize the jaws.

The teeth may not provide enough support for intermaxillary fixation. For example, it is impossible to wire jaws of patients who have lost most or all their teeth and who wear partial or complete dentures. In these instances, the denture itself, bound to the jawbone with wire loops, may be used as a splint, and connected in the usual fashion to a splint on the other jaw.

Severe fractures may require more extensive surgery. Sometimes pins are temporarily inserted through the skin into the fractured bones, to hold them in place until they knit together. Sometimes the fractured parts are held together with surgically inserted plates and screws, which are removed in a later operation after the bones have healed.

One of the advantages of inserting plates and screws is that the fractured jaw can be used almost immediately for speaking and eating. Otherwise the jaw must be immobilized for about six weeks, during which time

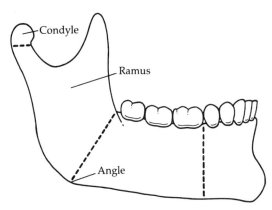

Parts of lower jaw most susceptible to fracture

you must remain on a liquid diet. Complete healing takes at least several months.

TREATMENT OF LACERATIONS

Oral surgeons, like plastic surgeons, may be called upon to repair lacerations of the skin of the face, caused by accident or violence. A major goal in such treatment is to prevent visible scarring. Thus, the surgeon will take special care in closing lacerations, making sure that the edges meet precisely and using very fine sutures.

APICOECTOMY AND ROOT RESECTION

Apicoectomy is a surgical operation ordinarily performed when root canal therapy fails to halt infection of a tooth root (see page 125). It may also be performed during removal of a cyst next to a root (see page 158).

To gain access to the root, the surgeon cuts through the gum and bone on the side of the jaw. The apex of the root is removed, along with any other infected tissue. The surgeon then seals off the remaining root like a cavity, with silver amalgam. The wound is closed by suturing the gum, and bone usually regenerates to fill in the empty space.

If one of the multiple roots of a back tooth (molar or premolar) is dead or diseased, it may be advisable to remove the whole root, rather than just the apex. This operation is called *root resection.* After cutting off the root, the surgeon seals off the remaining pulp chamber. Bone normally regenerates to fill the space left by the root. However, the remaining pulp is usually so contaminated that root canal therapy is required.

Sometimes not only the root, but part of the adjacent crown is removed as well. The pulp chamber is then sealed, and what remains of the crown is restored with an artificial crown.

PREPARATION FOR PROSTHETIC DENTISTRY

Before prosthetic restorations such as crowns, bridges, or dentures can be constructed, the soft tissues of your mouth or the bones of your jaws may have to be surgically reshaped. These procedures are often carried out by an oral surgeon.

RECONTOURING BONE RIDGES

If you have lost all or almost all your teeth, you are likely to suffer resorption of the ridges of alveolar bone that formerly contained the tooth sockets. Oral surgery may be needed to prepare these ridges so they can support dentures directly, or so they can receive *implants* (see Chapter 14) as a foundation for dentures or bridges.

It may only be necessary to make the bearing surfaces smooth and even. The surgeon cuts into the gums, peels away the soft tissues to expose the top of the ridge, and recontours the bone surface by removing any sharp or irregular protrusions before suturing the gums back together.

RIDGE AUGMENTATION

Resorption may have proceeded so far that there is too little bone left to support dentures or implants. The surface of the ridge can sometimes be surgically augmented with a *bone graft.*

Slivers of bone and marrow, "harvested" from other areas of your jaws or from a bone elsewhere in your body (such as a rib or a hip), are packed over the ridge before the gums are resutured. Eventually, these slivers will knit together with the ridge—in much the same way broken bones heal.

In recent years, *artificial* bone has come into wider use for this purpose. It is a mineral compound called *hydroxyapatite,* which is also a major component of natural bone.

VESTIBULOPLASTY

Complete dentures need an adequately sized ridge to rest on, if they are to be stable. One way to compensate for bone resorption is to enlarge the available surface of the soft tissues in the *vestibule* of the mouth—the space between the jaws and the cheeks and lips. This is accomplished by surgical procedures known collectively as *vestibuloplasty* (literally, "vestibule shaping").

One form of such surgery is *frenectomy.* One or more of the *frena,* the vertical membranes that connect the lips and cheeks to the jaws, are partly detached where they join the gums, thus enlarging the area of the vestibule. The vestibule can also be enlarged by removing fatty tissue underlying the mouth lining, or by grafting additional soft tissue at the base of the gums.

REMOVAL OF TUBEROSITIES, TORI, AND EPULI

The proper fitting of dentures, partial or complete, may require the surgical removal of a variety of extraneous tissues in the mouth.

When the bone ridges resorb, knobs of fibrous tissue, called *tuberosities,* may remain at the ends. And they may protrude far enough from the level of the resorbed ridges to make the fitting of dentures difficult. Tuberosities at the ends of the upper, or *maxillary,* jaw are most likely to interfere in this way. They are often surgically reshaped before dentures are constructed.

Some people have an overgrowth of bone inside the mouth known as a *torus* ("bulge"). Although a torus may appear within either jaw, the most common location is the roof of the mouth, the *hard palate* (see page 279). Or-dinarily, a torus is harmless and requires no treatment. But it is likely to interfere with the base of a denture and must usually be surgically removed beforehand.

For any of several reasons, dentures may cease to fit properly. They become unstable, and shift about from the pressures of chewing. The friction irritates the tissues underneath, and often causes the growth of a flabby soft tissue called *epulis.* The main remedy is to refit or replace the loose denture, but usually the epulis must be removed first.

IMPLANTATION

Oral surgeons often perform the surgical procedures needed for the installation of *implants* that are used to provide a firm foundation for dentures and bridges. These are described in detail in Chapter 14.

TEMPORARY DENTURES

All surgical procedures that prepare for prosthetic restorations require a period of postoperative healing, during which pressure on the affected tissues must be kept to a minimum. Thus, after surgery, the prosthodontist may install a *temporary* denture, especially shaped and padded to reduce pressure on the underlying ridge.

REMOVAL OF TUMORS AND CYSTS

Tumors are solid growths of extraneous tissue; *cysts* are hollow sacs of soft tissue, usually filled with fluid. For a variety of reasons—disease, irritation, heredity, developmental variation—and sometimes for no identifiable reason, tumors and cysts may form in either the bones or the soft tissues of the mouth (see pages 259 and 277). Some are essentially harmless, or *benign*. But others may threaten the health and function of the surrounding tissues and may require surgical removal.

Any tumor, and any cyst large enough to require removal, should be *biopsied*. A small sample of the tissue is taken for examination under a microscope to make sure the cells are not malignant (cancerous).

Tumors and cysts in soft tissue can usually be removed without further treatment, although the temporary installation of a *drain* (see below) may be necessary. A cavity created by a tumor or a cyst in bone may fill in naturally, but if it is very large, a bone graft may be necessary.

TREATMENT OF DISEASED SALIVARY GLANDS

Tumors or cysts may occur in the salivary glands, as in other soft tissues of your mouth, and are treated in the same way. Infections may also occur in the glands, and they are treated like other oral infections (see below). In addition, *salivary stones*, small but solid accumulations of minerals (such as calcium), may form in a gland and block the duct that carries saliva from the gland to the mouth. The usual symptom is swelling and discomfort from the blocked flow (see page 274).

Special X-ray studies called *sialograms* are often used in the diagnosis of stones and other disorders of the salivary glands. A dye opaque to X-rays is injected through the duct into the gland. The resulting films reveal obstructions and other irregularities.

Obstructive stones can be removed surgically. Should they recur, the surgeon may make an opening so that the duct is bypassed and the saliva flows directly from the gland into your mouth. In severe cases, the gland may have to be removed.

TREATMENT OF INFECTIONS

Infections of your mouth may result from disease or injury (see page 251 and page 262). The principal treatment is antibiotic therapy. But minor surgery may also be needed, if the level of infection has caused pus to collect, with resultant swelling and pain.

The surgeon opens up the site and inserts one or more flexible tubes, called *drains*. Sutures hold the drains in place until the infection subsides and no more pus forms. When the drains are removed, the wounds are usually small enough to heal without leaving a scar.

Infections are ordinarily treated in the office. But if they are severe enough to be life-threatening, hospitalization may be necessary.

TEMPOROMANDIBULAR JOINT SURGERY

Severe temporomandibular disorders such as displaced articular disks and restricted jaw movement may be treated surgically, if more conservative methods have failed. Such surgery must usually be performed in a hospital, under general anesthesia. The most common procedures are *arthroscopic surgery* and *open-joint disk plication* (see page 215).

ORTHOGNATHIC SURGERY

Some deformities of the teeth and jaws are too extreme to be remedied either by prosthodontic dentistry or by orthodontics. Generally, they result from basic malformations and mismatches of the bones of the jaws and face, sometimes caused by trauma, sometimes by disease, but most often by heredity. They can cause serious malocclusions and often

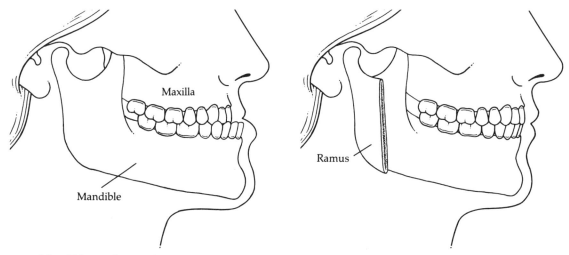

Mandible too large relative to maxilla

Mandible shortened by cutting and overlapping ramus

From Dale, B. G., and Aschheim, K. W., Esthetic Dentistry: A Clinical Approach to Techniques and Materials, © 1991, Lea and Febiger

contribute to temporomandibular disorders. They often very noticeably affect appearance. The most effective remedy for these severe defects is *orthognathic*, or "jaw-correcting," surgery.

The following are the most common kinds of defects needing surgical repair:

- The lower jaw, the mandible, is too large relative to the upper jaw, and to the size of the face, in general. The lower teeth jut forward beyond the upper teeth, producing a *Class III*, or *prognathic*, malocclusion.
- The upper jaw, the maxilla, is too small relative to the mandible and the face as a whole. The visual effect is similar to that of a mandible that is too large, and a Class III malocclusion is also likely.
- The mandible is too small relative to the maxilla. The visual effect is a receded, "weak" chin. A moderately severe condition is called *retrognathia*, or "backward jaw"; a very severe one is called *micrognathia*, or "small jaw." The teeth close in a *Class II* malocclusion. Sometimes the

upper teeth close entirely over those in the mandible, producing an *overclosed* bite.

- The maxilla is too long vertically, producing a *long face syndrome*. The whole face appears to be long and narrow. The line of the lips is high, so a smile reveals much of the upper gum. Sometimes the lips can't be completely closed, and the chin is flattened by muscles trying to bring the lips together.
- The maxilla is too short vertically, compared with the mandible and the face as a whole. Visually, the upper lip looks stunted, and too close to the nose.
- The bones on one side are larger (or smaller) than those on the other, producing *facial asymmetry*. The face looks lopsided, and the mandible may slide sidewise as it opens.

To correct these conditions, the bones must be surgically reshaped. Most orthognatic surgery is now performed entirely from within the mouth, so as to leave no visible scars.

ORTHOGNATHIC SURGERY

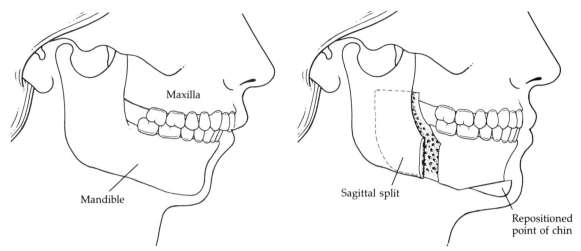

Mandible too small relative to maxilla

Mandible lengthened by sagittal split, and chin reshaped for greater prominence

From Dale, B. G., and Aschheim, K. W., Esthetic Dentistry: A Clinical Approach to Techniques and Materials,
© *1991, Lea and Febiger*

- If the mandible is too large, it can be shortened. On each side, the upright *ramus* is cut through, and some of the bone is trimmed off, or else the two pieces are made to overlap. Regrowth of bone eventually knits the pieces together.
- If the mandible is too small, it can be lengthened through a procedure known as a *sagittal split.* Just behind the teeth on each side, two shallow, parallel cuts are made in the mandible, an inch or so apart, one on the inside and the other on the outside. The bone is then sliced apart lengthwise between the cuts, and the front of the mandible is slid forward, so only a partial overlap remains. In healing, the pieces knit together, and new bone fills in the depressions beside the overlap.
- This procedure can be combined with others to reshape a micrognathic jaw. If the mandible is too narrow, segments of it can be cut apart and reassembled in a wider arch. The chin can be built up at the same time, by cutting off the point at a diagonal angle, and then sliding the

piece slightly forward and upward.
- To remedy long-face syndrome, the bones of the upper jaw can be reduced in depth. They are cut through horizontally across the whole width of the jaw, and the excess bone is removed before the cut pieces are drawn back together. To assure a proper bite, it is sometimes necessary to reshape the lower jaw and chin as well.
- If the maxilla is too small horizontally, it can be widened, and if the maxilla is too short, it can be repositioned downward. The first step in either case is to cut the bones free of the cranium. They are then placed in the desired position, and the gaps filled with bone grafts.
- Asymmetries in the bones of the jaws are remedied by using the same methods, often in combination.

All orthognathic surgery must be performed in a hospital, and requires very careful, very detailed planning. Intensive X-ray studies must be made, and the surgical procedures are often tried out first on casts of the

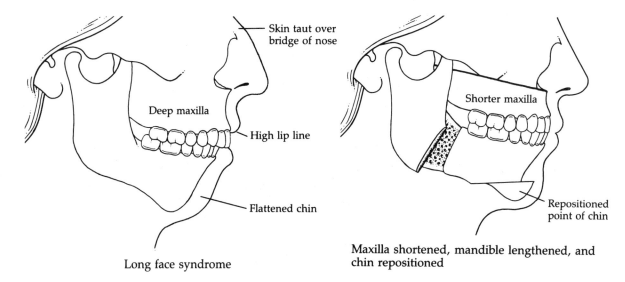

Skin taut over bridge of nose

Deep maxilla

High lip line

Flattened chin

Long face syndrome

Shorter maxilla

Repositioned point of chin

Maxilla shortened, mandible lengthened, and chin repositioned

jaws. Moreover, orthognathic surgery is usually not complete, definitive treatment in itself. It must often be accompanied—before or after or both—by restorative dentistry and orthodontics.

Procedures similar to those used for orthognathic surgery are used to repair developmental defects such as *cleft lip* and *cleft palate* (see pages 264 and 275), and to reconstruct jaws deformed by conditions such as oral cancer and radiation damage.

MAJOR ORAL SURGERY: WHAT TO EXPECT

Surgery for jaw malformations, developmental defects, cysts and tumors, fractures, or temporomandibular disorders is classified as major oral surgery. With few exceptions, it must be performed in a hospital, partly because the surgical procedures are themselves relatively complex, but partly so that facilities will be available if any unexpected complications occur. From your point of view as a patient, major oral surgery involves a basically similar sequence of procedures.

PREOPERATIVE TREATMENT

Surgery is almost always preceded by extensive consultations, examinations, and tests. Some of these preparations, such as recording your medical and dental history, physical examination, and X-ray studies, are office procedures usually conducted before you enter the hospital. But some findings will be verified after you are admitted.

In particular, you will be examined and tested to make sure that you are not likely to experience adverse physical effects from anesthesia or other aspects of the surgery. For this purpose, you may be admitted to the hospital several hours to a day before the scheduled operation. If you are to receive general anesthesia, you must fast for twelve hours beforehand, so that your stomach will be empty.

Just before the operation, you are likely to be given a sedative to make you feel relaxed and free of anxiety. Then you will probably receive a general anesthetic, administered at first through a mask that covers your nose and mouth. Once you are unconscious, the mask will be replaced with a tube passing through your nose and down your windpipe,

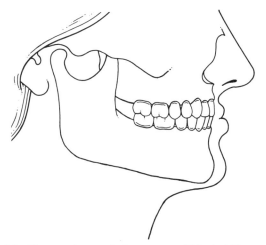

Maxilla too short relative to mandible (midface deficiency)

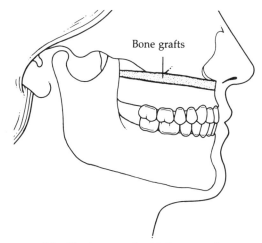

Maxilla deepened with bone grafts

through which the anesthetic gas, mixed with oxygen, is continuously delivered.

POSTOPERATIVE TREATMENT

Following the operation, you will probably be taken to a recovery area until the effects of the anesthesia have worn off, and your vital signs have largely returned to normal. While you are in the hospital, you will be given analgesics to control pain, anti-inflammatory medications to minimize swelling, and antibiotics to reduce the risk of infection.

Oral surgery patients can generally leave the hospital a day or so following the operation. The surgeon will probably prescribe further analgesics, and possibly antibiotics, for you to take at home. You will also receive instructions on how to control any bleeding that might occur. After three days to a week, you will go to the surgeon's office to have any surface sutures removed.

After most major oral surgery, a soft diet is recommended for about two or three weeks. The period may be longer if your jaws must be fastened together by *intermaxillary fixation* (see page 156).

Once your jaws are mobile, you will undertake a program of physical therapy—mainly gentle exercises to keep the muscles limber and to minimize the formation of scar tissue and *adhesions*. Adhesions are tough, fibrous tissues that are the by-products of internal bleeding. Left untreated, they can cause the jaw muscles and temporomandibular joints to become stiff and tender.

The recovery period varies widely, depending on the type of surgery. At one extreme is *arthroscopic* surgery, sometimes used for temporomandibular surgery (see page 215), which requires no more than a few days. At the other extreme is orthognathic surgery. Several weeks or months may be needed before the bones have knitted together sufficiently to be functional.

RISKS AND COMPLICATIONS

Compared with much other surgery, even major oral surgery is relatively safe. It is not inherently life-threatening, nor is there much danger of lasting harm from any of its procedures. Surgery poses risks mainly to patients who are *medically compromised*, that is, who suffer from other serious physical ailments (see Chapter 20).

There are slight but real risks in any procedure involving anesthesia, especially general anesthesia (see page 56). There is also a very slight risk of bacterial infection during the operation. This is controlled by aseptic techniques and the use of antibiotics.

Major oral surgery is often performed in areas close to, or even crossing, the facial nerves. In rare instances, a branch of a sensory or a motor nerve may be damaged during the operation, causing local numbness or loss of muscle control. The specific area will depend upon which branch is damaged. It may be located in the lower face, affecting one side of the chin, lips, or tongue. Or it may be located in the upper face, affecting the eyelids and forehead. Usually the damage is only temporary; during healing, the nerve fibers should eventually regenerate and recover their function.

S I X T E E N

ORTHODONTICS: MORE THAN STRAIGHTENING TEETH

The arrangement of the teeth in the jaws illustrated in Chapter 1 and the patterns of their development and eruption (see chart, pages 96–99) are only ideals. Real teeth in real jaws are seldom so evenly spaced or so well matched.

There are several basic reasons for irregularities. One of the most important is heredity. Just as the features of the human face vary enormously, so do the teeth and jaws. Moreover, the genes that control the shape and size of teeth differ from those that control those of the jaws, making a mismatch more likely.

There are also irregularities that may arise during the development and eruption of your teeth. Your teeth may not appear in the proper place or in the proper order. And after they erupt, they may become damaged or lost as a result of decay, disease, or injury. Or they may be forced out of position by habits such as thumb-sucking.

Your teeth may therefore be misaligned, and may not match your jaws or one another. The jaws themselves may not be well matched in size or shape. The results may not only be unsightly, but may also interfere with the effectiveness of the bite, contribute to periodontal disease, and otherwise threaten dental health.

Some of these problems can be treated with restorative dentistry, as described in Chapter 13. But the specialists most involved in treating them are orthodontists. In this country, at any given time, there are about four million orthodontic patients. According to a recent estimate, about half of all children have orthodontic problems that would benefit from treatment, and about 20 percent have severe disorders that need treatment urgently.

GOALS OF ORTHODONTICS

The word *orthodontics* comes from Greek words meaning "straight" or "correct," and "teeth." Many people indeed think of orthodontics as simply "teeth straightening." But there is much more to it than that.

Orthodontists do correct the positions of

the teeth. But they also treat one other major class of problems: abnormalities and discrepancies of the bones of the jaws. The main goals of treatment include the following:

- Improved *occlusion* so that when the jaws are closed the teeth mesh properly for chewing and swallowing.
- Reduced susceptibility to decay and periodontal disease, which can result from teeth that are crowded too close together, or otherwise badly aligned.
- Improved speech, since some 18 letter sounds require the assistance of the teeth for clear enunciation.
- Avoidance and alleviation of temporomandibular disorders (see page 203).
- Improved appearance, which, for many people, is the most important goal of all.

COMMON ORTHODONTIC DISORDERS

Most orthodontic disorders are described as *malocclusions*, or "bad bites." Malocclusions take two main forms: defects of the bones of the jaws, and defects of the teeth. There are also two main categories of causes: *hereditary*, which are genetically determined, and *functional*, which arise after birth, often as a result of neglect, injury, or faulty habits.

These forms and categories often overlap, and each includes several kinds of malocclusion.

HORIZONTAL MALOCCLUSIONS: THE ANGLE SYSTEM OF CLASSIFICATION

Most malocclusions are classified by a system devised by the "father of orthodontics," Edward H. Angle, around the turn of the century. He identified three basic classes of occlusion. All of these classes are based on relationships between the upper and lower

first molars. The relationships of these teeth, in turn, reflect *horizontal* relationships between the upper and lower jaws.

Class I

The normal relationship of the teeth and jaws is described as Class I occlusion. When the jaws are closed, the lower first molars are positioned slightly forward of the upper ones. The lower jaw is positioned directly under the upper one, and the lower front teeth rest lightly against the backs of the upper ones. The outer ridges of the lower back teeth meet the central valleys of the upper back teeth.

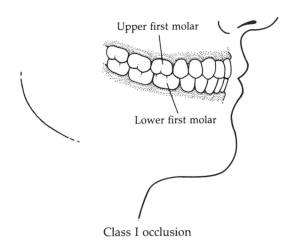

Upper first molar

Lower first molar

Class I occlusion

There are, nonetheless, malocclusions associated with Class I occlusion. The most prevalent one is *crowding* of the teeth, in one or both jaws. Crowding is sometimes accompanied by the *ectopic* ("out of place") eruption of the permanent teeth. Crowding and ectopic eruption are usually the result of *arch-length insufficiency:* There is not enough space in the arch of the jaw for all the teeth to fit properly.

Arch-length insufficiency is a hereditary

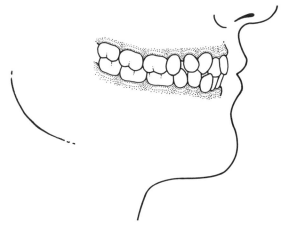

Crowding of teeth, due to arch-length insufficiency

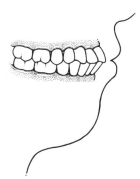

Bimaxillary protrusion

condition, and a very common one. Some biologists claim that it is an inevitable consequence of human evolution. Over the generations, human facial bones have become considerably reduced in size, but the size of human teeth has not diminished to the same extent.

Also, the genes controlling the size of bones are different from those controlling the size of teeth. It is quite possible to inherit small jaws from one parent and large teeth from the other, with crowding as the result.

There is another condition associated with Class I occlusion that can be a problem in some instances. It is called a *bimaxillary* ("both jaw") protrusion. That is, the front teeth in both jaws flare outward. Moreover, the natural flaring may become more pronounced with time, as chewing pressures tend to force the teeth forward.

Some people find this condition unattractive, and wish to remedy it for aesthetic reasons. But it can also lead to functional problems. In severe cases, the flaring front teeth meet at an abnormal angle, transmitting heavy, unbalanced chewing pressures to the supporting bones and ligaments. This repeated trauma can contribute to the development of periodontal disease.

Class II

In a Class II malocclusion, when the jaws meet, the lower first molars are either directly under, or to the rear of, the upper first molars. Thus, the lower jaw as a whole tends to close behind the upper one, and the upper front teeth protrude in front of the lower ones, a condition known technically as *excessive overjet*, and popularly as "buck teeth."

There are several types of Class II maloc-

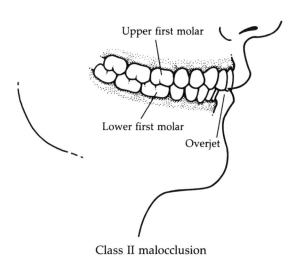

Upper first molar

Lower first molar

Overjet

Class II malocclusion

clusion. Sometimes just the upper front teeth protrude; sometimes the lower teeth are positioned too far back. The bones of the jaws are often mismatched in size: the upper jaw (maxilla) may be overdeveloped, with a normal lower jaw, or the lower jaw (mandible) may be underdeveloped with a normal upper jaw.

Furthermore, in one variety of Class II malocclusion—known as *Division 2*—the two central upper teeth don't protrude. Rather, these central incisors incline inward, and the *lateral* incisors, the teeth to either side of the central incisors, flare out.

Class II malocclusions pose one special problem: the protruding incisors are very susceptible to being accidentally knocked out, loosened, or fractured.

Class III

Whereas in Class I occlusion, the lower first molars are *slightly* forward of the upper ones, in Class III occlusion, the lower molars are positioned *far* in front of the upper ones. The mandible juts forward, giving the effect of a "bulldog chin" or a "Dick Tracy jaw." When the jaws close, the lower front incisors are in front of the upper front incisors, causing what is known as a *crossbite.*

A "true" Class III malocclusion is usually

caused by excessive bone growth in the lower jaw, a condition that is inherited. When it first appears during childhood the malocclusion is hardy noticeable, but it becomes more pronounced as the mandible grows during adolescence. More rarely, the mismatch in size is caused by underdevelopment of the upper jaw. This, too, is likely to be hereditary.

There are also *pseudo* Class III malocclusions. The lower front teeth close in a crossbite in front of the upper ones, but there is no serious mismatch in the size of the jaws. Sometimes the condition is caused by a habit of thrusting the chin forward when closing the mouth, or occurs when the primary upper front teeth fail to drop out on schedule and the permanent incisors erupt behind them (see page 171).

Sometimes these pseudo Class III malocclusions correct themselves; for example, when the primary teeth fall out, the pressure of the tongue may move the permanent incisors into the proper positions. In any event, these malocclusions are generally remediable.

True Class III malocclusions can be very hard to treat, and may require *orthognathic* surgery (see page 159).

VERTICAL MALOCCLUSIONS

The Angle system of classification is mainly based on the *horizontal* relationship of the jaws, from front to back. But malocclusions in these classes may be complicated by faulty *vertical* relationships between the lower and upper jaws.

Deep Bite or Overclosure

A *deep bite* is a condition in which the lower jaw closes too deeply under the upper one. There is an excessive *overbite* of the front teeth; when the jaws are closed, the lower

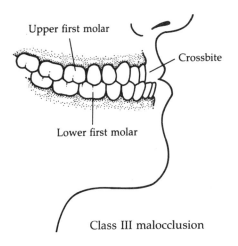

Upper first molar

Crossbite

Lower first molar

Class III malocclusion

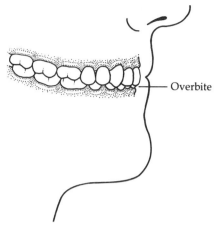

Deep bite (overclosure)

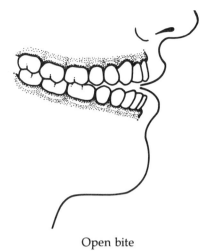

Open bite

teeth may be completely hidden. A severe form is sometimes called a *collapsed* bite.

This type of malocclusion has three main forms:

- Either the front teeth are naturally over-extended *(extruded)*, or the side teeth are underextended *(intruded)*.
- The side teeth are worn down through use, or have been restored by a dentist to an inadequate height.
- Several of the side teeth are missing or lost, through heredity, decay, or injury.

Open Bite

This condition is the opposite of a deep bite. When the jaws close, the molars meet, but a gap remains between the upper and lower front teeth. Sometimes the bones of the jaws simply grow in different directions, but the gap is more often the result of habits such as thumb-sucking and tongue-thrusting (see pages 170 and 171).

LATERAL CROSSBITE

Normally, the arch of the lower jaw, the mandible, is slightly smaller than the arch of the

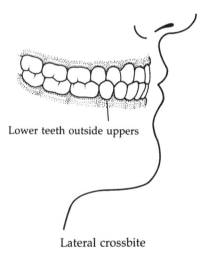

Lower teeth outside uppers

Lateral crossbite

upper jaw, so the lower front teeth close inside the upper ones, and the upper side teeth close on the inner edges of the lower side teeth (see page 9). But sometimes there are discrepancies in the sites of the jaws, so that some of the teeth of the lower jaw close outside, or *across*, the upper teeth. The result is called a crossbite, and there are two main types. If the lower jaw is too long in relation to the upper, a Class III malocclusion occurs, with an *anterior* crossbite (see above, page 168). If the lower jaw does not match the *width* of the upper, a *lateral* crossbite may occur. There are also two types of these:

- The lower jaw may be much narrower than the upper jaw. This condition tends to produce a crossbite on one side, as the lower molars seek purchase for chewing.
- Even more commonly, the upper jaw may be narrower than the lower jaw. The cause may be hereditary or a bad habit such as thumb-sucking or tongue-thrusting, which prevents the sides of the tongue from exerting enough pressure on the upper jaw and palate to make them expand to their proper width. The result is likely to be a lateral crossbite, on one or both sides.

ASYMMETRY

The malocclusions described here may occur on only one side because of an *asymmetry* (lopsidedness) of the teeth or jaws.

Asymmetry may result when some teeth on one side are lost or when they never grew in, or, more rarely, by uneven growth of the facial bones. It can also result from the habit in childhood of propping the head against the hand on one side, for extended periods. Asymmetry is often accompanied by a lateral crossbite, as the lower jaw shifts from side to side in an effort to accommodate the mismatch with the upper jaw.

SEVERE MALFORMATIONS

The malocclusions described here occur as part of the normal range of human traits. But there also exist several facial malformations, such as cleft lip or cleft palate, which radically affect the formation of the jaws and teeth (see pages 264 and 275).

FUNCTIONAL MALOCCLUSIONS

Many malocclusions are completely hereditary or have a strong hereditary component. But some are *functional* in origin, or at least they are aggravated by functional habits. Among the most common are harmful muscle habits.

Thumb-Sucking and Finger-Sucking

Sucking on a thumb or finger is a very common habit of early childhood (see page 94). It isn't likely to do any harm unless it persists to the time when the first permanent teeth are ready to erupt. Then it can seriously deform the teeth and jaws.

First, the pressure of the thumb in the mouth tends to push the upper front teeth upward and outward, while the lower front teeth are pushed downward and inward. This process is a major cause of open bite, and often aggravates Class II malocclusions.

Furthermore, the force of sucking causes the cheeks to press against the sides of the jaws. This process can seriously narrow either or both of the dental arches. The upper arch is especially likely to be affected, since the thumb displaces the tongue downward, and prevents it from exerting an effective outward counterpressure.

For methods of controlling thumb-sucking and finger-sucking, see page 174 and pages 94 and 95.

Sucking or Chewing the Lower Lip

This habit may occur alone, or it may accompany thumb-sucking. It tends to aggravate the outward flaring of the upper front teeth.

Tongue-Thrusting

Pressing the tongue against or between the front teeth while swallowing is a habit that often is the result of faulty nursing during infancy (see pages 87 and 91) or from thumb-sucking.

Tongue-thrusting is the most pernicious of all habits because it is not naturally outgrown and is difficult to correct. It can cause an open bite or a crossbite, or make these conditions worse. It also aggravates Class II malocclusions.

Sometimes tongue-thrusting is induced by *mouth-breathing*, which can result from asthma, sinusitis, allergic reactions, or similar disorders that block the nasal passages.

DEFECTS OF THE TEETH

Malocclusions result not only from defects and mismatches of the jawbones but also from defects of the teeth. Teeth may be incorrectly positioned *(malposed)*, irregular in shape or size, or missing. And like bone defects, tooth defects may be either hereditary or functional in origin.

Prematurely Lost Primary Teeth

For a variety of reasons, but usually because of decay or injury, one or more of the primary teeth may be prematurely lost. That is, the tooth falls out long before the permanent tooth is well enough developed to replace it. Such loss can cause at least two serious problems:

- The teeth on either side of the missing tooth are not stable. The six-year molars in particular are likely to tip and drift into an empty space, and may hinder or misdirect the eruption of other permanent teeth.
- The loss of a primary tooth may cause the succeeding permanent tooth to erupt too early, out of its proper order. The permanent tooth may then drift out of

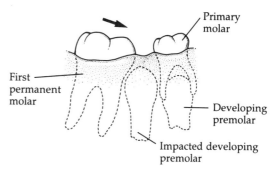

Drifting of first molar into space left by prematurely lost premolar

place, or erupt too far before meeting the resistance of a corresponding tooth in the other jaw.

Overretention of Primary Teeth

Primary teeth that exfoliate too late can cause problems just as severe as problems that are the result of premature loss of teeth. Such *overretained* teeth hinder the eruption of the succeeding permanent teeth, and may cause them to emerge out of place *(ectopic eruption)*. Common reasons for overretention include the following:

- One or more of the primary tooth roots may not resorb properly, when the succeeding permanent tooth is ready to erupt.
- The roots may have become *ankylosed*, that is, tightly fused to the bone of the jaw.
- The tooth may have become *impacted*, that is, wedged under or against one or both of the adjacent teeth.

Missing or Lost Permanent Teeth

It is not uncommon for teeth to be missing for genetic reasons. Certain permanent teeth are especially likely to be lacking: These include lateral incisors, second premolars (bicuspids), and third molars ("wisdom teeth").

Permanent teeth may also be lost through decay or injury. A lost or missing tooth can lead to tipping or drifting of the adjacent teeth into the empty space or overeruption of the opposing teeth in the other jaw. The loss of several side teeth may cause a collapsed bite.

Other Tooth Irregularities

Teeth naturally vary in shape and size, and sometimes the variation is great enough to cause orthodontic problems. For instance, one or more teeth may be misshapen. A common example is a "peg" lateral incisor, which is narrower and more pointed than normal. Or individual teeth may be considerably larger or smaller than the rest of the teeth. Large central incisors are especially common. Such variations may contribute to spacing problems with adjacent teeth, or prevent the teeth from meshing properly with the corresponding teeth in the other jaw.

ORTHODONTIC TREATMENT: APPLIANCES

Orthodontists use a wide variety of mechanical devices, called *appliances*, to direct the growth of the jaws, to alter muscle behavior, to move teeth, and to retain the position of the teeth after treatment. Most appliances are designed to apply steady but gentle pressure on the teeth and jaws; too much pressure can cause permanent damage. Appliances operate according to two basic principles:

- Bone growth tends to slow down when pressure is applied against the bone. Conversely, bone growth is accelerated when traction is applied upon the bone. This is the principle behind appliances that are used to control the growth of the facial bones.
- Similarly, pressure applied to a tooth changes the structure of the alveolar bone in which the tooth is embedded.

This pressure is transferred through the tooth and its ligament to the bone. On the compressed side, the bone tissue resorbs. At the same time, growth of new bone is stimulated on the opposite side, where the ligament is being stretched.

This is the principle behind appliances used to move teeth and to stabilize them in their new positions.

There are two main categories of appliances: *fixed* and *removable*. Each category has several subcategories. No one type of appliance solves all problems, any more than one type of shoe fits every foot.

FIXED APPLIANCES

These are appliances that are firmly fixed in the mouth for the duration of treatment. They are usually attached to the teeth by *bands*: metal cylinders that are shaped to fit snugly around individual teeth, and cemented in place. There are four main types of fixed appliance: *bracketed* appliances, *lingual archwires*, *habit-control* appliances, and fixed *space maintainers*.

Bracketed Appliances

These are the familiar "braces." They are used both to move teeth and to direct the development of the alveolar bone of the dental arches.

Many people dislike wearing braces—mainly on aesthetic grounds. But bracketed appliances are unsurpassed for the precise control of pressure applied to teeth and bone. Many conditions can't be treated successfully any other way.

A bracketed appliance is actually a system of several components:

- *Bands* used to be attached to all the teeth to be treated. Now they are usually placed only on *anchor* teeth at each end of the appliance. Before the bands are

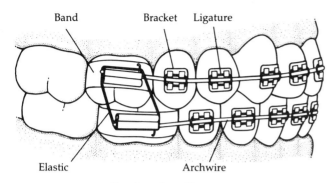

Bracketed appliances

inserted, *spacers*, small loops of wire or elastic, may be needed temporarily to separate the anchor teeth from the teeth adjacent to them.

- *Brackets* were formerly attached to the bands on the teeth, but are now usually bonded directly to the tooth surfaces. Their precise placement determines the direction of the force that will be applied to each tooth. Until recently, all brackets were made of metal, but transparent or tooth-colored brackets are becoming increasingly common.
- An *archwire* passes across the brackets around the arch of the teeth, from one banded anchor tooth to the other. It may be a single wire, or several light strands twisted together. Its ends pass through *buccal tubes* attached to the bands.
- *Ligatures* are wires or elastic loops that bind the archwire firmly to the brackets, to keep it from being dislodged by chewing.

Much of the pressure needed to move the teeth comes from the archwire itself. It is resilient—that is, it tends to retain its arched shape, and to pull or push misaligned teeth into the same arch. Building springlike loops into the archwire, or connecting the archwire to the bands with springs, can further increase its resiliency.

Any of several *auxiliary* components may be used to apply additional pressure upon a tooth or a group of teeth. Two types are especially common:

- *Elastics,* small rubber bands, may be attached to hooks on the bands or the archwire. The wearer must remove them before eating and replace them daily.
- *Headgear* may be used to provide *extraoral* ("outside the mouth") traction. It consists of an elastic strap around the head or neck, plus a metal *face bow* that attaches to *headgear tubes* on the teeth. Headgear uses the head and neck as a stable anchor for pressure on the teeth or jaws. It may be used to apply direct, backward pressure to the teeth. Or, in a reverse configuration, it may be used to pull the upper jaw forward.

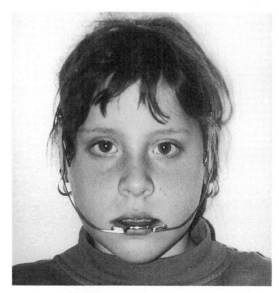

Headgear
Photograph by Gordon Gaynor

Lingual Bracketed Appliances

Recently, appliances have been developed that have their brackets and archwire mounted *inside* the dental arch. They are called *internal, invisible,* or *lingual* braces (*lingual* means "of the tongue"). Except for the

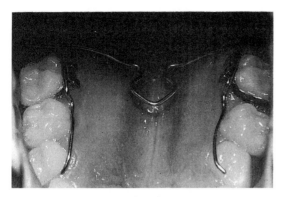

Lingual archwire

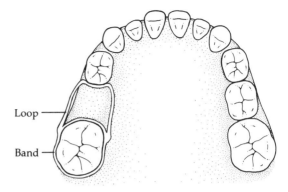

Fixed space maintainer

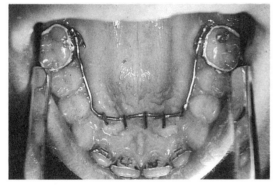

Habit-control appliance, with barrier, or "rake"
Photograph by Gordon Gaynor

bands on the molars, the appliances ordinarily can't be seen.

Internal appliances appeal to many patients on aesthetic grounds. But in several respects, they do not function as well as standard bracketed appliances. The internal brackets and archwire may irritate the edges of the tongue, and they interfere with normal speech. Treatment takes longer, and requires more effort; hence, it is considerably more expensive. Finally, external bracketed appliances may have to be used *after* internal ones, to achieve precise tooth alignment.

Lingual Archwires

These fixed appliances are attached to molar bands, but they are not bracketed to indi-

vidual teeth. They are often used to maintain the existing length and shape of the whole dental arch; and they are sometimes used to widen or to narrow the arch. Lingual archwires have been in use for a long time, and have none of the disadvantages of the lingual bracketed appliances mentioned above.

Habit-Control Appliances

Fixed *habit-control* appliances resemble lingual archwires. They are attached to bands or crowns on two upper molars. They have special barriers to help control harmful habits such as thumb-sucking and tongue-thrusting.

Space Maintainers

A relatively simple form of fixed appliance, often used by pediatric dentists and orthodontists, is the *space maintainer*. It holds open the space left by a prematurely lost primary tooth until the permanent tooth comes in.

A space maintainer often consists of a band or temporary crown attached to the tooth on one side of the space, plus a wire loop or spring to bridge the gap to the tooth on the other side. A lingual archwire (see above), which maintains the length of the whole arch, is sometimes used instead, especially when more than one tooth has been prematurely lost.

REMOVABLE APPLIANCES

All removable appliances can be at least partly taken out of the mouth by their wearers. Some are completely removable; others can be temporarily detached from fixed bands on the molars. Generally, they are most effective when worn nearly all the time, but they can be taken out for meals and special occasions.

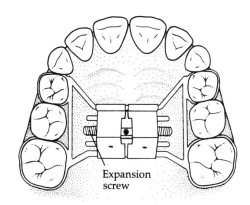

Palatal expander

Removable appliances appeal to many patients because they aren't fixed in the mouth, and are not particularly conspicuous. But they are *not* a complete substitute for fixed appliances. They are far less precise in controlling the teeth and jaws, and take more time to produce results. Also, they are more easily broken or lost. There are some conditions they cannot improve. Most important of all, they require the faithful, unfailing cooperation of the patient.

There are four main types of removable appliances; *"active"* appliances, *functional* appliances, *space maintainers and retainers*, and *headgear*.

"Active" Appliances

"Active" removable appliances are most similar to fixed appliances. They apply force directly to the teeth or the jaws or both. Typical examples include the following:

- *Palatal expanders* are used to widen the arch of a narrow upper jaw. The expander is a plastic plate that fits over all or part of the palate, the roof of the mouth. It is split down the middle, and screws or extraoral traction are used to provide outward pressure. The pressure forces open the lengthwise central joint, or *suture*, between the bones of the palate, and new bone grows to fill in the space. This procedure works best with younger children, whose bones are still growing rapidly. It is not effective past adolescence, when the suture becomes rigid.

- *Space regainers* are customarily used to expand the space between teeth in order to provide more room for teeth that haven't yet erupted. A space regainer, like a palatal expander, is an acrylic plate that fits inside the jaw. To it are attached extensions, such as screws or springs, that exert pressure to move the teeth or to extend the dental arch.

- *Tooth positioners* are made from a model of the complete dental arch. Casts of malposed teeth are cut off the model, and cemented back in the correct position. A soft plastic mold (rather like an athletic mouthguard) is made from the corrected model. When worn in the mouth, this mold gently encourages the malpositioned teeth to move into their proper positions. Tooth positioners are useful only for minor tooth movements, or as retainers after active treatment. They are not powerful or versatile enough to correct major problems.

Functional Appliances

Functional appliances are often completely removable. They change or harness the pressure of the muscles of the mouth, which, in

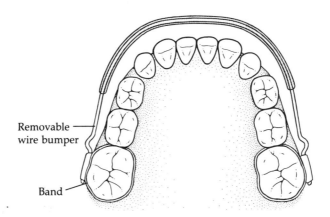

Removable wire bumper

Band

Lip bumper

turn, act on the teeth and bones. Sometimes headgear is attached to these appliances. Examples include the following:

Lip and cheek bumpers vary in design. Some simply hold the lips or the cheeks away from the teeth, relieving the teeth and jaws from the pressure of the lip and cheek muscles. The pressure exerted by the tongue is thus unchecked. Like lingual archwires and palatal expanders, they are useful in widening a narrow dental arch.

Some lip bumpers are attached by wires to bands on the molars; they use the transferred pressure of the lip muscles to move the molars backward.

Jaw-repositioning appliances are full or partial plastic plates that encourage the jaws to close

in a new and more desirable position than before. One of the most common is the *activator,* worn on the upper jaw. It brings the retruded lower jaw of a Class II malocclusion forward, and also stimulates its growth to bring about a better match with the upper jaw.

Removable Space Maintainers and Retainers

As with fixed space maintainers, removable space maintainers and retainers are used to hold open space between the teeth in the dental arch, or to stabilize the teeth following treatment with other appliances.

- *Space maintainers* resemble active plates. They fit inside the jaw, and have plastic

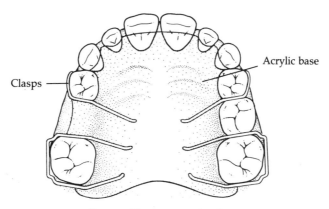

Clasps

Acrylic base

Removable space maintainer

HAWLEY RETAINER

Front view

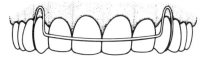

Hawley retainer

Occlusal view

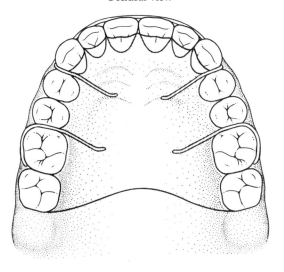

or metal extensions to keep the space between them open. They are essentially *passive* devices, that is, they exert enough pressure to hold the teeth in place, but not enough to move them.

• The most familiar retainer is the *Hawley* appliance. An acrylic plate that fits against the palate in the upper jaw, it holds the upper teeth in place following other treatment.

Hawley retainers are sometimes used to control habits such as thumb-sucking. They interfere with the sensory satisfaction of placing the thumb in the mouth, which often leads a child to abandon the habit. Like fixed devices, they can be supplemented with metal extensions that actually keep the thumb out of the mouth.

Headgear

As described earlier, headgear is generally used as an auxiliary for fixed, bracketed appliances. It is also used alone, or in conjunction with other removable appliances. Examples include:

• *Face masks*, which either restrain or encourage the growth of the upper jaw, depending on their form.
• *Chin cups*, which restrain excessive growth of the lower jaw. These are used more cautiously than they used to be, because it is suspected that sharply forcing the mandible backward can cause temporomandibular disorders.

ORTHODONTIC EXTRACTIONS

Orthodontic treatment sometimes requires the removal of teeth—primary, permanent, or both. The extraction of primary teeth is generally done to prevent later problems with the permanent teeth.

Badly decayed primary teeth may have to be removed so that infection won't harm the developing permanent teeth underneath. If primary molars are extracted, space maintainers may be needed until the permanent teeth erupt.

Overretained primary teeth, which delay or prevent eruption of permanent teeth, may also have to be removed. In some cases, a number of *serial* extractions is carried out, to assure the proper order of succession (see illustrated chart, pages 96–99).

Removal of permanent teeth is somewhat more controversial. Some practitioners extract teeth routinely; others believe that permanent teeth shouldn't be removed unless it is absolutely necessary. Extractions are most like likely to be performed in the following situations:

- Some people have extra, or *supernumerary*, teeth. When there is room in the jaw, supernumerary teeth are allowed to remain. But extraction is often required to prevent crowding or ectopic eruption.
- Severely crowded permanent teeth, resulting from dental arch-length insufficiency, may require the removal of teeth in one or both jaws.
- "Matching" teeth may have to be extracted. If a tooth in one jaw is missing or lost, the opposing tooth in the other jaw may have to be removed. In some cases, corresponding teeth on the *other* side of the jaws may have to be removed as well, for symmetry.

Whether primary or permanent, teeth may have to be extracted if they are ankylosed to the bone or impacted against other teeth.

PERIODS OF TREATMENT

Orthodontic treatment takes place during any of four main periods in life:

- *Early childhood,* before the primary teeth are lost.
- The period of *mixed dentition,* when the primary teeth are being succeeded by the permanent teeth.
- *Adolescence,* when most of the permanent teeth are in, but the facial bones are undergoing a "growth spurt."
- *Adulthood,* when growth is complete, but some movement of the teeth and of the nearby *alveolar* bone is still possible.

Treatment will vary considerably from one period to another.

EARLY TREATMENT

Orthodontic treatment of the jaws and teeth of children up to the age of about six is almost entirely preventive and interceptive, rather than corrective. It is often provided by a pediatric dentist, rather than an orthodontic specialist.

The dentist monitors the development of the teeth and gums, watching for decay or gum disease that might lead to premature loss of primary teeth and for infection or injury that might affect the development of the permanent teeth. The dentist carefully observes—directly and by X-ray—the primary teeth and the developing permanent teeth, watching for conditions such as the following:

- Close spacing between the primary teeth, which may foreshadow crowding of the permanent teeth.
- Pre-eruption evidence of supernumerary, missing, or badly positioned permanent teeth.
- Early signs of facial bone problems, such as a mismatch of size or shape, which will lead to malocclusion later.

If a child needs treatment at this age, it usually consists of training and persuasion to end harmful habits, such as thumb-sucking and finger-sucking, lip biting or sucking, tongue-thrusting, and mouth breathing. If nasal congestion and airway blockage seem to be factors, the dentist may refer the child to an ear, nose, and throat specialist, an allergist, or the like.

If the child loses one or more primary teeth prematurely, space maintainers, fixed or removable, may be inserted to assure sufficient room for the permanent teeth to erupt. These may not be needed for the front teeth, but they are often essential when primary molars have been lost, to prevent adjacent teeth from tipping or drifting into the empty space.

If the child has a malocclusion of the primary teeth, such as an open bite or a crossbite, it may be treated at this time with functional appliances. Such treatment, however, is more common during the period of mixed dentition.

Toward the end of the early period, individual primary teeth may need to be extracted, to assure that their permanent successors erupt properly.

TREATMENT DURING MIXED DENTITION

During the period when the permanent teeth are replacing the primary teeth, treatment is mainly preventive and interceptive, though it can sometimes be corrective as well. Treatment may be provided by an orthodontic specialist or a pediatric dentist.

The dentist pays special attention to two goals: assuring the proper eruption of the permanent teeth and controlling the growth of the facial bones to avoid later problems.

Harmful habits should be treated intensively during this period, since they can either cause or aggravate malocclusions, or render other treatment ineffective. At this stage, some practitioners supplement persuasion and education with habit-control appliances (see page 174).

If the child has lost primary teeth prematurely, the dentist may use a space maintainer to hold open the space of a single tooth, or an archwire to maintain the length and shape of the complete dental arch.

"Serial" extractions of primary teeth may have to be performed during this period to make sure that the permanent teeth erupt in the correct order and location.

Functional appliances may be used to assure that the jaws close correctly and to guide erupting teeth into their correct positions.

Other appliances may be used to intercept or remedy problems with developing facial bones. If one or both of the dental arches is too narrow, for example, fixed archwires or removable expanders may be inserted to widen them. Or such headgear as face masks

and chin cups may be used to control the growth of the jaws.

Though bracketed appliances (braces) are more commonly used during adolescence, they may be inserted at this time, to move malposed teeth, open or close spaces between the teeth, correct a crossbite, or control the growth of the bones.

TREATMENT DURING ADOLESCENCE

This is the period following the eruption of the second ("12-year") molars. Except for the third molars, which won't appear until about age 17, the permanent teeth are all in. Bone growth in the jaws continues, though at a slower rate. From this time on, any corrective treatment is usually entrusted to an orthodontic specialist.

The treatment of adolescents concentrates mainly upon correcting tooth problems. Treatment begun during the time of mixed dentition often continues into adolescence, and many of the same methods are employed.

The use of bracketed appliances is especially common at this period, to bring the teeth into alignment, to assure a good arch form, and to bring the jaws into normal occlusion.

One or more of the permanent teeth may need to be extracted to remedy severe crowding, or to remove ankylosed or impacted teeth that can't erupt properly. Such extractions are ordinarily followed by treatment with bracketed appliances.

Restorative dentistry may supplement orthodontic treatment. For example, missing teeth may be replaced with bridges, and small, "peg" teeth may be made larger with crowns or veneers.

ADULT TREATMENT

Adults used to be considered "too old" for orthodontics. Not anymore. A considerable improvement in both function and appearance can be achieved, to remedy both longstanding malocclusions and harmful changes (such as tooth loss) that have occurred over time. There are, however, certain limitations to adult orthodontics.

Once all the permanent teeth have erupted, and the facial bones have finished growing, orthodontic treatment must be almost entirely corrective. It is still possible to move the teeth, and such realignment is the most common form of treatment undertaken for adults. The alveolar bone next to the teeth can still be orthodontically reshaped to a certain extent, but not the basal bone of the jaws.

Orthopedic devices that influence bone growth are no longer useful. Any major changes in the size or shape of the jaws are likely to require orthognathic surgery (see page 159). This is often followed by orthodontic treatment to align the teeth and ensure that they occlude properly.

Adults are more susceptible to periodontal disease and loss of alveolar bone. To be effective and lasting, adult orthodontic treatment must sometimes be accompanied by periodontal treatment. Also, restorative dentistry is very often used in conjunction with adult orthodontics, mainly to remedy tooth damage or loss.

HOW—AND WHEN—TO FIND AN ORTHODONTIST

Orthodontics is one of the recognized dental specialties. It requires two years of postgraduate training in a recognized dental school. Most orthodontists then go into practice without seeking board certification. A majority of these orthodontists, however, join the American Association of Orthodontists.

Other dentists, especially pediatric dentists, may sometimes provide orthodontic treatment. For simple procedures, such as extractions of overretained primary teeth or insertions of space maintainers, treatment by nonspecialists is adequate. But for sustained or complex treatment, you should seek out a specialist in orthodontics.

Generally, the first warning of a need for orthodontics will come from a child's pediatric or general dentist, who may also recommend a particular specialist. The procedures described in Chapter 2 can be used to locate a qualified practitioner.

Orthodontic treatment is time-consuming, extensive, and relatively costly. It is crucially important for patients (and parents) to have a clear understanding of the diagnosis, the proposed plan of treatment, and its cost, and to establish a good working relationship with the orthodontist. Second opinions are quite common—the general dentist's counsel can be especially helpful.

Many orthodontists charge a fixed fee for a full course of active treatment, including appliances and retainers. Follow-up visits, however, may not be included. Comprehensive fees are often payable in installments as treatment progresses; the initial payment is usually the largest.

Orthodontic treatment may or may not be covered by dental insurance, since policies vary widely (see page 239). To reduce expenses, many orthodontic patients use dental school or hospital clinics. Advantages include the likelihood of high-quality treatment and the use of up-to-date materials and techniques. The disadvantages include less flexible scheduling, a longer time spent in the chair and waiting room, and a less personal relationship with treatment providers. Also, clinics are primarily intended for *teaching*, and patients are selected accordingly. Not all applicants are accepted.

UNDERGOING ORTHODONTIC TREATMENT

When orthodontic treatment begins, the first step is an extensive diagnostic process, which

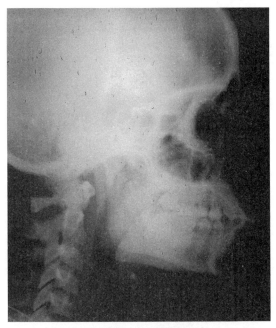

Cephalometric X-ray

usually requires at least two office visits. During the initial consultation, the orthodontist will take a complete history and thoroughly examine the patient's mouth and teeth.

An initial, tentative diagnosis may be possible, but at this first visit, or a subsequent one, the orthodontist will undertake further diagnostic studies. These will include X-rays, especially *cephalometric* views of the sides of the head, to show the jaws and their relationship to each other. The orthodontist will also take impressions of both jaws, and color photographs of the face and mouth.

The orthodontist may also consult with the patient's general dentist and physician to make sure that there are no dental or medical conditions that would interfere with or otherwise affect treatment.

Based on these studies, the orthodontist will arrive at a comprehensive diagnosis and plan of treatment. The patient (or parent) should receive answers to the following questions:

- What is the condition (or conditions) to be treated? What will happen if it is left untreated?
- What appliances, or other techniques, will be used?
- How long will each stage of treatment last?
- What is the result aimed for, in terms of both function and appearance, and what are the chances of success?
- What are the possible complications of treatment?
- What will the treatment cost?

After the last diagnostic visit, active treatment will begin. Treatment time varies widely. It usually continues for at least several months, and often for several years. Harmful habits such as thumb-sucking may lengthen the time considerably. Treatment with active appliances is often followed by a period of wearing a retainer until the softened bone of the tooth sockets becomes strong enough to stabilize the teeth.

THE PATIENT'S ROLE IN TREATMENT

The active cooperation of the patient is important in many aspects of dental care, but it is absolutely crucial in orthodontics, especially if removable appliances are used. Noncompliance, even for short periods, can significantly lengthen the treatment time, or sabotage the process completely. Some guidelines for success are shown here.

TROUBLESHOOTING MINOR PROBLEMS DURING TREATMENT

By and large, orthodontic treatment is painless and free of problems. But patients may experience some soreness, especially when appliances are first inserted. Also, their appliances may occasionally be damaged or broken.

DO'S AND DON'TS FOR ORTHODONTIC PATIENTS

- Diligently keep all appointments and follow all instructions. Wear appliances, elastics, retainers, etc., for the periods prescribed. Keep a daily written record of the hours you wear headgear or a removable appliance.
- Take good care of your appliances. Have a specific place to store removable appliances, elastics, etc., where they won't be lost or damaged. Don't fiddle with an appliance or bring it into contact with hard objects like pencils or hairpins. When taking part in active sports, take out removable appliances or headgear. Be especially careful to take out such an appliance before you swim, or you are very likely to lose it. Protect bracketed appliances with a mouth guard.
- Appliances readily trap food particles, so that tooth decay is more likely. Brush your teeth after every meal and snack, and if you are wearing a removable appliance, clean that, too. Irrigators do a good job of dislodging food particles, but they don't break up plaque. So brush thoroughly, especially the "danger zone" between the appliance and the gumline. Flossing may be somewhat difficult when bracketed appliances are being worn, but try at least to floss any unengaged teeth. Make a special effort to avoid sweets. See your regular dentist for examination and treatment of your teeth and gums. Your orthodontist may periodically remove the appliances for this purpose.
- Avoid hard or sticky foods that are likely to damage appliances. Such foods include nuts, bones, bagels and hard-crusted bread, caramels and other chewy candy, corn on the cob, corn chips and other crunchy snacks, and popcorn. Never chew gum, sugarless or otherwise. Never chew ice. Some hard fruits, such as apples, can be eaten if they are cut into small pieces.

Many removable appliances have a plastic plate that fits against the roof of the mouth. Some patients have trouble speaking clearly when they first wear such an appliance, but virtually everyone adjusts within a few days.

The teeth may become unusually sensitive to hot or cold, especially when appliances are first inserted. Some patients find it more comfortable to avoid ice cream and hot drinks, at least during the early stages of treatment.

The teeth may even feel a little loose during treatment. In fact, they are. But the patient shouldn't worry—they're not going to fall out.

Soreness

If an inserted appliance causes discomfort, a mouthwash of warm salt water often gives relief. So does a relatively soft diet for 24 hours or so. A mild analgesic, such as aspirin or acetaminophen (Tylenol), may be helpful as well. The orthodontist may supply pieces of a special wax to cover the brackets, so that the inside of the lips and cheeks are not irritated.

If the pain persists more than a couple of days, consult the orthodontist—the appliance may need adjustment. If the soreness is caused by a loose or protruding piece of the appliance, try to bend it gently away from the soft tissue, or cover it with wax. Again, see the orthodontist promptly for adjustment.

Damaged or Broken Appliances

Accidents do happen. If all or part of an appliance is loose, gently try to remove it. Try to bend back any protruding pieces, or cover them with wax, so they won't irritate the soft tissue.

If absolutely necessary, cut off the protruding part with nail clippers. Go see the orthodontist as soon as possible, and take all the broken parts with you.

POSSIBLE COMPLICATIONS AND FAILURES OF ORTHODONTIC TREATMENT

The success rate of orthodontic treatment is very high. Its techniques are well established, and of demonstrated effectiveness. Nonetheless, not every treatment is a complete success, and there are certain potential complications patients should be aware of.

Tooth decay and gum inflammation are somewhat more likely to occur during orthodontic treatment. Teeth may also become discolored, or lose some of their enamel. These problems can usually be headed off through diligent care by patient and dentist.

In rare instances, the roots of the affected teeth may resorb, and if this is severe, the teeth may never be fully stabilized in their new positions. If proper procedures are used, and if the patient is cooperative, this problem is extremely unlikely to occur.

The results of treatment may not last. Orthodontics essentially works against nature, and natural forces may eventually bring about a relapse. A late spurt of growth may alter or undo treatment performed in childhood or early adolescence. In later years, crowded lower front teeth are naturally apt to occur (see page 107), though the process doesn't usually cause occlusion problems.

If you have had orthodontic treatment, you should continue to monitor its results. In particular, you should consult the dentist or orthodontist if you notice any change in the bite. It may mean that the gums and the supporting tissues of the teeth are becoming weaker, or that some muscle habit is at fault.

S E V E N T E E N

AESTHETIC DENTISTRY: MAKING THE MOST OF YOUR SMILE

The foremost goal of dentistry is to preserve and restore oral health and function. But it serves another important purpose as well. As pointed out in earlier chapters, teeth that work well also tend to look good. And the techniques that dentists use to make your teeth healthy and efficient can also be used to make them more attractive.

The use of dental techniques for the specific purpose of improving appearance is known as *aesthetic dentistry*. Although it isn't one of the recognized dental specialties, aesthetic dentistry has become a major area of concentration for a growing number of practitioners and is becoming increasingly popular among patients.

Aesthetic dentistry can achieve dramatic, far-reaching changes. Your face is the part of your body that gets looked at longest and most often, and your mouth is a main focus of attention in your face. So improving the appearance of your mouth may greatly improve the whole visual impression you make.

But improved appearance is only one result—and often not the most important one. Defects of the teeth and mouth can cause great mental anguish, diminishing your self-confidence and sense of self-worth. You may develop the habit of hiding your mouth behind your hands, or you may avoid smiling entirely so you won't have to reveal your teeth. Aesthetic dentistry can have an enormous positive effect, improving not only your appearance but also your morale and outlook on life. Looking better can help you feel better about yourself and to deal more effectively with your social environment.

SPECIFIC AESTHETIC DEFECTS

A principal aim of dentistry is to correct specific defects that detract from the appearance of the teeth and mouth. A few of these defects are purely visual, but many of them cause functional problems as well.

DISCOLORED TEETH

Healthy, normal permanent teeth are basically light ivory. Several conditions may cause them to become noticeably discolored.

Surface Stains

Certain foods, such as coffee, tea, and red wine, can stain the surfaces of your teeth. So can tobacco, whether smoked or chewed. These stains are likely to be concentrated in areas that are hard to keep clean by brushing, such as the gumlines and the *interproximal* spaces between your teeth. Usually, such stains can be removed through regular professional cleaning. If you are a heavy tea or coffee drinker or a habitual smoker, you may need to have your teeth cleaned more often than usual to keep them looking presentable.

More troublesome are stains on tooth-colored composite fillings, of the kind used to restore the highly visible front teeth. Not only does the composite material discolor more readily than natural tooth enamel, but also stains are likely to work their way into the margins around fillings (see page 191). Even professional cleaning may not remove them.

Tetracycline Stains

Certain chemical substances, introduced into the body, may stain the inner layer, the dentin, of the teeth. These deep stains cannot be removed by cleaning. Among the most severe dentin stains are those caused by the antibiotic tetracycline.

Tetracycline and its various forms are useful against a wide range of infections. But if any one of them is taken by a woman during pregnancy, it may stain the developing primary teeth of her baby. And if it is taken by a child under the age of eight, it may be absorbed by the developing permanent teeth, staining them orange, brown, or gray (see pages 189 and 192). The stain may affect the whole tooth, or it may appear as parallel, horizontal "stripes" or "ribbons," alternating with more normal coloration.

Fortunately, the danger of tetracycline staining is widely known, and most obstetricians and pediatricians now avoid prescribing this antibiotic whenever possible.

Fluorosis

In some geographical areas, the water supply naturally contains rather large concentrations of fluorides. Drinking the water may cause a mottled grayish or brownish staining of the teeth, called *fluorosis*.

Incidentally, fluorosis is *not* caused by the artificial fluoridation of water—or by professional fluoride applications or fluoride toothpaste or mouthwash, when used as directed. In all these uses of fluoride, its concentration is too low or exposure to it is too limited to cause staining.

Developmental Defects

Sometimes disease or other health problems will interfere with the development of the teeth in childhood. The enamel of the teeth may develop irregularly, or improperly (see page 251). Or some of the enamel on individual teeth may be deficient in calcium and develop chalky-white spots popularly known as "headlights."

Diffusion from Amalgam Fillings

Silver amalgam, the most common material used for fillings, is largely a mixture of silver and mercury, plus small proportions of other metals. Chemical reactions in your mouth may cause a slight corrosion of those materials, to produce a gray stain that diffuses into the surrounding tooth enamel (see page 195).

Damaged Pulp

In teeth that have been subjected to trauma (accident or violence), or that have had root canal treatment, the blood vessels of the pulp may bleed into the surrounding dentin. Blood contains iron, which can darken teeth to a grayish or brownish color (see page 189).

Tooth Wear

Though tooth enamel is the hardest substance in your body, it is not totally resistant to wear. With advancing years, parts of it may be worn thin, so that the darker dentin underneath becomes more visible (see page 190). Several factors may be involved. Habitual grinding, or *bruxing*, of your teeth may wear off the tops of the crowns, exposing the dentin. Improper brushing may *abrade* the tooth surfaces. Or strong acids may *erode* them (see page 192).

Exposed Roots

Periodontal disease or advancing age may cause your gums to recede from the necks of your teeth. This tends to expose the roots of the teeth, below the enamel. The protective cementum that covers the roots is thinner and more transparent than enamel, and reveals the darker dentin underneath.

MALPOSED TEETH

Many factors may cause your teeth to become crooked or misaligned. They are discussed in detail in Chapter 16 (page 165). Severe malpositions are likely to cause functional problems, but even rather slight deviations may affect your appearance, especially if several teeth are involved.

SPACES BETWEEN TEETH

Gaps or notches between adjacent teeth may result from tooth loss or a naturally occurring malposition. Such empty spaces, particularly between your upper teeth, create distracting "holes" in the dental arch.

Particularly common and noticeable are natural gaps (*diastemas*) between the upper central incisors (see pages 192 and 193). Also relatively common are small "peg" lateral incisors, with prominent notches on one or both sides (see page 192). Congenitally missing permanent teeth will often create spaces in the dental arch.

Teeth that are tipped, rotated, or moved from their correct positions will often produce gaps or notches. When teeth are lost, not only do they leave a gap in the dental arch, but also the teeth that were adjacent to a lost tooth may drift into the empty space, creating additional gaps (see page 134).

Periodontal disease and its treatment may cause the gums to recede from teeth, exposing their roots and leaving triangular gaps. And when periodontal disease becomes advanced, it erodes the alveolar bone of the sockets, depriving the teeth of support. Pressure from the tongue and opposing teeth may then cause the front teeth to splay outward, opening up spaces between them.

TEETH OF IRREGULAR SIZE

Individual teeth may be noticeably larger or smaller than their neighbors. Especially distracting are overlong canines ("vampire fangs"), oversize upper central incisors ("buck teeth," "bunny teeth," or "barn doors"), and undersized "peg" lateral incisors (see pages 190 and 191).

CHIPPED TEETH

The front teeth, especially the upper central incisors, are susceptible to fracture. Even if only a small part is broken off, and the life of the tooth is not threatened, the jagged, irregular contour is likely to be unsightly (see pages 189 and 190).

WORN TEETH

When teeth are worn down by natural use or by habitual bruxing, the edges in each arch form a straighter, flatter line. In addition, the worn upper teeth tend to "hide" behind the upper lip, giving the impression that they are missing. These consequences of wear form part of the stereotype of old age (see page 104).

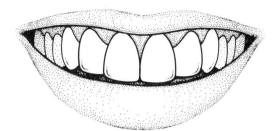

The attractive smile

"COLLAPSED" BITE AND LOSS OF THE VERTICAL DIMENSION

If many back teeth are lost or severely worn, the bite may "collapse," and your face may lose some of its *vertical dimension*—the distance separating the nose and the chin. Loss of vertical dimension accentuates facial wrinkling and reinforces the stereotype of old age.

Furthermore, when back teeth are lost, the tongue tends to be forced forward against your front teeth—particularly the upper front teeth. The additional pressure may cause these to splay outward, opening up gaps between them.

SEVERE IRREGULARITIES OF THE JAWS

Mismatched or otherwise irregular jaws may not only cause significant functional problems but may also detract seriously from your appearance. These conditions are described in detail in Chapter 15 (page 151).

THE ATTRACTIVE SMILE

Aesthetic dentistry seeks not only to remedy specific visual defects but also to achieve an "attractive smile." This cannot be defined exactly; there is no fixed, universal ideal. Nonetheless, there do exist a few criteria, based generally on healthy, unworn young teeth:

- The teeth—especially the conspicuous front teeth—should be relatively even in

color, with a slight yellowing near the gumline. They should be slightly translucent, especially near the biting edges and neither dead white nor darkly discolored.
- The upper front teeth are the most visible teeth in the mouth. The open smile should reveal most of their surfaces. Lips should not sag so far, nor the teeth be so worn, that the biting edges can't be seen. A smile, however, shouldn't be so high that it exposes large areas of the upper gums.
- The teeth in each jaw should be fairly straight, and shouldn't tip or overlap. The biting edges should form a fairly smooth contour, a *smile line,* that curves gently upward to parallel the line of the smiling lower lip.
- The biting edges of the front teeth should be slightly curved at the corners, and not ground flat. The upper central incisors and canines should be slightly (but only slightly) longer than the lateral incisors.

PROCEDURES OF AESTHETIC DENTISTRY

To correct unsightly defects and to make a smile attractive, dentists use techniques and materials like those used for functional restoration. The most important include *bleaching, contouring, bonding, veneering,* and *replacing fillings,* and inserting *artificial crowns* or *prosthetic teeth. Orthodontics* and *orthognathic surgery* may also be required.

BLEACHING

The most conservative way to remove penetrating stains from the teeth is by bleaching. This technique can be used on any tooth, but is most often used to lighten the highly visible front upper teeth.

Bleaching teeth is rather like bleaching laundry. The dentist applies oxygen-releasing chemicals that react with the discolorations and oxidize them out. The chemicals used to bleach the outer surfaces usually have hydrogen peroxide as their main ingredient. Those applied within teeth (see page 189) may contain sodium perborate as well.

When outer surfaces are to be bleached,

the dentist first isolates the teeth to be treated with a rubber dam, to protect the gums. It used to be customary to etch the surfaces with acid before applying the bleach, and to use heat to accelerate the bleaching process, but the bleaching gels now available make both those steps unnecessary. Once the gel is applied, it is allowed to remain on your teeth for half an hour or so, and then rinsed off. Many dentists then polish the surfaces, just as they do after routine cleaning. Repeated treatments over several weeks may be needed until the desired degree of lightening is achieved.

Careful, controlled bleaching doesn't harm your teeth, but it may make them temporarily more sensitive. Anesthesia is not used during treatment. If you feel any discomfort, the dentist can simply stop the process by removing the gel.

Sensitivity may persist a day or two after treatment. The bleach used must be quite

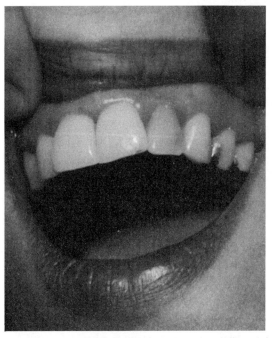 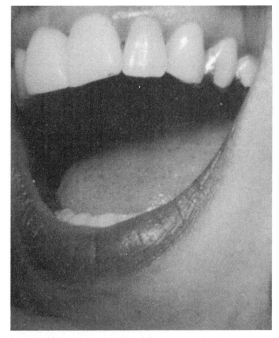

Stain of lateral incisor, caused by iron diffused from damaged pulp. Remedied by internal bleaching. *Photographs by Herbert F. Spasser*

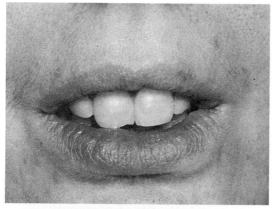

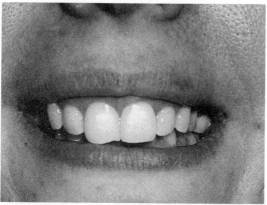

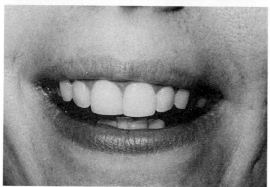

Fluorosis from excessive fluorides in the water supply. Also oversize incisors, one of them chipped. Remedied by bleaching and contouring. *Photographs by Barry Dale*

strong—far stronger than household products—and it must penetrate the enamel to reach the discolored dentin. There it may irritate the nerves in the pulp. You can usually alleviate lingering sensitivity with mild analgesics such as aspirin or acetaminophen (Tylenol). About two weeks are allowed to pass before treatment is repeated; this gives the tissues time to recover.

Children and adolescents, whose teeth have relatively large pulps, may experience more pronounced discomfort. For this reason, it may be preferable to delay treatment. But young people are often very sensitive about their appearance, and may quite willingly endure some discomfort in order to improve the color of their teeth.

If a tooth is discolored from damaged pulp or from root canal treatment, it may be bleached from *within*. For example, if a tooth turns dark after an injury, the change is evidence that the pulp is damaged or dead. During root canal therapy (see page 120), the dentist will apply a mild bleach as part of the standard procedure to clean and sterilize the pulp chamber and canal. Often this will oxidize, and remove, the stain in the surrounding dentin.

If the stain persists, or appears after root canal treatment, a *walking bleach* can be applied. The dentist reopens the pulp chamber and partly empties it of gutta percha. Bleaching liquid is inserted, and sealed under a temporary filling. You then "walk around" for a few days, while the bleach diffuses into the dentin, oxidizing the stain. When the desired level of lightening is achieved, the dentist removes the temporary filling and bleach, and inserts a permanent filling.

The results of bleaching vary widely. Some stains, such as the mottling caused by fluorosis, usually come out without difficulty—often with a single treatment. Mild tetracycline stains and the natural darkening of teeth in later years can also be reduced with considerable success.

Severe tetracycline stains, however, may resist even repeated treatments. Teeth stained gray, even when bleached lighter, tend to remain gray.

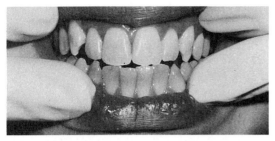

Tetracycline staining. Remedied by bleaching (top teeth only).
Photograph by Barry Dale

Some discolorations cannot be corrected by bleaching. For example, teeth with dead-white "headlights" can't be bleached to match the areas of deficient calcium. Bleaching is also ineffective on the stains caused by diffused amalgam fillings, unless the fillings themselves are removed and replaced (see page 195).

Bleaching is ordinarily an office procedure. So-called "whitening" toothpastes do not work well on deep stains, and some contain abrasives that can harm teeth. Over-the-counter bleaching compounds work slowly and unpredictably, but their most serious drawback is that their safety, especially if they are used for a long period, has not been established.

Somewhat more reliable are bleaching systems that are used at home, but under professional supervision. The dentist takes an impression of the teeth to be treated, from which a soft appliance—rather like a mouth guard—is fabricated. At home, you line this appliance with a relatively mild bleaching gel, and you wear it for a few hours each day. Compared with bleaching in the dentist's office, this process, too, is rather slow, and not always predictable. More and more dentists are now using *both* office and supervised home methods, for faster and more reliable results than either accomplishes by itself.

Bleaching may not be permanent. Dentin stains, such as those caused by tetracycline, are especially likely to return. Later "touch-ups" may be desirable. Sometimes bleaching is undertaken as a first step in trying to remove discoloration. If it doesn't produce satisfactory results, more elaborate methods, such as bonding or the application of veneers (see below), may be required.

AESTHETIC CONTOURING

The enamel of healthy permanent teeth is ordinarily more than thick enough for its two main functions—withstanding the forces of chewing and protecting the underlying dentin from decay. Dentists take advantage of this fact when they perform *occlusal equilibration*, selectively grinding the enamel chewing surfaces so the opposing teeth mesh properly (see page 79).

The same principle can be used to adjust the shape of your teeth to make them more attractive. The process is known as *aesthetic contouring*. The dentist selectively grinds off small areas of enamel of each tooth to be re-shaped. The process is painless and, if it is done carefully, it won't harm the tooth. But it can often substantially change the way the tooth looks—by itself, and in relation to the other teeth.

An obvious function of contouring is to reduce teeth that are too large, in comparison with their neighbors. The teeth most often contoured for this reason are overlong canines, which give the face a predatory, vampire look. Slightly rounding their pointed edges can make them far more harmonious with the rest of the teeth in the arch.

Other teeth that are frequently contoured include upper central incisors that have erupted well below the level of the adjacent teeth ("buck" or "bunny" teeth). Trimming the bottom edges can make the smile line more even and harmonious. To look natural, though, these teeth, like the canines, should be allowed to remain *slightly* longer than the lateral incisors next to them.

Sometimes one of these incisors is wider

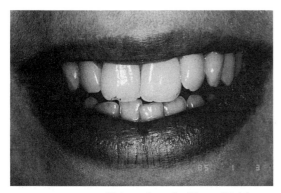 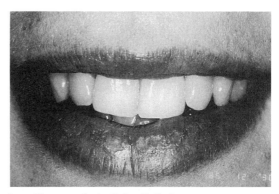

Chipped teeth. Remedied by contouring. *Photographs by Brian Pollack*

than the other, an especially noticeable irregularity. Slightly reducing the outer edge of the larger tooth may create a better match. But it may be necessary not only to make the larger incisor smaller but also to make the smaller one larger, by bonding or by adding a veneer.

With the exception of the upper central incisors and canines, the smile lines of both your jaws should be relatively even. Teeth that are tipped, overlapping, or erupted to varying levels can produce a line that looks unattractively jagged and "sharklike." Contouring can sometimes remedy the most obtrusive of these irregularities.

The edges, however, shouldn't simply be ground flat. This makes them look worn and old. Indeed, worn, flattened front teeth can sometimes be made more attractive and youthful-looking by rounding off their sharp outer corners. If your teeth are badly worn, though, contouring usually isn't satisfactory—restoration or replacement may be needed.

Ordinarily, teeth with chipped edges must also be built up or covered over to restore their original contours. But if the chip is very small, contouring may successfully conceal it, without further restoration.

For tipped, misaligned, or overlapping teeth, contouring is sometimes a compromise solution, undertaken as a less demanding, less expensive alternative to orthodontics or restoration. Contouring can't change the *actual* position of a tooth, but it can affect the *apparent* position. Slightly contouring the protruding side of an overlapping tooth, for example, can make it look much more closely aligned with its neighbor.

Contouring, like bleaching, is followed with polishing, to smooth the reshaped surface. Fluoride is often applied as well, to protect the newly exposed enamel from decay.

COMPOSITE BONDING

When cavities occur on highly visible tooth surfaces, the material often chosen to fill them is a composite, made of fine glass particles in a resin binder. Its chief advantage is that it can be tinted to match virtually any natural tooth enamel. Well-made composite fillings can be practically indistinguishable from the teeth in which they are inserted.

In aesthetic dentistry, the same material is used for *bonding*, to change either the color or the shape of individual teeth. It is usually applied to tooth surfaces to mask deep stains or to build up inadequate contours or both.

The composite is available in a wide variety of colors; and the dentist can also selectively tint it with dyes after it is applied. It is ordinarily translucent—like natural tooth enamel—but it can be made more opaque if necessary to cover deep stains. The dentist

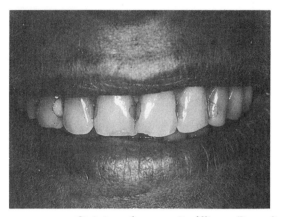 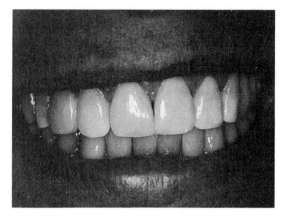

Staining of composite fillings. Remedied by bonding. *Photographs by Barry Dale*

often uses two or more shades, so the tooth surface will be *characterized,* that is, it will have the same subtle variations in color that natural teeth have.

The bonding process is similar to the insertion of composite fillings. Usually no anesthetic is required, and the procedure can be completed in a single office visit.

First, the dentist etches the tooth enamel slightly with acid, and brushes on a liquid *bonding agent* to which the composite will adhere. Then the composite itself, which is about the consistency of putty, is spread over the surface. It is often applied in thin successive layers, and carved while it is still soft to achieve the desired contours. When the tooth being bonded is next to highly visible front teeth, the dentist may retract the gum slightly before applying the layers, so that the edge of the composite will subsequently be hidden behind it.

As with composite fillings, the material is then hardened, or *cured.* Some composites are self-curing, but may require a strong light to activate the process.

Whereas bleaching lightens stains, bonding covers them. It tends to be more satisfactory than bleaching for tetracycline stains. Unlike bleaching, it is often effective in concealing calcium-deficient white "headlights"

and the dark stains caused by diffusion from silver amalgam fillings. It is also useful in masking stains on earlier composite fillings, and smoothing their surfaces.

Bonding can be used to build up the contours of teeth to a limited extent. The material used is not strong enough to withstand heavy chewing pressure, or repeated contact with opposing teeth. Bonding is especially helpful in restoring the edges of chipped or worn teeth. It is also used to enlarge unusually small teeth, such as "peg" lateral incisors, thus minimizing the size of minor gaps between teeth. And it can both cover and build up the necks of teeth exposed by receded gums.

Bonding is often combined with contouring, to give teeth a more desirable shape. For example, if one of the upper central incisors is broader than the other, contouring may reduce its width. The other incisor may then be built up with bonding, to make a more perfect match in size, and to close any gap caused by the contouring.

Bonding has definite limitations. Even opaque layers will not completely cover some very strong stains. The material is subject to scratching and chipping, and can itself become permanently discolored by coffee, tea, tobacco, and sometimes lipstick. It is likely to

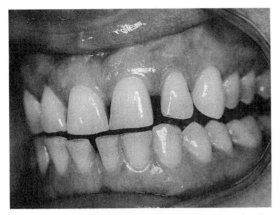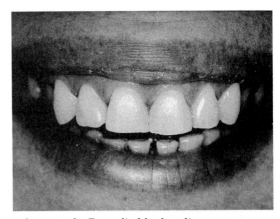

Gaps (diastemas) between undersize upper front teeth. Remedied by bonding.
Photographs by Alfred Carin

last from three to ten years before it must be replaced. Moreover, bonding may not be effective if your teeth are badly worn or eroded, though bonding agents now in use adhere better to enamel than to dentin.

Bonded teeth require a certain amount of special care. They will probably need to be professionally cleaned more often than once every six months. They may also need occasional polishing and touch-ups to remove scratches, cracks, or stains.

If you have bonded teeth, scrupulous home care is also important. You must brush and floss regularly and thoroughly. You should avoid or minimize contact with materials likely to cause stains—tobacco, in particular. To keep the bonding composite from chipping off, don't chew on ice, pencils, fingernails, or other hard objects. Don't pick your teeth with a fingernail or a hard toothpick. If the edges of your front teeth have been built up, try to avoid biting directly into hard foods such as apples, corn on the cob, hard rolls, and meat on bones; try to use your side teeth instead.

Despite its limitations, bonding is a relatively quick and conservative way to improve the appearance of your teeth. It is less expensive than veneers, and far less expensive than restorations such as crowns.

VENEERS (LAMINATES)

Whereas composite is applied soft and then hardened on the teeth, veneers are rigid shells that are prefabricated in the laboratory and then bonded, or *laminated,* to the teeth.

The veneering process requires at least two office visits. At the first visit, the dentist *reduces* the enamel, removing a little of its surface, so the added veneers won't make the teeth look too bulky. Then the dentist takes impressions of the prepared teeth, from which models will be cast.

In the laboratory, the veneers are fabricated to fit the models. At the second visit, the prepared surfaces are etched, and the veneers are firmly attached with a bonding agent. Properly fabricated, they look like natural teeth.

Several materials are used for veneers. The most durable, stain-resistant, and (in the view of many) natural-looking material is porcelain—like the porcelain used for fillings, onlays, or artificial crowns. Veneers may also be made of acrylic plastic or of composite, but they are far weaker and less durable than porcelain.

Veneers can be made more opaque than composite bonding. They are especially effective in covering front teeth that are chipped, worn, severely stained, or eroded at the

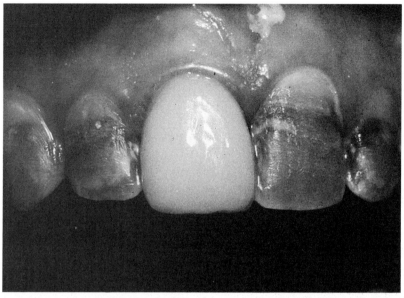

Severe tetracycline staining. Left and right: teeth reduced for veneers.
Center: veneered incisor. *Photograph by Kenneth Aschheim*

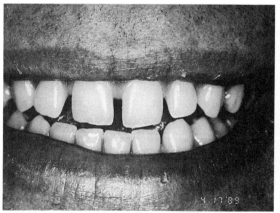
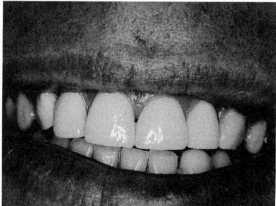

Gaps (diastemas) between upper front teeth. Remedied by veneers. *Photographs by Brian Pollack*

gumline. They can also be used to mask gaps
(diastemas) caused by undersized teeth.

They are not completely resistant to chipping or cracking, however, and they do not
hold up under heavy chewing pressures as
well as artificial crowns do. The same precau-

tionary guidelines for bonded teeth should be
followed for veneers.

The strongest veneers, those made of porcelain, have been in use for only a few years,
and it is too early to assess their long-term
reliability. Teeth with veneers made of acrylic

or composite are not likely to hold up as well as teeth with composite bonding.

REPLACEMENT OF DISCOLORED FILLINGS

As mentioned earlier, composite fillings are susceptible to staining from food and tobacco—especially around their edges—and silver amalgam fillings are likely to cause a gray mineral stain in the surrounding enamel.

Such stains can often be concealed, by covering the visible tooth surfaces with bonding or veneers. This is sometimes the best solution for stained but otherwise sound composite fillings. For amalgam fillings, though, the best solution may be replacement.

One alternative is to replace old amalgam fillings with new ones. The filling may be relatively small, and the stain may extend only a little way into the enamel. In such cases, when the old filling is removed, and the cavity slightly enlarged, the discoloration may disappear. Before inserting the replacement filling, the dentist applies a new liner or varnish (see page 67) to minimize future staining from the replacement and to minimize further penetration of the old stain.

Amalgam fillings can also be replaced with cast metal or porcelain inlays. These will not cause stains, but they are considerably more expensive than silver amalgam.

In some instances, amalgam fillings can be satisfactorily replaced with tooth-colored composite fillings. Materials now in general use are not as strong or as permanent as silver amalgam, and are not suitable for restorations that must withstand heavy chewing pressures. But new composites are becoming available that show promise even under these conditions.

It isn't always practical to replace old, extensive fillings in molars or inaccessible fillings at the proximal edges of any teeth. Molars, furthermore, are often so inconspicuous that stains on them are not worth trying to remedy. In general, the treatment of stains is reserved for the front teeth, from the incisors to the premolars.

It must be emphasized that it is rarely necessary to replace silver amalgam fillings for functional reasons. Amalgam is long-lasting and durable. Even more important, amalgam fillings should not be replaced out of concern for the mercury they contain. There is no evidence that amalgam fillings cause mercury poisoning.

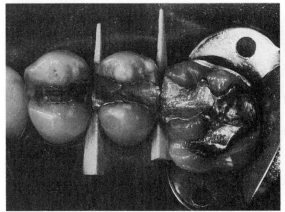 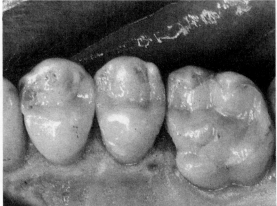

Stain caused by minerals diffused from silver amalgam fillings. Remedied by replacement with composite fillings. *Photographs by Kenneth Aschheim*

ARTIFICIAL CROWNS

Artificial crowns are used to replace the natural enamel of teeth that are too badly damaged to be restored with fillings or onlays. Thus, their purpose is primarily functional. The process of preparing the teeth, and of fabricating and inserting these restorations, is described in Chapter 13 (page 127).

But artificial crowns, or *caps*, also improve the appearance of the teeth they cover. Porcelain crowns in particular can be almost indistinguishable from natural teeth. Moreover, caps can be made in almost any size or shape, so they can effectively cover teeth that are undersize, malposed, misshapen, or severely worn.

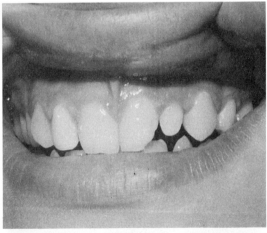

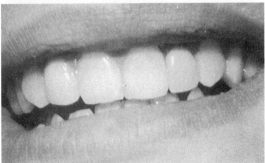

"Peg" lateral incisor. Remedied by artificial crown. *Photographs by Barry Dale*

Caps are stronger and last longer than bonding or veneers, and they withstand heavy chewing pressures. They are more expensive, however.

PROSTHETIC TEETH

Prosthetic teeth, in fixed bridges or removable dentures, are inserted, as are artificial crowns, mainly to maintain dental function. Even so, they too may significantly improve appearance, especially by filling gaps between teeth and increasing the vertical dimension of the bite. These restorations are described in detail in Chapter 13 (page 127).

ORTHODONTICS

Moving the teeth with orthodontic appliances has both a functional and an aesthetic purpose. For many patients, aesthetic improvement is the more important goal. Orthodontics is discussed in detail in Chapter 16 (page 165).

ORTHOGNATHIC SURGERY

Surgical reshaping of the jaws is not usually undertaken for aesthetic reasons alone. Nonetheless, the results almost always produce a dramatic improvement in appearance. Orthognathic surgery is described in detail in Chapter 15 (page 151).

UNDERGOING AESTHETIC TREATMENT

Aesthetic dentistry is not a separate dental specialty. Virtually all dentists use at least some of its techniques. Nonetheless, some dentists concentrate their practice in this area, and those who do are likely to have more experience than the average dentist. Your regular dentist may refer you to such a practitioner, or word-of-mouth recommendation from friends may be helpful.

Before you undergo aesthetic treatment, the dentist will probably insist upon first correcting any functional problems you may have. Decayed or badly fractured teeth should be restored, and periodontal disease must be treated. Some restorations, such as crowns, bridges, and dentures, have both a functional and an aesthetic purpose, as does orthodontics.

As in other forms of dental treatment, the dentist should prepare a comprehensive treatment plan, and should explain it to you fully before actual treatment begins. The dentist may apply tooth-colored wax to models of your teeth, in order to model the visual effects of bonding, veneers, or artificial crowns. Or you may be shown before-and-after photographs of patients who have been treated for conditions similar to yours.

Some dentists now use video and computers to illustrate the effects of aesthetic procedures. An image of your smile taken either directly, or from a photograph, is projected on a video screen. Then computer-generated graphics are used to superimpose images that approximate the proposed changes.

If you are undergoing aesthethic dentistry to correct adverse changes that have occurred over time—severe tooth wear, tooth loss, or the like—you should, if possible, provide the dentist with closeup photographs that show how your face used to look. Within limits such photographs can indicate to the dentist what your goals should be.

It is very important for you to reach an agreement with the dentist as to what these goals should be. On the one hand, absolutely optimum results may be more than you desire—or more than your time and budget allow. For example, you may decide that a conservative program of selective bonding and contouring will be a satisfactory compromise solution for misaligned or misshapen teeth, rather than more time-consuming, expensive orthodontics or restoration by insertion of artificial crowns.

On the other hand, it is not realistic or desirable to insist upon absolute perfection—especially at very close range. Few people will scrutinize your smile as closely as you do when you look in the mirror. Many imperfections (such as stained molars) aren't noticeable under ordinary circumstances. And it is unrealistic—not to mention unaesthetic—to try to make the teeth of an older adult look like those of an 18-year-old.

Moreover, your smile is an important element of your individuality. Some irregularities in tooth size, color, and shape are natural, as is a slight facial asymmetry. All these con-

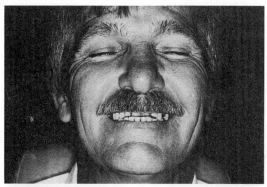

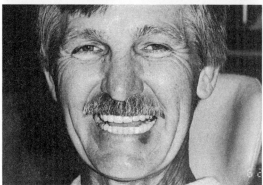

Face deficient in vertical dimension due to tooth wear and loss. Remedied by replacement of missing molars and by artificial crowns over worn teeth. *Photographs by Fred B. Abbott*

tribute to your unique personal appearance. Trying to remove all irregularities, in the hope of achieving a "movie-star" smile, is likely to produce a lifeless, artificial result.

THE COST OF AESTHETIC DENTISTRY

Before starting treatment, you should also discuss how much it will cost. This will vary widely, since every patient is unique, and no two courses of treatment will be exactly the same. Moreover, it is not always possible for the dentist to know in advance how extensive the treatment must be.

For example, it may be impossible to predict whether deep staining can be remedied by bleaching, or whether it will need to be masked by bonding or veneers. And if you insist upon absolutely perfect results, rather than just noticeable improvement, more time and effort may be required—at greater expense.

Nonetheless, the dentist should be able to give you at least a range of what treatment will cost. Some dentists have fixed fees for specific procedures. You should also be made aware of the costs of treatment alternatives. As mentioned above, conservative, relatively inexpensive procedures may be satisfactory substitutes for more intrusive and expensive ones.

By definition, aesthetic dentistry is elective. Unless treatment corrects a functional problem as well, it will not be covered by dental or medical insurance (see page 238).

Despite its cost, more and more people are taking advantage of aesthetic dentistry to improve their appearance. The reasons lie deeper than vanity. An attractive, youthful-looking smile has demonstrable social benefits, and conveys an impression of healthy self-confidence. It also helps turn that impression into reality. When people feel better about the way they look, they often feel better about themselves as well.

EIGHTEEN

TEMPOROMANDIBULAR DISORDERS AND THEIR TREATMENT

When you open and shut your mouth, only the lower jaw, the U-shaped *mandible*, moves. At each end of the mandible is a joint with one of the *temporal* bones of the cranium. It is called a *temporomandibular joint*, or *TMJ*.

The temporomandibular joints are more complex than most joints in the body. When the mouth opens and closes, the ends of the mandible don't simply rotate like hinges. As the jaw opens, the knob-like ends, or *condyles*, of the mandible first rotate, but then they slide forward, or *translate*, along the curving lower edges of the temporal bones.

To facilitate this movement, a separate piece of cartilage, called an *articular disk*, is mounted like a slippery cushion on top of each condyle (see page 201). The disk moves with the condyle as it rotates and translates. It is flexible enough to conform to the varying space between the condyle and temporal bone.

Each joint is enclosed in a sheath, or *capsule*, which is mainly ligament. The inner surface of the capsule is a membrane called the *synovial lining*, or *synovium*. It produces *sy-*

novial fluid, which lubricates the joint. The motion of the joints is controlled by the chewing muscles, known formally as the *muscles of mastication*. And the joints are greatly affected by the teeth, which largely determine the relationship of the jaws when the mouth is closed.

Probably because of their complexity and flexibility, TMJs are subject to a variety of disorders. In a recent change of nomenclature, these are now called *temporomandibular disorders*, or *TMDs*. They may afflict the joints themselves or the muscles and other tissues adjacent to them. Since the teeth are so intimately involved, diagnosis and treatment are usually provided by dentists. But the collaboration of specialists such as physical therapists, orthodontists, oral surgeons, and even psychologists is often needed as well.

SYMPTOMS OF TMDS

Temporomandibular disorders are often hard to diagnose. Symptoms are not simple or

BONES OF THE TEMPOROMANDIBULAR JOINT (TMJ)

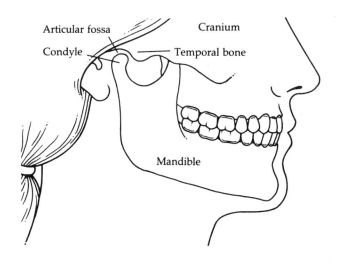

Articular fossa

Condyle

Cranium

Temporal bone

Mandible

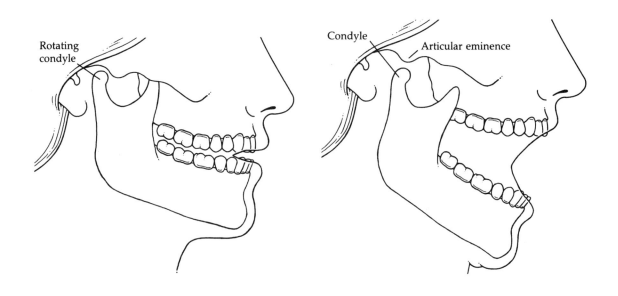

Rotating condyle

Condyle

Articular eminence

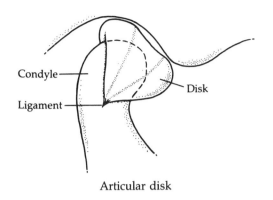

Articular disk

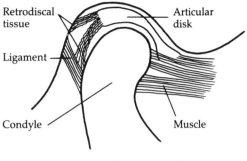

Interior of joint capsule

clear cut and can easily be attributed to other problems. The most common symptoms are the following:

- *Headaches,* often severe and recurrent. They occur more commonly on one side than on both sides, and in areas around the eyes, the cheeks, and the temples. But they can also occur at the top or the base of the skull.
- *Toothaches* that cannot be traced to decay, nerve damage, or other causes.
- *Burning, tingling sensations,* especially in the tongue, but sometimes in the mouth or throat.
- *Earaches,* or "stuffed" sensations in the ears, sometimes accompanied by dizziness or by ringing or rushing noises.
- *Neck aches, shoulder aches, or backaches,* sometimes accompanied by numbness in the arms or hands.
- *Tenderness and swelling,* sometimes near the joints themselves, sometimes more generally in the sides of the face.
- *Clicking, popping, or grating noises* when the jaw is opened and closed.
- *Inability to open the mouth freely,* either because of pain or because something seems to "lock" the jaw at a certain point. If the problem occurs on one side only, the jaw may not open straight up and down but rather deviates to one side.

TYPES OF TMDS

There are three main types of temporomandibular disorders: *myofascial pain, joint inflammation,* and *displacement of the articular disk.* They may occur separately or together, and one disorder may provoke another.

MYOFASCIAL PAIN

Myofascial pain occurs in the muscles (*myo* means "muscle") and in the connective tissue (*fascia*), that binds muscle fibers together. Myofascial pain may be chronic, or it may occur as an acute attack called *myofascial pain dysfunction.*

The pain may be concentrated in the chewing muscles that directly control the TMJs. But it may also be *referred,* through the nervous system, to other muscles of the head, neck, or shoulders. As noted above, severe headache is a common symptom.

JOINT INFLAMMATION

The soft tissues within the joint capsule can be inflamed. There are two main forms of inflammation, and they often appear together. The first is *capsulitis,* or *synovitis:* an inflammation of the *synovium,* the membrane lining the capsule. The second is *retrodiscitis:* an inflammation of the *retrodiscal tissue,* which is located behind the articular disk, and which connects the disk to the temporal bone.

DISPLACEMENT OF THE ARTICULAR DISK

The articular disk is attached to the condyle by ligaments on each side, and further stabilized by soft tissue such as the retrodiscal tissue. For a variety of reasons, to be discussed below, the disk may be squeezed forward, so that it slips either partly or entirely in front of the condyle. This condition is known as *an-terior displacement* or *internal derangement.*

In the process, the retrodiscal tissue is likely to become stretched and irritated, a process that results in retrodiscitis. Moreover, as the disk migrates forward, it can "escape" the condyle, producing the symptom of *clicking.*

When the jaw is closed, the "escaped'" disk is situated entirely in front of the condyle. As the jaw is opened, the condyle translates forward and rides over the relatively thick, posterior section of the disk. It then lands, or *reduces,* on the thinner center section, and clicks or pops.

Then, when the jaw is closed, the condyle

ANTERIOR DISK DISPLACEMENT WITH REDUCTION

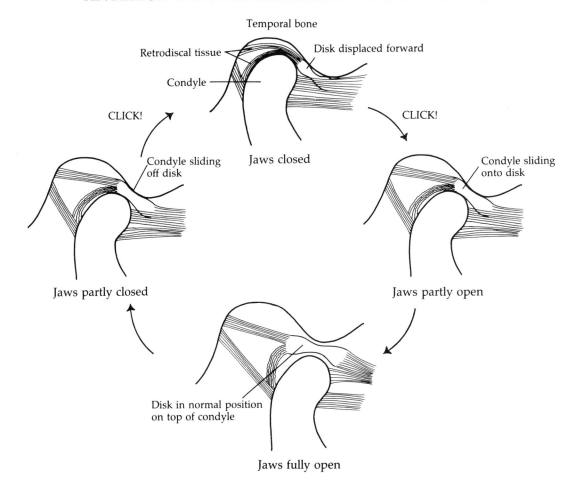

Temporal bone

Retrodiscal tissue

Disk displaced forward

Condyle

CLICK!

CLICK!

Condyle sliding off disk

Jaws closed

Condyle sliding onto disk

Jaws partly closed

Jaws partly open

Disk in normal position on top of condyle

Jaws fully open

DISK DISPLACEMENT WITHOUT REDUCTION

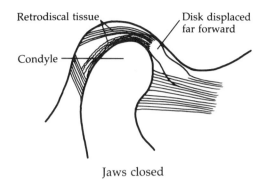

Jaws closed

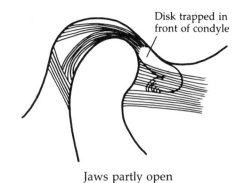

Jaws partly open

rides back over the thicker ridge and off the disk again. The result is a second click or pop. This condition is known as anterior displacement *with reduction.*

Clicking by itself may not be painful and often requires no treatment. But it may indicate more serious disorders to come. For example, the disk may continue to migrate forward until the condyle will no longer "reduce" on it. Instead, as the condyle translates forward, the disk rolls or folds up in front of it, and prevents the jaw from opening past that point. This is called *closed locking,* or internal derangement *without* reduction.

At first, locking tends to occur periodically. But the intervals between episodes may become shorter, and the condition may eventually become permanent. Furthermore, friction on the disk and retrodiscal tissue may *perforate* them or even destroy them.

Without the protection of the disk, the surfaces of the bones themselves may become worn and damaged, as they rub against each other. The final result is bone degeneration, or *osteoarthritis.*

CAUSES OF TMDS

Just as temporomandibular disorders often produce multiple symptoms, they often have multiple causes. These causes are not com-

pletely understood. Nevertheless, two factors, which are often interrelated, appear to underlie many TMDs: malocclusion of the teeth and psychological stress.

Other factors may not cause the disorders in themselves, but often contribute to them: these include faulty habits of posture and breathing. And finally, trauma (direct physical injury, as from an accident or a blow) may cause a temporomandibular disorder.

Symptoms *like* those of TMDs can also be produced by systemic disease, such as rheumatoid arthritis, temporal arteritis, or trigeminal neuralgia. A dentist must consider such possibilities when making a diagnosis.

MALOCCLUSION

Malocclusion—literally, "bad bite"—(see page 167) can throw the whole chewing mechanism out of balance. Some of the chewing muscles may have to work harder than others, and their fatigue may cause myofascial pain.

Also, over time, small areas of hypersensitivity may form within the fatigued muscles. These may or may not be painful themselves, but they serve as *trigger points* that set off the *referred pain* described earlier.

Moreover, pain can radiate from the chewing muscles through the process of *muscle guarding.* For example, if you sprain your ankle, your uninjured muscles tend to "guard" the injured tissues. You limp, to avoid putting painful pressure on the injured part. Similarly, when the chewing muscles are fatigued and painful, other muscles in the head and neck may guard them from further stress. Then these muscles, too, may become fatigued and painful.

Malocclusion can cause joint inflammation as well as myofascial pain. The unbalanced bite may cause one or both of the condyles to exert heavy pressure against the temporal bones every time the jaw closes. This is called *loading* the joints, and it produces *microtrauma*—literally, "little injury"— to the soft tissue. Repeated microtrauma can result in capsulitis or retrodiscitis or both.

Repeated loading of a temporomandibular joint may also squeeze its articular disk forward. This may result in disk displacement.

PSYCHOLOGICAL STRESS

Psychological stress can be defined as the effect upon the central nervous system of a powerful, disturbing stimulus from the environment. People respond to stress in many different ways. But there is one specific, physical response that profoundly affects the TMJs: habitually clenching or grinding (*bruxing*) the teeth.

Some people only clench; some only grind; some do both. Many are unaware of the habit, and may even clench or grind their teeth while they are asleep.

Clenching and grinding wear down the teeth, and should be discouraged, if only for that reason. But they also fatigue the chewing muscles, which can cause myofascial pain and the formation of trigger points. But the most serious long-term consequence is likely to be disk displacement.

When you chew food, the pressure of the bones upon each disk is not severe. But when your mandible clenches or grinds upon nothing except the opposing teeth, the joint becomes "loaded," and over time the disk tends to be squeezed forward between the bones. The result is displacement, accompanied by retrodiscitis as the retrodiscal tissue is pulled forward over the condyle.

FAULTY HABITS

Certain postural habits of the head and neck are likely to aggravate TMDs. The head weighs some 12 or 13 pounds, and carrying it is a considerable burden—especially if it is not centered on the neck bones (the *cervical spine*).

The most harmful of these postural habits is the *forward-positioned head:* The head is thrust forward, and the chin is tilted up. It is common among people who are near-sighted and thrust their heads forward to read. It can also be due to vanity. In our society, a receding, or "weak," chin is considered unattractive. Some people who have a naturally small mandible tend to thrust it forward to make it look larger.

This forward position puts too much pressure on the neck and back muscles, and is likely to tire them. It can also strain the temporomandibular joints, risking inflammation of the soft tissues.

Other positions that can aggravate TMDs, if they are habitual, or assumed for long periods of time, include the following:

- Cradling a telephone between the shoulder and the cheek.
- Propping the chin on one or both hands.
- Reaching high overhead for heavy burdens. Also painting, hammering, or doing other work on high walls or ceilings.
- Carrying a heavy shoulder bag with the strap over the same shoulder for a long period of time.
- Wearing high-heeled boots or shoes.

Two other faulty habits, though not strictly postural, are closely related:

- *Mouth breathing,* breathing through the open mouth rather than through the nose, is a habit that may develop early in childhood. Mouth breathing tends to be rapid and shallow, and it utilizes the muscles of the neck and upper chest, rather than the diaphragm under the lungs. Fatigue in these muscles can aggravate TMDs.
- *Tongue-thrusting* is also a habit of early childhood (see page 87). The tongue presses against the front teeth, and its tongue muscles are overworked.

These oral habits are best resisted by keeping the mouth in the "healthy resting position" (see page 211).

TRAUMA

The factors underlying temporomandibular disorders already discussed—malocclusion, response to stress, postural habits—originate essentially *within* the body. One important factor comes from *outside:* mechanical injury, or trauma. In our mobile society, trauma often results from motor vehicle accidents.

Collisions cause two main types of TMJ injuries.

- Injury from a *direct blow* to the lower jaw, usually the result of a front-end or side collision.
- Indirect injury, or *whiplash,* resulting from a rear-end collision.

Injury from a Direct Blow

A direct blow to the lower jaw is likely to move it suddenly and sharply backward. The strain on the joint capsule may then produce capsulitis, and the pressure of the condyles

upon the retrodiscal tissue may cause retrodiscitis.

Such inflammations can, in turn, lead to muscle guarding, myofascial pain, and the formation of trigger points. A common symptom is a severe, recurrent headache, appearing days, weeks, or even months after the accident and seemingly unrelated to it.

Furthermore, the injury may cause bleeding in the retrodiscal tissue. After the blood clots, it may form hard, fibrous tissue in the joint, causing permanent stiffening *(ankylosis).*

Whiplash Injury

Whereas a direct blow to the jaw leaves visible signs—bruises or contusions on the skin—a whiplash injury, from a rear-end collision, may cause no visible damage. But the internal damage can be severe.

In a rear-end collision, the impact drives the car seat and the rider's body abruptly forward, but inertia tends to keep the head where it was. The head "whips" backward on the flexible column of the neck. Then, when the impact ends, inertia works in the opposite direction, and the head "lashes" forward.

Much of the damage is caused by the reactions of the neck muscles. At the moment of impact, in just a millisecond, the muscles tense to protect the head from bobbing uncontrollably. These tensed muscles are highly susceptible to strains and tears.

The same tensing also damages the TMJs. When the cranium is whipped backward, the lighter, smaller mandible is held by these tensed muscles, and the mouth is suddenly opened far wider than usual. In extreme cases, the mandible may be completely dislocated, or *luxated,* out of the joints. Usually, though, it is only partially dislocated, or *sub-luxated.* In either case, as the condyles are suddenly thrust forward, one or both articular disks may be squeezed forward and dis-

WHIPLASH INJURY

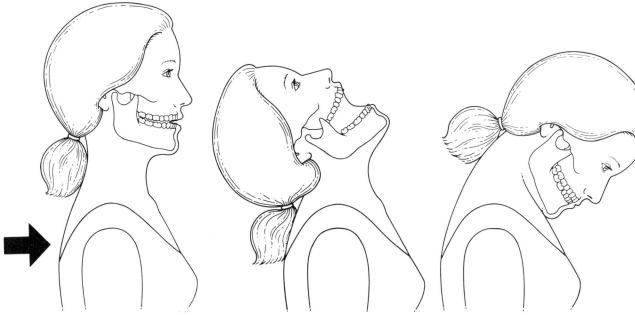

Impact forces body forward. Inertia holds head in place.

Head "whips" backward. Jaws open too wide.

Head then "lashes" forward. Jaws slam shut.

placed, and the retrodiscal tissue may be stretched or torn.

Then, when the head lashes forward, the jaw tends to close so hard that one or both condyles are rammed backward, stretching the capsule, and further damaging the retrodiscal tissue.

As with symptoms of injury from a direct blow, whiplash symptoms may be delayed in appearing, or they may be temporarily masked by other injuries.

Other Traumatic Injuries

Trauma can also result from overly wide jaw opening of any kind. This can sometimes occur during dental and medical treatment, such as the extraction of a deeply rooted "wisdom tooth," or surgery under general anesthesia (see page 56).

Trauma may also result when the jaw is forced upward and backward. This can occur during orthopedic treatment of the spine. If the head is put into *traction*, using a sling under the chin, the pressure may cause loading of the TMJs, with resulting microtrauma and inflammation.

DIAGNOSIS OF TMDS

If you have one or more of the symptoms described earlier, you may have reason to suspect a temporomandibular disorder. To obtain further evidence, you can administer some simple *palpation* tests:

- Place the first two fingertips of each hand directly in front of each ear. The TMJs are directly underneath, and you can feel them move as you open and close your mouth. If even the light pressure of the fingertips causes pain, on one or both sides, joint inflammation may be the cause.

- Place the fingertips against the lower jaw on each side of the face. As you open and close your mouth, you will feel the movement of one pair of chewing muscles, the *masseters*. If even light pressure provokes tenderness, the cause may be myofascial pain.
- Press the fingers lightly against the temples, above and in front of the ears. If opening and closing the mouth produces pain, one or both of the fan-shaped *temporalis* muscles may be fatigued and sore.

Resistance tests will also help identify fatigue and soreness of less accessible muscles inside the mouth:

- With the mouth partly open, press three fingers against the biting edges of the lower front teeth—firmly, but not hard. Then close the jaw against this resistance.
- With the jaw closed, press a fist against the chin, and open against this resistance.
- Finally, press an open palm against one side, and then the other side, of the lower jaw, and each time move the jaw sideways against this resistance.

THE TMJ EXAMINATION

If you have symptoms typical of temporomandibular disorders, and if other possible causes have been ruled out, then it is appropriate to have a special examination of the joints.

You may be referred to a TMJ practitioner by your regular dentist or physician. If you have to find one on your own, you can use the methods for finding specialists in other dental fields (see Chapter 2 and Appendix).

The first step of the examination should be a complete medical and dental history, and a history of your symptoms, including any previous examination or treatment. The examiner may ask permission to consult physicians or dentists who have treated you earlier; it is, in fact, desirable to do so.

A thorough physical examination is likely to follow. It probably won't be limited to your head and neck, but may include an evaluation of your posture and an examination of your neck, upper back, shoulders, arms, and hands. Pain or tenderness in these areas may be referred from a TMD.

A standard dental examination will be included, if it hasn't already been performed by the referring dentist. Your occlusion (bite), will be checked, and impressions may be taken of your upper and lower teeth.

The examiner will perform palpation and resistance tests, similar to those described above, to locate areas that may be stiff and sore or that may serve as trigger points for pain referred elsewhere.

The *range of motion (ROM)* of your lower jaw will be checked. For example, it should be possible to insert three fingers of the hand between the upper and lower front teeth. If four will fit, the jaw may be opening more than it should, and may become dislocated. If no more than two fingers can be inserted, the range of motion is said to be *restricted*, and normal eating is likely to be difficult.

The examiner will also look for *deviations* in jaw movement. If your mandible deviates to one side as it opens, there may be a problem in the muscles or the joint on one side.

All these procedures put additional strain on the joints and the chewing muscles. As a result, they may temporarily become more tender than before the examination.

Finally, the examiner may ask questions designed to assess the level of psychological stress in your life, especially if there is physical evidence that you clench or grind your teeth.

Imaging Techniques

The examiner may use a variety of *imaging techniques*, most of which involve X-rays, to assess the condition of the joints:

- *Transcranial and Panoramic (Panorex) X-rays* (See page 22). These show the general condition of the jawbones and teeth, to make sure that no other pathological conditions, such as cysts, tumors, or arthritic degeneration, are present.

- *Tomography*. The term means "picture of a slice." The X-ray beam is focused, somewhat the way a light camera is focused, so that only one thin layer of the subject is "sharp." Tomograms provide a clearer view of the bones; however, no information about the disk and other soft tissue can be obtained.

- *Arthrography*. This term means "picture of the joint." A liquid dye, opaque to X-rays, is injected into the capsule. On X-ray film, the dye-filled cavity appears as a well-defined light area. From the shape of this area, a specialist can deduce whether the nearby articular disk is displaced or damaged.

- *Computerized tomography*, or *CT* (formerly called a "CAT scan"). X-rays are directed sequentially in a circle all around one body part (such as the head), and the results are translated by a computer into a single, cross-sectional image. CT is sensitive enough to reveal subtle details of both bone and soft tissue.

- *Magnetic resonance imaging (MRI)*, also called *nuclear magnetic resonance (NMR)*. Like CT, this technique produces images of great sensitivity, but it does not use radiation. It is sophisticated and expensive, but its advantages make it the method of choice for assessing the condition of a disk and other soft tissues.

The Final Diagnosis

Once the examination is complete—a process that may require more than one appointment—the examiner should be able to arrive at a diagnosis and treatment plan. You should receive answers to the following questions:

- *What's the matter?* Is it a TMD, and, if so, what type?
- *What's to be done?* What course of treatment is proposed? How many steps are involved, and how long are they likely to take? What is treatment likely to cost—both in money and in time? What is likely to happen if the condition is *not* treated?
- *What can be achieved?* What is the *aim* of treatment? A complete cure? That may not be realistic or practical. Alleviation of pain? Reaching a particular level of activity or comfort? And what are the chances of success or failure?

The TMD practitioner may not be able to provide precise answers to all these questions, but you should be given at least a range of alternatives. If you have any doubts, you can (and should) obtain a second opinion.

TYPES OF TREATMENT: PHASE ONE, PHASE TWO, AND SURGERY

There are three main types of treatment for temporomandibular disorders:

- *Phase-one* treatment is primarily intended to relieve symptoms, such as pain. It may not provide permanent relief from, or recurrence of, the underlying disorder. Its procedures are *reversible*—nothing is done that can't be undone later.
- *Phase-two* treatment (see page 214) aims to provide a more definitive solution to

the underlying cause (or causes) of the problem. Its procedures are largely *irreversible.* The consequences can't be altered without great difficulty, if at all.

• *Surgery* (see page 215) is used to remedy or alleviate certain specific TMDs, such as a severely displaced disk.

There are important distinctions between these forms of treatment, in terms of priority. Under ordinary circumstances, phase-one treatment should always be tried first, at least to bring the symptoms under control. Often this is enough to provide satisfactory long-term relief, and in any event, the procedures are reversible. Phase-two treatment should only be undertaken when the acute symptoms are under control and there is evidence that its irreversible procedures will correct a specific, identifiable condition. Surgery, finally, is a solution of last resort, which will alleviate only a few specific conditions, and which should be undertaken only after phase-one treatment has failed.

PHASE-ONE TREATMENT

Many of the techniques of phase-one treatment weren't developed specifically for TMDs, but have been adapted from those used by physicians, chiropractors, osteopaths, and physical therapists to relieve muscle pain and joint inflammation in many parts of the body.

Treatment may require a team effort. A dentist serves as overall coordinator but must often rely on other specialists, such as physical therapists, for assistance.

"WALKING-CANE" THERAPIES

When you sprain an ankle, you may use a cane or crutch to avoid putting unnecessary

weight on it. In the same way, you can use some of the following techniques to avoid putting unnecessary pressure on inflamed TMJs or fatigued chewing muscles.

Limiting Movement

Avoid opening your mouth wide. Open the lower jaw only as far as is comfortable. Restrict yawning by pressing a fist under your chin.

Adopting Healthy Resting Position of the Mouth

To overcome habits of clenching and grinding, try to keep your mouth in what is called the *healthy resting position.* Open your jaws slightly, so the upper and lower teeth are separated. Rest the tongue lightly against the roof of the mouth, without pressing it against the front teeth. Keep your lips shut, and breathe through your nose. Your teeth should not make contact except when you are chewing and swallowing.

Following a Soft Diet

You don't have to switch entirely to liquids or baby food. But avoid foods like raw vegetables, nuts, hard rolls, and chewy meat such as steak.

Eliminating Caffeine

Caffeine increases muscle tension and sensitivity to nerve signals, including pain. Avoid foods containing caffeine, such as coffee, tea, cola drinks, and chocolate, until your symptoms subside.

MEDICATIONS

Since medications can have undesirable side effects and become habit-forming, they should be used only in moderation and for limited periods of time. But they can be very helpful, at least for patients who are starting a course of treatment and are in pain. Medications fall into five basic categories, several of which are discussed in more detail in Chapter 7.

Painkillers

The most familiar painkiller, or analgesic, is aspirin, but there are several others. Analgesics help relieve both myofascial pain and inflammation. Only very seldom is a narcotic, such as codeine, necessary or desirable.

Anti-inflammatory Medications

These are used mainly to relieve joint inflammation. There are two main groups: *corticosteroids* (often called *steroids*), and *nonsteroidal* anti-inflammatory drugs (commonly known as *NSAIDs*).

The NSAIDs are the more commonly used of the two groups. They must be taken regularly for periods up to three weeks before results are apparent. Their effectiveness varies widely from patient to patient, as do such side effects as an upset stomach.

In cases of severe, acute inflammation, corticosteroids may sometimes be appropriate. These are usually administered by injection, often directly into the inflamed joint. They must be used sparingly; frequent injections can lead to the destruction of joint tissue.

Local Anesthetics

The same anesthetics used in other forms of dental treatment are also used to treat TMD symptoms. They are injected to relieve muscle pain and to eliminate trigger points. They are also used in *inject-and-stretch* massage (see page 212).

Muscle Relaxants

Medications that relax tense muscles can be used to relieve myofascial pain. Examples include *methocarbamol (Robaxin)* and *orphenadrine citrate (Norgesic).*

Some *antianxietal* drugs also act as muscle relaxants. They include *diazepam* (best known as *Valium*) and *chlordiazepoxide (Librium).* They are used as sedatives in dental anesthesia, and in smaller doses, they are often effective for treating TMDs in which psychological stress is a factor. Some patients are prescribed such a drug to be taken at bedtime to reduce grinding while they sleep.

Antidepressants

These were originally developed to fight emotional depression. One of the better known is *amitriptyline (Elavil).* They are given to myofascial-pain patients in very small doses; the dose is gradually increased until the desired pain relief is obtained.

Physical Therapy

Phase-one treatment commonly includes several forms of physical therapy. Physical therapy has two main goals: the relief of pain and the restoration of function, particularly the function of movement. Reducing pain usually comes first. A wide variety of techniques are used.

Heat and Cold Therapy

Heat and cold are among the oldest remedies for pain and are still among the most effective.

They work in rather different ways. Cold tends to slow down the activities of living cells. It makes inflamed cells, such as those in the capsule of the TMJ, less hyperactive, and it helps relax muscle spasms. Cold also serves as an anesthetic, dulling pain, and is used for this purpose following many dental procedures.

Heat tends to work more indirectly. Pain, especially muscle pain, is often caused by a relative shortage of oxygen, an *oxygen debt,* in the tissue. Heat applied to the tissues dilates the blood vessels passing through them, increasing the blood flow and introducing more oxygen. As the oxygen debt is reduced, the pain diminishes.

Cold tends to be used particularly to relieve inflammation, and heat to relieve myofascial pain. But there is no fixed rule—some patients simply respond better to one or the other. They can also be used together—cold to diminish pain sensations, followed with heat to bring more oxygen to the tissues.

There are several ways to apply heat:

- A *moist compress.* This can be a towel soaked in hot water or a moist towel wrapped around a hot water bottle or a waterproof heating pad used with a dampened sponge.
- A *hydrocolator.* This is a scarflike wrapper made of soft fabric, with a pocket for a bag filled with a heat-retaining substance.
- An *ultrasound* generator. This produces high-frequency sound waves that heat soft tissue deep under the skin.
- *Electrogalvanic stimulation (EGS).* A mild electric current is passed through the tissues to produce the *effects* of heat therapy by stimulating muscle fibers to contract and increasing blood flow.

There are also several ways to apply cold:

- *Ice.* The simplest and commonest cold therapy, ice is easily applied by sealing it in a plastic bag, which is then wrapped in a damp towel.
- A commercial *cold pack.* This pack, usually of plastic, contains a cold-retaining substance. It remains flexible even after it has been chilled to a temperature below that of ice.
- A *snap-pack.* This product doesn't require chilling. Striking it on a hard surface sets off a chemical reaction that makes it cold.

Ice and other cold materials can damage your skin if they are used for too long at a time. The usual rule is no more than 20 minutes in an hour. If your skin looks unnaturally pale (*blanched*), cold therapy should be immediately discontinued.

Transcutaneous Electrical Nerve Stimulation (TENS)

Another useful tool to relieve TMD pain is *transcutaneous electrical nerve stimulation,* or *TENS.* Like ice, it is used as an analgesic following a variety of dental procedures (see page 57). TENS usually gives only temporary relief, but it requires no drugs, and sometimes works when other methods don't.

Massage

Massage is a very old therapy for relieving pain, particularly myofascial pain. Like heat, it encourages the flow of blood through tissues, and reduces oxygen debt. Massage also helps cramped, spastic muscles regain mobility.

Physical therapists often massage muscle tissues both longitudinally (along the fibers) and transversely (across the fibers). Simple massage is often combined with *contract-and-stretch* massage. A specific set of muscles is induced to contract, allowed to relax briefly, and then stretched out to full extension.

Trigger Point Therapy

Muscle trigger points refer pain to other parts of the body. Several techniques are used to locate these areas and eliminate them:

- *Stretch and spray.* The therapist sprays a highly volatile liquid, often ethyl chloride, on the skin over a set of muscles. It immediately evaporates, chilling the area and partly numbing it. The therapist then slowly stretches the muscles to full extension.
- *Anesthetic injection.* Only physicians and dentists can perform this technique. A muscle with one or more trigger points is injected with a local anesthetic. The injection, combined with muscle stretching, sometimes eliminates trigger points.
- *"Blank" injection.* For a trigger point close to the skin, a dry needle may be inserted directly into the hypersensitive area. Sometimes this counterirritation is all that's needed to eliminate it.

Exercises for Mobility

Physical therapy ordinarily includes a program of exercises to restore muscle function, or *mobility*. Mobility has two aspects: suppleness, the capacity for smooth, unobstructed movement, and strength, the capacity to do work.

In the treatment of TMDs, exercises to maintain suppleness in the head and neck muscles are especially important. Instructions for a short series of these exercises appear on the following page.

Posture Correction

Poor posture strains the muscles of the head and the neck. It is at least a contributing factor in TMDs. Physical therapists not only train patients to avoid harmful positions and activities but also to develop healthy habits of standing, sitting, and lying down.

SPLINTS

Unlike many other forms of phase-one therapy, the use of *splints* requires dental training, experience, and equipment.

A splint is usually a U-shaped piece of plastic, which fits over your teeth in either the upper or the lower jaw. Its main purpose is to keep the jaws from closing completely, which can serve at least three useful functions:

- Resting and relaxing fatigued chewing muscles.
- Discouraging the clenching and grinding of the teeth.
- Reducing the "load" on the articular disk and other soft tissues of each joint, by holding the condyles apart from the temporal bones.

Splints come in two main forms, *flat-plane* and *repositioning*.

Flat-plane Splints

A flat-plane splint is sometimes called a *bite plate*, or, if it is to be worn only at night, a *night guard*. It is constructed to conform closely to the teeth in one jaw. The biting surface is smooth and *flat*, hence the name.

The splint separates the jaws, but the flat biting surface allows you to close your lower jaw in whatever position feels comfortable. Thus, the appliance is also called a *permissive* splint.

Flat-plane splints are made in a variety of forms. Some fit over the top teeth, some over the bottom. Some cover all the teeth in the jaw, some only a few. There is no consensus on which form works best.

The very simplest splints are made of soft rubber or plastic—similar to the protective mouthpieces used in athletics. They are not recommended for patients who habitually clench or grind their teeth—a soft, yielding surface appears to encourage these habits.

Most practitioners favor hard acrylic splints. These are made in a dental laboratory, over a cast of the teeth, and then fitted and trimmed to fit snugly and comfortably.

Splint therapy can last anywhere from three to six months. At first you wear the splint all the time except when you are eating. As symptoms subside, use can taper off, until the splint is worn only at night, and then not at all. You may find that you need the splint for a longer period of time or that you must return to it from time to time.

Wearing a splint may take a while to get used to. The appliance can be quite inconspicuous visually, but at first it may feel "foreign" in your mouth. It may be difficult to speak clearly, especially if the splint is installed over your upper teeth. Usually, though, the tongue learns to adjust to its new environment within a week or so.

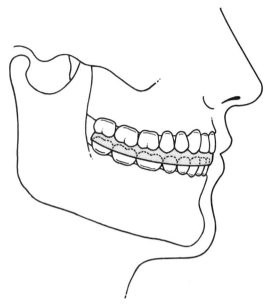

Repositioning splint, inserted between the jaws

REPOSITIONING SPLINTS

Flat-plane splints are not effective for all patients. In particular, two groups aren't likely to be helped.

The first group consists of patients with myofascial pain caused by severe malocclusion, especially patients who have lost many teeth and whose bite lacks its normal *vertical dimension*, and is *overclosed* or *collapsed* (see page 168). The second group consists of patients with severely displaced articular disks. To relieve the pressure on inflamed soft tissue, the condyles may have to be repositioned relative to the temporal bones.

For some of these patients, a *repositioning splint* may give relief. A repositioning splint, like a flat-plane splint, may be fitted over either the upper or lower teeth. But the surface facing the other teeth is not smooth. Instead, it contains shallow impressions of the opposing teeth. When the jaws close, the teeth are directed into the impressions on the splint, which specifically repositions the mandible relative to the upper jaw.

There is no universal agreement over

EXERCISES FOR THE HEAD AND NECK MUSCLES

Repeat each of the following five times.

1. Tuck in your chin sharply, hold the position two or three seconds, and relax. (This exercise helps overcome the postural fault of thrusting the head forward.)

2. With arms folded, rotate your head to the left, and your arms to the right. Hold the position for two seconds, and then rotate your head to the right and your arms to the left. Hold that position for two seconds, and relax.

3. Stretch your chin toward each shoulder, in turn, for five seconds.

4. Gently roll your head and upper neck above your shoulders, in a wide shallow oval.

where the mandible should be repositioned. But most experts agree that the condyles should be repositioned somewhat *forward* and *down* from their customary location, so they won't "load" the backs of the joints.

A repositioning splint, like a flat-plane splint, is usually worn for a period of up to six months, and its use can be tapered off as symptoms subside. But there is a major difference between the two. A repositioning splint distinctly *changes* your customary bite. Once you stop wearing it, and your bite returns to its usual position, the symptoms may return.

You may then have to choose between two alternatives. One is to wear a *permanent* repositioning splint, most of the day, for an indefinite period of time. This splint is like a standard splint but has a heavily reinforced metal framework, with stainless steel plugs at the points of greatest wear.

The other alternative is to undergo phase-two treatment, to establish the bite permanently in the new position (see below).

COPING WITH PSYCHOLOGICAL STRESS

Psychological stress may lead to habitual clenching and grinding of the teeth, which can lead to TMDs. Breaking these habits often requires learning to cope more effectively with the underlying stress, through some form of behavioral therapy.

Relaxation Exercises and Biofeedback

A main goal of behavioral therapy is teaching your body to relax, or rather teaching it new habits of relaxation. The most common techniques are the same as those used in the treatment of dental fear: *progressive relaxation* exercises and *guided imagery* (see page 47).

To reinforce these exercises, therapists also use the mechanical technique called *biofeedback.*

A biofeedback machine amplifies electrical signals produced by muscles when they contract. Thus it "feeds back" information concerning the general muscle tension of the body. Regular use of this monitoring machine leads to a greater awareness of stress, and improves your ability to relax.

PHASE-TWO TREATMENT

As mentioned earlier, phase-one treatment is intended primarily to relieve symptoms. If the underlying disorder remains, recovery may not be complete or long lasting. Phase-two treatment aims at a more definitive solution, particularly of malocclusion, which may be the cause of the problem.

What often makes phase-two treatment necessary is the use of a repositioning splint to bring forward the mandible. Once the splint has relieved your symptoms, the dentist will then attempt to "walk back" your lower jaw toward its former closing position. But this process may cause the symptoms to return. It then becomes necessary to establish an effective bite with your jaw in the *new* position.

To accomplish this goal, or to correct other types of malocclusion that may underlie a TMD, there are three main forms of phase-two treatment.

EQUILIBRATION

If the malocclusion is not severe, and if your teeth are basically sound, the dentist may be able to balance your bite by selectively grinding and smoothing the surfaces of individual teeth (see page 79).

RESTORATIVE DENTISTRY

Malocclusion, especially in older people, is often the result of worn, damaged, or missing teeth. These losses can be corrected by dental restorations, ranging from onlays to dentures (see Chapter 13).

ORTHODONTICS

If your teeth are relatively sound and your gums are healthy, the best solution for malocclusion may involve moving your teeth into better positions, by means of orthodontics (see Chapter 16).

SURGERY

There are some conditions that phase-two treatment cannot cure. For instance, some defects of the jaws are too severe to be corrected by even the most extensive restoration or orthodontics. In these instances, the only alternative may be surgery.

The three basic criteria for determining whether surgery is appropriate for a temporomandibular disorder are as follows:

- The disorder is *severe*. It is not only painful but is also greatly debilitating, and prevents you from leading a normal life.
- The disorder is *structural* rather than simply functional. It arises from observable abnormalities in or around the joint, such as a dislocated disk, osteoarthritis, or a serious mismatch in the size or shape of your jaws.
- Other treatment has *failed*, and there is no reasonable alternative.

Surgery is not a substitute for phase-one or phase-two treatment. You must often settle for something short of a complete and perfect cure. Usually, the goal is simply a measurable improvement in comfort and the ability to function.

ARTHROSCOPIC SURGERY

Increasingly, oral surgeons are using the recently developed technique of *arthroscopic* surgery as the procedure they use first in treating TMDs.

Arthroscopic surgery utilizes an *arthroscope*—an instrument that "looks into the joint." It is basically a miniature microscope, and resembles a hypodermic syringe. At the end of the "needle" is a small magnifying lens, with optical fibers that cast light into the area being viewed.

This apparatus is inserted into the joint through a cylindrical metal sheath. The sheath has such a small diameter—no more than two-and-a-half millimeters—that it can be inserted through a puncture that requires no sutures and leaves almost no scar. There is nonetheless enough room in the sheath for a salt water (saline) solution to be pumped through it, to bathe and open up the joint space.

The image can be viewed directly by the eye, but a special video camera is generally used instead. Often the image is videotaped.

The arthroscope gives a highly detailed view of joint structures. It isn't customarily used alone but rather is used to monitor surgery. A second cylindrical sheath is inserted into the joint a short distance from the first. It is used to introduce miniature surgical instruments; the surgeon then operates while watching through the arthroscope.

The technique is used mainly to clean out extraneous tissue from the joint spaces. When the disk is displaced or damaged, nearby blood vessels often rupture and bleed. When the blood clots, it forms fibrous scar-like tissues in the joint spaces. These fibrous tissues may cause *adhesions* between the disk and the temporal bone, which keep the disk from moving freely. Some experts believe that such adhesions are a major cause of restricted jaw movement, or *ankylosis*. The miniature surgical instruments are used to scrape or cut them loose, and the fragments are then flushed away with the irrigating solution.

Arthroscopic surgery is ordinarily performed in a hospital, under general anesthesia. But since the incisions are so small, and the "insult" to the joint tissues is so slight, recovery is relatively fast and easy. Ordinarily, no stitches are required, and the small punctures are covered with a bandage until they heal.

Complications after surgery seldom occur, though there are minor risks in any procedure involving general anesthesia (see page 56). As in all surgery on the jaws, there is a slight danger of damaging one of the facial nerves, which cause at least temporary numbness or loss of muscle control. In addition, there is the chance that the needle-like end of the arthroscope or one of the fine surgical instruments will break off in the joint, hit a blood vessel, or even perforate the inside of the joint and enter the cavity of the skull. The patient must agree in advance to let the surgeon proceed immediately to *open-joint* surgery (see below) to treat any such complications should they arise.

Because the instruments and working space are so small, arthroscopic surgery is usually limited to clearing away superfluous fibrous tissue and adhesions. For some patients, this procedure is sufficient to restore mobility and relieve pain. For others, however, the results may be unsatisfactory or temporary. More extensive, open-joint surgery may be advisable. Even then, the "advance look" and the videotape record provided by the arthroscope allow the surgeon to plan the operation with much greater precision than would otherwise be possible.

OPEN-JOINT SURGERY: DISK PLICATION

If the articular disk is "dislocated" in front of the condyle (see page 203), it may be necessary to open up the joint surgically to gain access to it. The disk is then pulled back and sutured in its correct position. The procedure is called *disk plication*, which means a "binding of the disk."

Disk plication is major oral surgery, performed in a hospital under general anesthesia. To enter the joint, the surgeon makes an L-shaped incision in front of the ear. The modest size and placement of the incision make the resulting scar all but invisible.

The surgeon then opens the capsule of ligaments surrounding the joint. If the bone surfaces of the condyle or the eminence have become worn or roughened, they may be filed smooth, and if bony spurs *(osteophytes)* have formed, they may be removed. Some surgeons file off part of the temporal bone so that there is more space between it and the condyle.

Sometimes the articular disk has become *perforated*—torn open or worn through. A perforation can sometimes be repaired by sewing it shut, but some surgeons prefer to remove a perforated disk entirely, replacing it

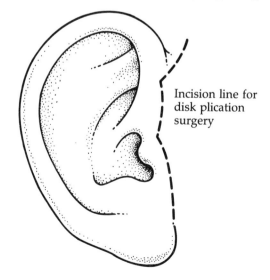

Incision line for disk plication surgery

with a piece of pliable plastic. But such substitutes have a poor record for long-term durability.

If the disk can be salvaged, it is pulled back over the condyle and sutured in place. If the retrodiscal tissue has been stretched, some of it may be removed, and the tissue is sutured to the disk. Extraneous fibrous tissues and adhesions are removed from the joint spaces.

Recovery after disk plication is similar to that from other oral surgery (see page 163). An important part of postoperative treatment is physical therapy, to minimize the formation of scar tissue and adhesions. You may also be fitted with a splint (page 212), to avoid "loading" the joint while it heals.

For from 10 to 20 percent of all patients, disk plication doesn't produce satisfactory results. The range of movement of the lower jaw may not be significantly improved. Some patients experience temporary relief from pain, since cutting through the small nerve endings in the capsule numbs the joint for a while. But the pain may return when the nerves regenerate. And if the disk must be removed, no artificial replacement is likely to be permanent.

Possible complications of disk-plication surgery include the slight but real risks in any operation involving general anesthesia, as well as damage to one of the facial nerves.

ORTHOGNATHIC SURGERY

Some basic defects in the bones of the jaws call for more drastic treatment: *orthognathic*, or "jaw-correcting" surgery (see page 159). Four such conditions are particularly associated with TMDs:

- The mandible is too large, relative to the upper jaw, and juts forward beyond it. This condition doesn't necessarily cause a temporomandibular disorder. However, some patients themselves, and

some dentists or orthodontists as well, try to force the lower jaw backward into a normal bite. The condyles may then press against the back of the joints and "load" them, which results in retrodiscitis or disk displacement.

- The mandible is too small, relative to the upper jaw. The visual effect is a receded, "weak" chin. Sometimes the upper teeth close entirely over those in the mandible, producing an overclosed or collapsed bite. The condyles may then "load" the tops of the points, which again results in retrodiscitis or disk displacement.

- The bones of the upper jaw grow downward to such an extent that *long face syndrome* results. The mandible is shifted to a less efficient position, and the chewing muscles may become fatigued, which results in myofascial pain.

- The bones on one side of the jaw are larger (or smaller) than those on the other side, producing *asymmetry*. The face may look lopsided, and the mandible may slide sideways as it opens. The muscles are unbalanced, resulting in myofascial pain.

COSTS AND BENEFITS OF TMD TREATMENT

Treatment for TMDs is expensive. It requires the skills of highly trained professionals—often a team of them—working over an extended period. And the procedures and materials involved are themselves expensive. The cost of tomograms, MRI, and other sophisticated diagnostic procedures is several times that of ordinary dental X-rays. The cost of a splint is comparable to that of a denture or a bridge.

If you seek to reduce the financial burden, there are a few alternatives. Perhaps the best, if it is available, is a clinic at a university dental school or teaching hospital (see page 242). Or treatment may be available through a health-maintenance organization (HMO), but many such programs specifically exclude treatment for TMDs.

Coverage under either medical or dental insurance is at present uncertain. Some policies exclude payment for such treatment altogether, or attach so many conditions and exceptions that it is virtually impossible to make a successful claim. In recent years, the principle that phase-one treatment should be covered by medical insurance, and phase-two treatment by dental insurance has won growing acceptance. But if you plan to have a TMD treated and expect your insurance to pay for it, you should check your policy carefully to see whether you have coverage. For further information about insurance see page 235.

The high cost of treatment must be measured against potential benefits. The most important benefit, for most patients, is relief from pain—the chronic, often severe pain that is the most prevalent symptom of temporomandibular disorders. It usually doesn't subside on its own, and can get worse if not treated.

Structural disorders, such as disk dislocation, can also get worse if not treated, and they may lead to problems such as disk perforation or osteoarthritis. Early treatment of TMDs is likely to be less costly and less drastic than the treatment of more severe problems later on.

NINETEEN

THE "MEDICALLY COMPROMISED" PATIENT: MEDICAL CONDITIONS THAT AFFECT DENTAL TREATMENT

The dental treatments discussed in this book are most often performed upon people who are healthy and unimpaired. But not everyone is. Many people have medical conditions that can affect their dental treatment. These conditions may require the dentist to take special precautions, adopt special procedures, or even avoid certain forms of treatment altogether.

This is one reason why your dentist must keep your medical history complete and up to date. You should alert the dentist to any health problems you may have and any medical treatment you may be receiving. In particular, you should inform the dentist about any changes in your health or any new medical treatment since your last visit. And you should permit—indeed, encourage—your dentist to consult and collaborate with your physicians in your treatment.

Some of the more common conditions that require special dental care are described here.

DISORDERS OF THE HEART AND BLOOD VESSELS

Disorders of the heart and its related blood vessels include a wide array of conditions, of which the following are especially common:

- Defects of heart structure, congenital or acquired.
- Obstruction (*atherosclerosis*) or hardening (*arteriosclerosis*) of the coronary arteries.
- Ballooning enlargements (*aneurysms*) of artery walls.
- Disorders of heart function such as *congestive heart failure* and irregular heartbeat (*arrhythmia*).

Virtually all these disorders pose problems and potential risks that require special attention by the dentist.

RISK OF INFECTION

Your mouth is full of bacteria and other microorganisms, and there is no way of making it completely sterile. During and after dental treatment, the risk of contamination cannot be eliminated. Moreover, conditions such as deep tooth decay and advanced periodontal disease are likely to be accompanied by a proliferation of bacteria, and produce a higher risk of infection.

When infective organisms invade one part of your body, they may be carried into other parts through the bloodstream, to cause *systemic* infection. Ordinarily, your body's own defenses, supplemented by antibiotics, should be enough to prevent systemic infection or to minimize its consequences. But if you suffer from a disease of the heart or blood vessels, the risk of infection rises.

Conditions that roughen or deform the inner surfaces of the heart and related blood vessels, for example, provide places for bacteria to lodge and multiply. Chief among these are defects of the heart valves, which can be congenital or the result of diseases such as rheumatic fever. Surgery on the heart or blood vessels also produces rough tissue surfaces, at least temporarily. Bacteria growing on these surfaces may cause an inflammation of the heart lining called *infective endocarditis*, which further damages the heart valves, and raises the risk of heart failure.

You also run a much larger risk of infection if you have received a heart transplant. To prevent rejection of the replacement heart, your normal immune system is suppressed with drugs, which makes infection far more likely.

If you are at special risk for infection, your dentist is likely to prescribe a special regimen of antibiotics. You will be given several relatively large doses, *before* as well as after treatment.

After surgery, the dentist may adjust the *timing* of your treatment. Except in emergencies, procedures such as tooth extraction, root canal therapy, and gum surgery should be delayed for several months.

Home care is also important in reducing the risk of infection. You cannot completely eliminate bacteria and other microorganisms from your mouth, but you can reduce the risk of invasion by way of decayed teeth or diseased gums, by brushing and flossing regularly and thoroughly.

You should be especially careful to use a soft toothbrush, to avoid injuring the gums. Similarly, you should floss gently between the teeth, especially near the gumline. If you use a mechanical irrigator, it should be set at low power, so as not to drive bacteria or viruses into the gums. If you wear a removable denture, you should clean it daily, and unless advised otherwise by the dentist, you should remove it periodically from your mouth.

DISORDERS AGGRAVATED BY STRESS

Dental treatment inevitably causes stress, both physical and psychological, which may aggravate existing disorders of the heart and blood vessels, or cause dangerous symptoms to appear.

For example, a natural and virtually universal response to stress is an increase in the production of *adrenaline*, which causes your heart to beat faster, and to pump more blood through its chambers. Adrenaline also constricts the blood vessels, which raises your blood pressure. The sudden rise in heartbeat and blood pressure can increase the risk of heart attack if you suffer from atherosclerosis or congestive heart failure. And if you have *hypertension* (high blood pressure), the additional rise also raises the risks of stroke or the rupture of an *aneurysm* (a thin-walled, weakened ballooning of an artery wall).

To avoid these problems, your dentist may

take special precautions to reduce the inevitable stress of treatment. Treatment may be scheduled over several short appointments, rather than a few extended ones. Stressful forms of treatment may be postponed following a heart attack, or until hypertension can be brought under control. The dentist may also make special efforts to reduce the psychological component of stress, using techniques of relaxation training and desensitization before treatment, and sedatives during treatment (see pages 46 and 52).

A common ingredient of the local anesthetics used in dentistry is a synthetic form of adrenaline, *epinephrine*. In the past, there has been concern that such use might contribute to high blood pressure or other heart disorders. It is now generally believed that the amount of epinephrine in local anesthetics is too small to be harmful. However, if you have a heart disorder, your dentist should consult with your physician before using any formulation containing epinephrine.

RISK OF FAINTING

If you have a heart or a blood-vessel disorder, you may be especially susceptible to *orthostatic hypotension*—a tendency toward fainting (*syncope*) when standing or sitting up suddenly (see page 55). The cause is not so likely to be the disorder itself, but rather medications you may be taking for it (see table, pages 231–233). There are a few simple techniques the dentist can use to help you avoid fainting after getting up from the chair.

Perhaps the simplest thing you can do is remain in the chair for a "recovery period" after treatment, and then get up slowly. If you feel giddy or faint, the dentist may place you temporarily in the *Trandelenberg position*: lying down, with the feet raised slightly higher than the head. The dentist may also administer pure oxygen or use spirits of ammonia ("smelling salts") to stimulate respiration.

RISK OF PROLONGED BLEEDING

If you have a disorder such as atherosclerosis, or are recovering from heart surgery, you may be taking an *anticoagulant* medication, which keeps dangerous blood clots from forming in the heart or blood vessels. However, such a medication may also contribute to prolonged and excessive bleeding after dental treatment (see below).

INTERFERENCE WITH PACEMAKERS

To correct an irregular heartbeat (*arrhythmia*), you may have had a temporary or permanent electronic pacemaker installed.

Electrical currents or electromagnetic fields can damage a pacemaker or interfere with its performance. Such interference may be produced by unshielded electrical appliances, including certain dental equipment. These include the Cavitron machine used for cleaning teeth and TENS devices used to relieve muscle pain. If you have a pacemaker, your dentist should turn such machines off, and use alternative equipment.

BLEEDING DISORDERS

Blood cells called *platelets* or *thrombocytes* are produced in the bone marrow and are essential to blood clotting. Bleeding disorders may reduce the number of platelets or interfere with their function. As a result, wounds or bruises tend to bleed excessively, and to heal slowly. Since even routine dental treatment may cause bleeding, your dentist must take special precautions if you suffer from any of these disorders.

THROMBOCYTOPENIA

Thrombocytopenia means, literally, a "shortage of thrombocytes." The bone marrow produces too few platelets for effective clotting. *Primary* thrombocytopenia is thought to be a hereditary *autoimmune* disease (see page 259). More common is acquired, or *secondary* thrombocytopenia, which has a wide range of causes, including the following:

- *Leukemia.* Cancer of the blood (see page 273).
- *Multiple myeloma.* Cancer of the bone marrow (see page 280).
- *Aplastic anemia.* This form of anemia is often a consequence of radiation therapy and chemotherapy used to treat cancer (see page 272).
- *Polycythemia.* The bone marrow produces too many red blood cells, compared to other blood cells (see page 272).
- *Bacterial* and *viral* infections, and the drugs (such as antibiotics) used to treat them.
- *Surgery* or *trauma* causing significant loss of blood and requiring multiple transfusions.

HEMOPHILIA

This hereditary disease cannot be cured, but excessive bleeding can be controlled with injections of replacement clotting factor (see page 272).

LIVER DISEASE

Most of the clotting factors necessary for coagulation are produced in the liver. Liver disease such as *hepatitis* and *cirrhosis* can disrupt this process (see page 224).

DISORDERS TREATED WITH ASPIRIN

A side effect of aspirin is the disruption of platelet production. If you suffer from an inflammatory disease such as rheumatoid arthritis, you may be taking aspirin routinely and in large doses, and you may bleed excessively.

DISORDERS TREATED WITH ANTICOAGULANTS

If you have undergone surgery, are recovering from stroke, or require kidney dialysis routinely, you are likely to be given *anticoagulant* medications, such as *dicumarol, heparin,* and *warfarin,* to prevent the formation of dangerous clots inside the blood vessels. But a side effect of these medications is a tendency toward prolonged and excessive bleeding.

If you suffer from any of the above bleeding disorders, your dentist should work closely with your physician, to coordinate dental procedures with medical treatment of the disorder. The lack of clotting factor caused by hemophilia, for example, can be at least temporarily remedied with injections of replacement factor. So if you have hemophilia, your dentist should check with your physician to determine whether you should receive replacement factor before such treatments as tooth extraction or other oral surgery.

If you have thrombocytopenia from an infection or medication, your dentist should try to postpone treatment until the underlying problem is brought under control. If, however, you are scheduled for radiation therapy or chemotherapy, any needed dental treatment should be completed first if possible (see also pages 223 and 228).

Some types of thrombocytopenia can be temporarily alleviated with transfusions, either of whole blood or of platelets. Medications such as *aminocaproic acid* can stimulate clotting, and *vasopressors* such as *Desmopressin* can help reduce bleeding. Doses of anticoagulant drugs can be temporarily reduced, or the drugs can be discontinued for a short period, before dental treatment.

Several bleeding disorders also pose a high risk of bacterial infection, which itself requires special precautions (see below).

There are also techniques the dentist can use to prevent or control bleeding during treatment. For example, the dentist will avoid certain areas of the mouth when injecting local anesthetics, to minimize the risk of nicking a blood vessel.

To control bleeding from wounds inevitably caused in treatment, the dentist may apply the clotting agent *thrombin*, or a gelatin sponge (*Gelfoam*), to encourage at least local clotting of blood. The socket of an extracted tooth may be packed with *microfibrillar collagen* (*Avitene*), to form a temporary artificial clot. The dentist may also construct a soft plastic splint, rather like an athletic mouthguard, to fit over the jaw from which teeth have been extracted. This helps control bleeding by exerting pressure on the soft tissues and by protecting the wound.

Since aspirin has anticoagulant activity, the dentist will prescribe some other analgesic (such as acetominophen) to reduce discomfort following treatment.

By planning in advance and by taking precautions, most patients with bleeding problems can be treated in the dental office. If you have a severe disorder such as hemophilia, however, you may have to be hospitalized for even minor procedures that might cause bleeding.

OTHER BLOOD DISORDERS

Disorders of the blood may affect the red blood cells, the white blood cells, or both. Their main impact upon dental treatment is increased susceptibility to infection (see page 220).

ANEMIA

Anemia is a general term for several disorders involving the red blood cells. Either the number of red cells is reduced or their active ingredient, *hemoglobin*, is abnormal. In either case, the ability of the blood to carry oxygen is diminished. Common forms include the following:

- *Iron deficiency anemia, folic acid deficiency anemia*, and *vitamin B$_{12}$ deficiency anemia* (*pernicious anemia*) (see page 269).
- *Sickle cell anemia* and *thalassemia*. Hereditary diseases, caused by defective forms of hemoglobin.
- *Aplastic anemia* (see page 222).
- Anemia caused by *chronic renal failure* (see page 224).

In addition to delayed wound healing and the higher risk of infection, anemia also poses problems with inhaled anesthetics, since the ability of the blood to carry oxygen is impaired. If general anesthesia is required, the patient should be hospitalized, and ordinarily nitrous oxide should not be used.

WHITE BLOOD CELL DISORDERS

Various kinds of white blood cells (*leukocytes*) comprise the body's chief defense against infection. Hence, diseases that affect white blood cells greatly raise the risk of infection following dental procedures. Among the most prevalent disorders are leukemia (see page 273) and *leukopenia*.

The most common form of leukopenia is called *neutropenia* or *agranulocytosis*. One cause is an adverse reaction to a wide range of medications, including those used in chemotherapy for cancer. Thus, dental procedures that carry the risk of infection should usually be scheduled either well before or well after chemotherapy. Indeed, if a patient is to undergo chemotherapy, a complete dental examination should be performed beforehand, to identify and treat existing oral infections, or conditions such as tooth decay.

LUNG DISORDERS

Diseases of the lungs, such as *tuberculosis, emphysema, lung cancer,* and the hereditary disorder *cystic fibrosis,* significantly affect breathing and the body's ability to obtain enough oxygen.

If dental treatment requires general anesthesia, patients suffering from lung disorders should probably be hospitalized. Sedative medications that affect breathing, such as barbiturates and narcotics, must be used with great caution, or avoided altogether. Rubber dams must also be used with care, to make sure that they don't obstruct the breathing passages. Finally, if you have a lung disorder, you may find that you breathe with less difficulty if seated upright rather than lying down.

LIVER DISORDERS

The most common diseases of the liver are *cirrhosis,* usually resulting from alcoholism, and the various forms of *viral hepatitis.* Hepatitis is extremely infectious, and requires the dentist to take special antiseptic precautions (see page 226).

Otherwise, the dentist must be mainly concerned over the use of certain medications, which are processed in the liver. These include local anesthetics, many analgesics, sedatives such as Valium and the barbiturates, and the antibiotics ampicillin, erythromycin, and tetracycline. Sometimes substitutions can be made, but often the best solution is simply to reduce the dosage as much as possible.

KIDNEY DISEASE

Kidney disease, of which the most prevalent form is *chronic renal failure,* adversely affects the dental patient several ways:

- It may cause anemia. The kidneys produce a hormone that stimulates the formation of red blood cells in the bone marrow. Kidney disease may disrupt this process.
- It may lead to excessive bleeding, from the use of anticoagulant medication (see page 222) if you are undergoing dialysis. Thus, you shouldn't have dental treatment on the same day you undergo dialysis.
- The risk of infection is greatly increased if you have received a kidney transplant, since you must take immunodepressant drugs to prevent your body from rejecting the transplant.
- It can lead to problems with medications that are normally excreted by the kidneys. These include most analgesics, and certain antibiotics. These should be avoided, or used only in small doses.

PEPTIC ULCERS

Peptic ulcers are accompanied by the overproduction of hydrochloric acid in the stomach, which is in turn intensified by stress. Acid analgesics such as aspirin should be avoided or used in low doses. The dentist should also try to reduce the level of psychological stress during treatment (see page 220).

ENDOCRINE GLAND DISORDERS

DIABETES

Diabetes, in either its hereditary or acquired form, lowers the body's resistance to infection, and slows the healing of wounds. It can, however, be kept under control through diet or insulin administration or both. Before beginning treatment, therefore, the dentist may request a test of blood sugar to see whether the diabetes is under control, and may use antibiotics and other measures to minimize the risk of infection.

ADRENAL INSUFFICIENCY

The outer, or *cortical*, layers of the adrenal glands produce *steroid* hormones involved in the function of many body organs. Adrenal insufficiency—the failure of the glands to produce enough corticosteroids—may be *primary* or *secondary*.

Primary insufficiency, known as *Addison's disease*, is far less common than secondary insufficiency, which is usually caused by the administration of *synthetic* corticosteroids, which are widely used to treat inflammatory diseases such as rheumatoid arthritis (see below).

One effect of adrenal insufficiency is to suppress the body's immune system, which increases the risk of infection. It is often advisable to *increase* the amount of corticosteroid medications just before dental treatment, to replace the hormones that the adrenal glands would normally produce. The dentist may also try to minimize psychological stress during treatment (see page 220).

HYPERTHYROIDISM

Hyperactive thyroid glands produce excessive thyroid hormones, which, in turn, overstimulate several body functions. If not treated and controlled, hyperthyroidism can cause a life-threatening *thyroid storm* under the stress of dental treatment.

Symptoms include high fever, racing and irregular heartbeat, severe weakness, and mental confusion. Emergency treatment, with hospitalization, is required.

HYPOTHYROIDISM (MYXEDEMA)

If the thyroid fails to produce enough thyroid hormone—a condition called *hypothyroidism* or *myxedema*—many body processes are slowed. Usually this disorder can be controlled with synthetic thyroid hormones. It is sometimes advisable, however, for the dentist to avoid the use of sedatives that in themselves slow down body processes, such as barbiturates, narcotics, and tranquilizers.

INFLAMMATORY DISEASES OF THE JOINTS

The principal diseases causing inflammation of the joints are *rheumatoid arthritis* and *osteoarthritis*. Others include *multiple sclerosis*, *polymyositis*, and *sarcoidosis*. Sometimes joint diseases affect the temporomandibular joints, limiting the range of motion of the jaws. But the chief problems they create for dental treatment arise from the side effects of the drugs used to treat them. Among the most common of these are the following:

- *Aspirin.* The most widely used analgesic for arthritic pain. Taken in large doses, it can lead to bleeding disorders.
- *Phenylbutazone.* A powerful nonsteroidal anti-inflammatory drug (*NSAID*). Occasionally it will disrupt the bone marrow's production of red blood cells, to produce *aplastic anemia* (see page 222).
- *Corticosteroids.* Synthetic adrenal hormones, widely used to reduce inflammation. They diminish natural adrenocortical function, greatly increasing the risk of infection. It is often advisable to alter the usual dosage of these

medications shortly before dental treatment (see above).

ARTIFICIAL JOINTS

Joints badly damaged by rheumatoid arthritis or osteoarthritis are often surgically replaced with artificial joints of metal or plastic. A disadvantage of such artificial joints is the susceptibility of adjacent tissues to bacterial infection. Since such infection can result from oral surgery or other dental treatment, prophylactic antibiotics are indicated (see page 275).

SKIN DISEASES

Diseases that can cause skin inflammation, such as *erythema multiforme* and *lupus erythematosus*, are ordinarily treated with corticosteroids; such treatment raises the risk of infection following dental treatment.

Severe, systemic lupus erythematosus may also be accompanied by a reduction in blood *platelets*, causing a bleeding disorder.

BACTERIAL AND VIRAL INFECTIONS

Recent concern over the possible spread of the AIDS virus by dental treatment has led to increased awareness of the dangers of infection and the need for precautions by medical and dental practitioners. But the problem is not a new one. Many diseases caused by bacteria and viruses are far more infectious than AIDS—doctors can readily catch them from their patients, and can, in turn, transmit them to other patients. The diseases that are especially significant to dental treatment include *infectious mononucleosis*, various types of *hepa-*

titis, and sexually transmitted diseases such as *syphilis* and *gonorrhea*.

Of these, probably the most insidious is hepatitis. Patients who have recovered from the symptoms may remain *carriers* of the virus, and they can easily transmit it to others. In rare instances, people exposed to the virus may become carriers without exhibiting any symptoms at all. For these reasons, you should be careful to inform your dentist if you have had hepatitis, or have been exposed to it since your last visit.

To prevent the spread of infection, dentists are increasingly using the following precautionary measures:

- Disposable latex gloves.
- Face masks and eye protection.
- Single-use needles and syringes, and special containers for their disposal.

ACQUIRED IMMUNE DEFICIENCY SYNDROME

Much of the concern over infection during medical and dental treatment has been provoked by the recent appearance and the spread of the HIV virus that causes AIDS. This virus is, in fact, far less robust, and harder to transmit, than many others. But its effects are so devastating that it has led to the widespread adoption of precautions such as those listed above.

In treating patients with AIDS and AIDS-related complex (ARC), these precautionary measures do indeed hinder transmission of the virus. But they are far more important in preventing the spread of other infections—viral, bacterial, and fungal—from dentists to patients who lack immune protection.

ALLERGIES

An allergy is a hypersensitivity toward specific substances that enter the body. These substances, called *allergens* or *antigens*, provoke the body's immune system to react as it would to an infection. A variety of symptoms result, such as headaches, skin eruptions (*eczema* and *hives*), localized swellings (*angioedema*), asthmatic attacks, and hay fever. In rare instances, an allergic reaction may produce *anaphylactic shock*, a dangerous condition in which blood pressure drops too low to maintain body functions, and which requires immediate emergency treatment.

Allergies affect dental treatment in two principal ways:

- Medication, anesthetics, and other dental material may act as allergens for some patients.
- Severe allergic reactions, such as angioedema of the throat or anaphylactic shock, may cause an emergency during treatment.

It is very important to tell the dentist any allergies you have, especially if adverse reactions have occurred previously during treatment. But be precise in describing your symptoms. Not all adverse reactions are true *allergic* reactions. Stomach upset from aspirin or other anti-inflammatory drugs, for example, is not. Your dentist will adopt different strategies depending on the nature of your problem. And if there is any doubt whether you are allergic to specific substances, your dentist may recommend testing by an allergist.

ALLERGIES TO MEDICATIONS AND ANESTHETICS

Allergies to medications are uncommon; allergies to anesthetics even rarer. The medication most likely to produce an allergic reaction is penicillin. If you are allergic to penicillin, and an antibiotic is needed to prevent or treat infection, your dentist can usually substitute some other form (such as erythromycin).

Similarly, if a particular local anesthetic has provoked an allergic reaction (such as angioedema) in the past, the dentist can usually offer a substitute.

CONTACT STOMATITIS

Some people are allergic to specific metal alloys, plastics, or other materials used in dental treatment. Prolonged contact with these materials may inflame the mouth's soft tissues (*contact stomatitis*). Once such material is identified as an allergen, the dentist can usually use something else in its place.

The material most often implicated in contact stomatitis is the acrylic plastic used for dentures and other prosthetic devices. The problem is most likely to arise if the plastic has not been allowed to cure thoroughly before it is inserted into the mouth. Unevaporated solvents may pass from the plastic to the soft tissues, and cause a reaction.

ASTHMA

The main symptoms of an asthmatic attack include a narrowing and thickening of the airway passages, and an increased production of mucus. The patient experiences "air hunger," and in extreme instances may be in danger of asphyxiation.

If you suffer from asthma, your dentist will take precautions to avoid precipitating an attack during treatment. In particular, since attacks are often triggered by stress, the dentist will use techniques designed to keep stress and anxiety to a minimum (see page 220). Sedative drugs that depress the central nervous system, such as morphine, should be avoided. You will be advised to bring with you any medications you may be taking to avoid or control attacks.

Also, since asthma impairs breathing capacity, the dentist will follow the same guidelines used in treating patients with lung diseases (see page 224).

ALLERGIC REACTION EMERGENCIES

On rare occasions, despite your dentist's precautions, you may experience a severe allergic reaction during dental treatment. An asthmatic attack or angioedema of the tongue or throat may be extensive enough to threaten asphyxiation. Anaphylactic shock may lead to loss of consciousness, breathing difficulties, irregular heartbeat, and death.

If such a situation arises, your dentist should be prepared to take emergency measures. First, you are placed in a supine position, and pure oxygen is administered. To control the allergic reaction, you may be given medications such as antihistamines, corticosteroids, or epinephrine (a synthetic form of adrenaline). Sometimes cardiopulmonary resuscitation (CPR) is necessary, and you will be transferred to a hospital.

ORAL CANCER

If you have cancer of the mouth, you will require special dental treatment, not so much because of the disease itself but rather because of the side effects of the therapy—particularly radiation and chemotherapy (see page 273). They greatly reduce your body's defenses against infection, and so make necessary the use of antibiotics and other special measures.

Infection following irradiation of the mouth can lead to *osteomyelitis*, in which the bone tissue of the jaw is attacked and destroyed. To reduce this risk, it is important for the dentist to restore your teeth and treat your gums thoroughly before radiation ther-

apy. Sometimes it is advisable to extract diseased teeth, rather than to try to save them.

It is also important for your dentist to work closely with your physician and general surgeon when surgery is necessary to remove cancerous tissue from the jaws. Possible disfigurement and disruption of function can often be minimized with dental prostheses or orthognathic surgery.

MOTOR NERVE DISORDERS

A number of disorders involving the motor nerves cause special problems in dental care, mainly because of the loss of muscle control. The most common of these disorders are *cerebrovascular accident* (*CVA, stroke*) and *Parkinson's disease*. Others include *muscular dystrophy, cerebral palsy, amyotrophic lateral sclerosis, peripheral neuropathy, Bell's palsy, tardive dyskinesia,* and *senile tremors*.

If you suffer from any of these disorders, your dentist will try to avoid unnecessary stress during treatment (see page 220), and will use sedatives sparingly. Sometimes special equipment can be used to help support you in the dental chair or to maintain you in an immobile position. There is equipment available to facilitate your transfer from a wheelchair or stretcher to the dental chair, and there are even attachments that make it possible for the dentist to treat you while you remain seated in a wheelchair. If you are subject to severe tremors or other involuntary movements, you may have to receive most dental treatment under sedation or general anesthesia.

Involuntary jaw movements may damage your natural teeth, or may cause you to bite your cheeks, lips, or tongue. The dentist may fabricate a plastic *splint*—rather like an athletic mouth guard—that you can wear at night to hold the teeth slightly apart.

Inability to control movements also makes the retention of dentures and other prosthetic devices more difficult. Such appliances should be examined frequently and refitted promptly if they work loose. Sometimes it is possible to add clasps and other devices that will give a denture greater stability, or *implants* (see Chapter 14) can be used to provide a firmer foundation for the appliance.

A major problem arising out of neurological impairment is the difficulty, or even impossibility, of self-care. Sometimes a toothbrush can be made easier to manage by enlarging or extending its handle (see page 110). An electric toothbrush and mechanical irrigator may also be helpful. Floss can be placed in a floss holder for easier manipulation, especially with one hand. Often, however, the most effective solution is for someone else to take over the duties of brushing and flossing.

If anything, home care becomes even more important under these conditions. Many of the medications used to treat neurological disorders tend to cause mouth dryness, or *xerostomia*, which in turn can lead to increased tooth decay and periodontal disease.

EPILEPSY

Epilepsy may or may not be accompanied by neurological impairment. The chief problem for the dentist is to avoid provoking a seizure during treatment. Precautions will be taken to minimize stress (see page 220). Sedatives may also be useful in inducing relaxation beforehand. Any procedure requiring general anesthesia should be performed in a hospital.

If an attack should occur during treatment, most dentists are trained to manage it, and to know when special help is needed.

The dentist may also collaborate with the physician in trying to avoid or control the *gingival dysplasia* (overgrowth of the gums) that

is often produced by anticonvulsant drugs such as phenytoin (see page 271). Scrupulous home care and office care appear to help prevent this condition. Changing the medication or lowering the dose is also sometimes effective, but surgery is sometimes necessary.

MENTAL IMPAIRMENT

Due to congenital mental retardation, or to Alzheimer's disease or other forms of senile dementia, patients may be mentally impaired. These conditions make both home and office dental care more difficult, and neglect of dental health more likely.

Patients with severe mental impairment cannot be expected to attend to their own dental health. Others must brush and floss for them. Special efforts must be made to avoid the loss of dentures and other removable appliances. Dental office visits must be kept short and as free of stress as possible. It must be emphasized, however, that maintaining dental health is as important for mentally impaired patients as for anyone else, and deserves the continuing attention of those responsible for their care.

ALCOHOLISM

Excessive use of alcohol has many harmful effects on health, some of which have an impact on dental treatment. They include the following:

- Liver damage and disease (see page 224).
- Bleeding disorders, resulting from damage to both the liver and the bone marrow (see page 221).
- Reduced resistance to infection.
- Increased likelihood of tooth decay and

periodontal disease, as a result of poor oral hygiene and mouth dryness (*xerostomia*).

- A higher risk of oral cancer (see page 228).

In addition, alcohol can interact harmfully with several medications commonly used in dental treatment. These include the following:

- Sedatives, such as barbiturates and tranquilizers. Alcohol intensifies their depressant effect on the nervous system. During treatment, there is a higher risk of deep sedation and unconsciousness. Following treatment, the ability to drive may be impaired.
- Medications used to control high blood pressure (such as *guanethidine*) and angina (such as *nitroglycerin*). These dilate the blood vessels, an effect intensified by alcohol. The result is a higher likelihood of *orthostatic hypotension* and fainting (see page 221).
- Aspirin. This widely used analgesic may disrupt platelet formation and cause excessive bleeding. Alcohol intensifies the effect.

- Narcotic analgesics, such as codeine. Like sedatives, these intensify depression of the central nervous system.

NARCOTIC ABUSE

Narcotic abusers require special dental treatment for two reasons. First, the abuser is more likely to be a carrier of bacterial or viral disease. Second, narcotics used for pain relief may interact harmfully with the drugs being abused.

The most serious form of narcotic abuse is the intravenous injection of heroin. The chief danger to health comes from the injection process itself. Unsterilized, shared needles greatly increase the risk of transmitting infections such as hepatitis and AIDS. The dentist must take special care to avoid such infection (see page 226).

Analgesics containing narcotics, such as codeine, should be avoided by present or recovering narcotics abusers. The addition of prescription drugs to the illegal drugs taken by a present user can produce a dangerous overdose. Taken by a recovering abuser, prescription narcotics can renew cravings for the drugs or lead to withdrawal symptoms.

DRUGS WITH SIDE EFFECTS THAT AFFECT DENTAL TREATMENT OR DENTAL HEALTH

DRUGS THAT CAUSE OR CONTRIBUTE TO MOUTH DRYNESS (*XEROSTOMIA*)

Amphetamines and related compounds: (detroamphetimine (Bimetamphetamine, Dexedrine); methamphetamine (Desoxyn); phentermine (Fastin, Ionamin).

Analgesics (used to relieve pain): aspirin; acetaminophen (Tylenol); meperidine (Demerol); propoxyphene (Darvon).

Antianginals (used to relieve causes or symptoms of angina pectoris): diltiazem (Cardizem); erythritil tetranitrate (Cardilate); nifedipine (Procardia); nitroglycerin.

Antianxiety medications: See *Minor tranquilizers*, below.

Antiarrhythmics (used to control irregular heartbeat): disopyramide (Norpace); lidocaine (Xylocaine); procainamide (Procan, Pronestyl); quinidine (Cardioquin, Quinaglute, Quinidex, Quinoral); verapamil (Calan, Isoptin).

Anticancer drugs (antineoplastics, cytotoxics): See *Drugs that contribute to infection by candida albicans* below.

Anticonvulsants (used to prevent epileptic seizures, and to treat stroke): phenytoin (Dilantin); carbamazepine (Tegretol); ethosuximide (Zarontin).

Antidepressants (used to alleviate mental depression): amitryptiline (Elavil, Limbritol, Triavil); amoxapine (Asendin); desiparmine (Norpramin, Pertofrane); doxepin (Sinequin); imipramine (Tofranil); loxapine (Loxitane); matrotiline (Ludiomil); trazodone (Desyrel).

Antiemetics (used to counteract dizziness, nausea, and vomiting; some *antihistamines*, *antispasmodics*, and *major tranquilizers*, see below, are used for the same purpose): diphenidol (Vontrol); domperidone; droperidol (Inapsine); dronabinol (Marinol); metoclopramide (Reglan); trimethobenzamide (Tigan).

Antihistamines (used mainly to reduce allergic reactions and inflammations; also used as *antiemetics*, see above, and *minor tranquilizers*, see below): azatadine (Optimine); brompheniramine (Dimetane); buclizine (bucladin-S); chlorpheniramine (Chlor-Trimeton, Teldrin, Contac); clemastin (Tavist); cyclizine (Marezine); dimenhydrinate (Dramamine); diphenhydramine (Benadryl); hydroxyzine (Atarax, Vistaril); meclizine (Antivert, Bonine); promethazine (Phenergan); terfenadine (Seldane); trimeprazine (Temaril); triprolidine (Actidil, Myidil, Actifed).

Antihypertensives (drugs that reduce blood pressure by decreasing stimulation of the heart by the nervous system; many *diuretics*, see below, are used for the same purpose): atenolol (Tenormin); captopril (Capoten); clonidine (Catapres); enalapril (Vasotec); guanabenz (Wytensin); hydrazaline (Apresoline); methyldopa (Aldomet); prazosin (Minipress); metropolol (Lopressor); nabetolol (Normodyne, Trandate); nadolol (Corgard); pindolol (Visken); propranolol (Inderal); reserpine (Serpesil).

Anti-Parkinsonian drugs (used to control the tremors and rigidity of Parkinson's disease): benztropine (Cogentin); biperiden (Akineton); ethopropazine (Parsidol); levodopa (Dopar, Larodopa, Sinemet); procyclidine (Kemadrin); trihexiphenydil (Artane).

Antispasmodics (relax smooth muscles, such as those in digestive tract; used to treat diar-

Continued on next page

rhea and irritable bowel syndrome, and sometimes as *antiemetics* for motion sickness, see above): belladonna; dicyclomine (Bentyl); isopropamide (Darbid); hyoscyamine and scopolamine (Donnatal); propantheline (Pro-Banthine).

Bronchodilators (used in treatment of asthma, to widen air passages in lungs): atropine; epinephrine (Primatene); isoproterenol (Isuprel); ipratropium (Atrovert).

Decongestants (used to relieve colds, allergies, and other respiratory inflammations; often contain *antihistamines*, see above): oxymetazoline (Afrin, Dristan); phenylephrine (Neo-Synephrin); pseudoephedrine (Sudafed, Actifed); xylometazoline (Neo-Synephrine II, Otrivin).

Diuretics (stimulate excretion of fluids from body; used to relieve *edema*—swelling of tissues from excess fluids—and to reduce hypertension): amiloride (Midamor); chlorothiazide (Diuril); chlorthalidone (Hygroton, Thalitone, Regroton); furosemide (Lasix); hydrochlorothiazide (Esidrix, Hydrodiuril, Hydromal, Oretic, Thiuretic); metolazone (Diulo, Zaroxolyn); polythiazide (Minizide); spirolactone (Alatone, Aldactone); triamterene (Dyrenium, Dyazide).

Major tranquilizers (antipsychotics, neuroleptics) (used to control psychotic disorders and mental confusion; lower concentrations are also used as *antiemetics*, see above): chlorpromazine (Thorazine); Haloperidol (Haldol); Flufenazine (Prolixin); prochlorperazine (Compazine); perphenazine (Trilafon); promazine (Sparine); thioridazine (Mellaril); thiothixene (Navane); trifluoperazine (Stelazine).

Minor tranquilizers (antianxiety medications) (act upon the area of the brain that controls emotions; used to relieve anxiety, diminish pain, and relax spastic muscles; some forms are also used as sleeping medications: alprazolam (Xanax); chlordiazepoxide (Librax, Librium, Limbitrol); clorazepate (Tranxene); diazepam (Valium); flurazepam (Dalmane); lorazepam (Ativan); meprobamate (Equanil); oxazepam (Serax).

Muscle relaxants (relax fatigued and spastic muscles; used to relieve muscular pain): chlorzoxazone (Paraflex); cyclobenzaprine (Flexeril); orphenadrine (Norflex, Norgesic).

DRUGS THAT CAUSE OR CONTRIBUTE TO GAGGING OR OTHER SWALLOWING DISORDERS (*DYSPHAGIA*)

Antispasmodics: See drugs that cause or contribute to mouth dryness, above.

Major tranquilizers (antipsychotics): See drugs that cause or contribute to mouth dryness, above.

DRUGS THAT INDUCE FAINTNESS UPON STANDING UP, AS AFTER DENTAL TREATMENT (*ORTHOSTATIC HYPOTENSION*)

Antianginal drugs: See drugs that cause or contribute to mouth dryness, above.

Antihypertensives: See drugs that cause or contribute to mouth dryness, above.

Diuretics: See drugs that cause or contribute to mouth dryness, above.

Major tranquilizers (antipsychotics): See drugs that cause or contribute to mouth dryness, above.

Minor tranquilizers: See drugs that cause or contribute to mouth dryness, above.

Narcotics: (opium derivatives, used as anesthetics during dental procedures and as analgesics afterward): codeine; meperidine (Demerol); morphine.

DRUGS THAT CONTRIBUTE TO INFECTION BY *CANDIDA ALBICANS* (*CANDIDIASIS*, OR *ORAL THRUSH*)

Antibiotics (used to fight bacterial infections): aminoglycoside; cephalosporin; metronidazole; penicillin; sulfonamide; tetracycline.

Anticancer drugs (antineoplastics, cytotoxics). (used in chemotherapy to kill cancer cells or to prevent their growth): alkylating agents (Chlorambucil, *cis*-Platin); cyclophosphamide (Melphalan); antimetabolites (Fluorouracil, Mercaptopurine, Methotrexate); cytotoxic antibiotic (doxorubicin).

Corticosteroids (used to treat inflammatory disorders of many kinds; reduce resistance to all forms of infection): beclomethasone (Beclovent, Vancenase, Vanceril); betamethasone (Alphatrex, Diprolene, Diprosone, Lotrisone); cortisone (Cortone); dexamethasone (Decaderm, Decadron, Dexone, Hexadrol); fluocinolone (Fluonid, Synalar, Synemol); hydrocortisone (Cortaid, Hytone); methylprednisolone (Medrol); prednisolone (Prelone, Metimyd); prednisone (Deltasone, Steropred); triamcinolone (Aristocort, Kenalog, Tynex).

Immunosuppressants (used to counteract autoimmune reactions and transplant rejections; anticancer drugs, see above, are also used for this purpose): antilymphocyte globulin; azathioprine; cyclosporin.

DRUGS THAT CAN LEAD TO BLEEDING PROBLEMS DURING SURGERY OR PERIODONTAL TREATMENT

Analgesics: Aspirin.

Anticoagulants (medications that reduce blood clotting; used in the treatment of strokes, and heart disease): heparin; warfarin (Coumadin); dicumarol; dipyridamole (Persantine).

DRUGS THAT CAUSE OR CONTRIBUTE TO GUM SWELLING (*GINGIVAL HYPERPLASIA*)

Anticonvulsant: phenytoin (Dilantin).
Anti-arrhythmic: nifedipene (Procardia).

DRUGS THAT CAUSE OR CONTRIBUTE TO *BROWN HAIRY TONGUE*

Antibiotics: See above.

DRUGS THAT CAUSE OR CONTRIBUTE TO *TASTE LOSS* OR *ALTERED TASTE SENSATIONS*

Antidepressants: See above.
Antihistamines: See above.
Antibiotics: D-penicillamine; tetracycline. Thiamine, Methimazole, Lithium.

TWENTY

THE ECONOMICS OF DENTAL CARE

Regular professional dental care is cost-effective, but it isn't cheap. It is cost-effective because its basic procedures are *preventive*—they help you avoid more expensive treatment later on, saving money in the long run. For example, the costs of office visits for examination and cleaning, even over several years, are likely to total less than the cost of extensive prosthetic dentistry. Moreover, the value of retaining your natural teeth and keeping them functional and presentable goes beyond what can be measured in dollars and cents.

At the same time, the costs of regular treatment do add up. You cannot assure your dental health with home care alone, however conscientious you may be. Office visits at least twice a year are also necessary. And the cost of these visits takes into account your dentist's extensive professional training, and the necessity of maintaining an able staff, up-to-date equipment, and an office that is reasonably accessible to you and other patients.

The costs are significantly higher for complex, specialized treatment. It is impossible to list precisely and in detail what these costs are likely to be—there is simply too much variation among them, not only in different parts of the country, but also within the same area. Suffice it to say that wherever you live, the costs of dental treatment are likely to be comparable to the costs of similar levels of medical treatment.

YOUR RIGHT TO KNOW

Whatever you pay for dental treatment, it is in your interest to know, *in advance*, approximately what the costs will be. It may not be possible for a dentist to give you a precise estimate—emergencies and other contingencies cannot always be predicted. Nonetheless, the dentist should be able to tell you the customary charges for specific services and procedures, and to provide you with at least a *range* of possible costs for a specific course of treatment.

You have a right to this information. Many dentists will provide it without your asking—

but you shouldn't hesitate to ask. Neither should you hesitate to consult more than one dentist, especially if you may need expensive, sophisticated procedures. You will have to pay a consultation fee to each practitioner you visit, but the cost of these fees is likely to be low compared to the complete cost of treatment.

Moreover, you shouldn't hesitate to inquire about *alternative* forms of treatment. As is explained in the earlier chapters of this book, dental treatment often requires making choices among different possible procedures, and these choices involve many factors—cost among them.

If you do consult more than one dentist, however, be careful not to compare "apples with oranges." Don't simply ask for cost estimates, but make sure you understand the complete *treatment plans* on which they are based. The costs of treating a specific condition may vary widely, according to the techniques and materials used, and the basic goal of treatment. For example, a silver amalgam filling is far less expensive than a metal and porcelain crown, but for the restoration of a severely decayed tooth, a crown may be a more reliable and long-lasting solution.

HOW TO COMPLAIN

If you are dissatisfied with the dental treatment you have received, or dispute the charges for it, there are ways of seeking redress. First, you should discuss the matter directly with your dentist, in the hope of arriving at a mutually agreeable solution.

If you reach no settlement, you can file a complaint with your state or local dental society, which may have a *peer-review panel* examine your case. The panel may decide that the treatment and charges are appropriate, or that you are entitled to receive a refund for any payment you have made. You will not,

however, be awarded any *compensatory damages* for harm done to you by treatment, or to make up for any pain or inconvenience you may have suffered. Neither will you be awarded *punitive damages*, to deter the dentist from similar behavior in future. To recover such damages, you must bring a lawsuit.

In some states, you can also file a complaint with the department responsible for licensing dentists. The function of the licensing department in such a dispute is essentially disciplinary. That is, it may determine either that your complaint is not justified, or that the dentist should be disciplined, by sanctions ranging from formal rebuke to suspension of the license to practice. You will not receive either compensatory or punitive damages.

DENTAL INSURANCE

Most people nowadays have some form of medical insurance. Many have dental insurance as well, and their number is growing rapidly. Almost all dental insurance is supplied through *group plans* provided by employers, by labor unions, or by other organizations or institutions. Such sponsors may contract for a group plan from an insurance company or a *dental service corporation* (such as Delta Dental Plan), to which premiums are paid. Some employers and organizations "self-insure"—finance and administer their own plans.

Group plans usually provide insurance coverage only to subscribing members and their immediate families (spouses and children). A few cover *all* dental costs. Far more limit coverage in some respects. Also, most group plans are *contributory*—they require at least partial contribution by their members, at least for advanced services.

Few insurers offer *individual policies*. Even when available, such policies are expensive, and tend to contain many exclusions and limitations (see page 238).

Because most dental insurance is provided by employers or other institutions, you may not have much choice concerning the particular plan available to you. Nonetheless, you *are* likely to be given a choice whether to become a subscriber, especially if you must bear at least part of the cost. Moreover, some plans offer members "cafeteria-style" choices among coverage and benefit options. In any event, you should be familiar with the basic elements of your plan and know how it compares with other kinds.

REIMBURSEMENT PLANS

Insurance plans are of two basic types: *reimbursement plans* and *service plans* (see page 238). Some plans combine features of both.

Reimbursement plans are the more common of the two. Sometimes called *indemnity* or *fee for service* plans, they provide payments for specific dental procedures. To qualify for reimbursement, either you or your dentist submits a *claim*, often on a special form, which specifies the treatment received and the charge for the service.

The reimbursement payment is made either to you or to the dentist. It is made directly to you if you have paid for the service. It is made directly to the dentist if the dentist has *accepted assignment*—has agreed to accept as full payment the amount assigned by the plan. It must be pointed out that no dentist is obliged to accept assignment without a prior agreement to do so. Thus, the total charge by your dentist may be greater than the assigned amount.

Closed Panels, Open Panels, and Preferred Providers

Some plans will make payments only to members of a *closed panel*—dentists who are specifically affiliated with the plan. Usually these will be practitioners who have agreed to accept assignment. Other plans will reimburse claims from an unlimited *open panel*—that is, from any practitioner—but payments may not cover the total charges, and you'll have to make up the difference.

Preferred provider plans give you a choice. On the one hand, you can receive treatment from one of their preferred providers—dentists affiliated with the plan. The service will be provided either at no cost or at a substantial discount. On the other hand, you may choose a practitioner who is not affiliated with the plan. You will be reimbursed at least in part for the cost of treatment, but the level of reimbursement is likely to be considerably lower, and your share higher, than if you went to a preferred provider.

Scheduled versus Non-scheduled Plans

The benefits paid under reimbursement plans may be *scheduled* or *non-scheduled*. Scheduled benefits are fixed, uniform payments for specific procedures, such as routine examination and cleaning, filling a cavity, root canal therapy, tooth extraction, or inserting a crown or bridge.

Non-scheduled benefits are not fixed, but are instead based on "usual, customary, and reasonable" charges. That is, they represent an average of the charges made by dentists working in your area.

Some *combination* plans offer both scheduled and non-scheduled benefits. Often, the benefits for routine preventive treatment are non-scheduled, to encourage subscribers to take maximum advantage of them. Benefits for advanced procedures, by contrast, are scheduled, to place a limit on their cost.

As noted there is no guarantee that either scheduled or non-scheduled payments will fully cover what your dentist will charge for a particular procedure. This is one of the reasons that you should discuss the cost of treatment fully and frankly beforehand.

Deductibles

Some reimbursement plans require the deduction of a fixed amount from the total payments made within any given year. This is intended not so much to reduce the cost of benefits as to control the administrative cost of managing small claims.

If a deductible is required, the amount is likely to be modest. Most dental insurance plans are designed to encourage routine preventive care, so they are not likely to require a substantial deductible that might keep subscribers from obtaining such care.

Maximums: Annual and Lifetime

Most reimbursement plans have an *annual maximum*—a maximum benefit that will be paid for all treatment within a given year. There may be a maximum for each family member, or for all family members collectively, or both.

If a member of your family requires expensive treatment that will push you over the annual maximum, your dentist may be able to "pace" treatment—alter the schedule so that treatment extends over more than one year. It is unethical and dishonest, however, for a dentist to put false treatment dates on a claim in order to avoid the annual limit. Similarly, a dentist must not alter a treatment schedule in ways that would harm a patient's health.

Some plans have a *lifetime plan maximum* as well. This limit may apply only to certain procedures, such as orthodontics (see page 239).

Percentage Limits, Copayments, and Incentives

Plans that offer non-scheduled benefits may reimburse only a percentage of the cost for certain procedures, rather than the total "usual, customary, and reasonable" charge. Under some plans, only a fixed percentage (such as 80 percent) is reimbursed for *any*

charge. The other 20 percent is a *copayment* that must be made by the subscriber.

It is not uncommon, however, for the costs of routine, preventive care to be paid in full, and for advanced procedures to be partially reimbursed. The aim is to encourage preventive care, so as to avoid more expensive treatment made necessary by neglect. *Elective* procedures (see pages 238 and 239) are especially subject to percentage limits.

Some plans use a sliding scale of percentages to provide an *incentive* for preventive care. For example, the standard limit might be 80 percent, and would apply to all claims during your first year as a subscriber. The second year, the limit might rise to 90 percent, if your claims demonstrated that you and your family received regular preventive treatment. If you and your family do not receive such treatment, however, the percentage for the following year might drop to 70 percent.

Coinsurance

You may not be the only member of your family covered by a reimbursement plan. Your spouse or other family member may also be covered, under some other plan. You may then be able to take advantage of *coinsurance*. For any specific claim, or for all claims, one member may be established as the *primary* subscriber, whose plan is mainly responsible for payments. But claims may also be made under the plan of the other family member, the *secondary* subscriber. Payments under the secondary plan may be enough to cover deductibles, percentage limits, or other costs not covered under the primary plan.

Termination of Employment and Family Limitations

Most reimbursement plans are group plans provided by employers to employees, present and retired. If your employment terminates before retirement, you will no longer be a member of the group or its plan. The plan may accept claims for a brief period after termination, but then your coverage will end.

Current federal law, however, allows you to extend your coverage at the same group rate. A former employee is entitled to extended coverage for up to 18 months, as long as the premiums continue to be paid. The surviving spouse (widow or widower) of a deceased employee is entitled to coverage for up to 36 months.

Group plans ordinarily cover not only the individual subscriber, but members of the immediate family—spouses and children. Not covered, however, are children above a certain age (anywhere from 18 to 23), or children who are no longer dependents.

Divorced spouses are not covered, and neither are stepchildren, unless they are entirely the dependents of the subscriber. No other adults are covered, even if they are dependents.

SERVICE PLANS

Service plans differ from reimbursement plans in one central respect: they provide actual dental *care*, instead of money to cover the *cost* of care. In return for a fixed periodic fee (monthly, quarterly, annual, or the like), the subscriber receives at least basic professional care without further cost, plus substantial discounts for advanced procedures. Technically speaking, service plans do not provide insurance but rather treatment that is paid for in advance. For this reason, they are often known as *prepaid care* plans.

The main limitation to a service plan is that you do not have a completely free choice of dentists. You must accept treatment from a *closed panel*—the dentists participating in the plan. Some plans operate their own clinics, staffed with dentists they employ. Others have contracts with individual dentists, or

with an *individual practice association* of dentists. You can then choose from among these *affiliated* dentists, and you will be treated in the dentists' own offices.

Service plans, like reimbursement plans, may be provided by employers to employees. But in some areas, such plans are available to individuals as well. Some of these plans are known as *group practice* plans. That is, a group of dentists, often including specialists as well as general practitioners, will affiliate to offer a plan to subscribing individuals and their families.

Among the major providers of dental service plans are the nonprofit health-insurance corporations Blue Cross and Blue Shield. Increasingly active in this field are *health maintenance organizations* (*HMOs*), which provide subscribers with comprehensive health services. In many communities, there are HMOs available to individuals as well as to groups.

Many dental service plans, especially those associated with HMOs, are *capitation* plans. The affiliated dentists are not paid for specific office visits or procedures. Instead, they are paid a fixed amount *per capita* for each subscriber. It then becomes the dentist's responsibility to provide care as economically as possible.

EXCLUSIONS

Very few plans, whether reimbursement or service, provide complete coverage for all dental treatment. Some make outright *exclusions* of particular kinds of procedures. Especially likely to be excluded are *elective* procedures, which may significantly improve appearance and function, but which are not absolutely essential to health.

Just about universal is the exclusion of purely *aesthetic* treatment—treatment that has no other purpose than to improve appearance. However, even though some dental procedures are indeed simply aesthetic (see Chapter 17) most have functional benefits as well, and will not be excluded on this ground.

Several plans now exclude surgical *implants* (see Chapter 14). As these procedures become more common, and their benefits more apparent, coverage for them is likely to become more widely available.

Some plans completely exclude coverage for orthodontics, temporomandibular disorder therapy, or treatment of what are called *pre-existing conditions*. More commonly, however, coverage for these procedures is merely limited, rather than excluded outright (see below).

Dentists may find it necessary to charge patients who fail to keep appointments. Such charges are always excluded from coverage.

PRE-EXISTING CONDITIONS

Dental insurance, like medical insurance, is basically intended to reduce *risk*—the risk of incurring high expenses for treatment. A group plan reduces the risk to individual members by spreading it out among all members. But if you have a condition that already needs treatment when you join a plan—a *pre-existing* condition—the cost is not a potential risk, but a virtual certainty. For this reason, some insurance plans exclude coverage for treatment of pre-existing conditions such as missing teeth.

If such coverage is not excluded, it may be limited. For example, your *eligibility* may be controlled. For example, when you first become employed, you may not be eligible to join your employer's plan for several months. Or the plan may cover only preventive care and minor restorations for the first year, and may then gradually extend coverage to pay for advanced procedures in succeeding years. Another, related limitation applies to prosthetic devices (crowns, bridges, and dentures) that break, wear out, get lost, or

otherwise need replacement. Many plans refuse to pay for replacing an appliance that is less than five years old, on the ground that it is essentially defective, and should be replaced by the dentist without additional charge.

This policy can be unfair, since the need for replacement may be caused by changes in the mouth or by an accident—both beyond the dentist's control. If your plan has such a limitation, a letter from your dentist explaining why the replacement is necessary may persuade the plan administrators to accept the claim.

If an appliance needs replacement because you have lost it, however, your claim will almost certainly be denied.

TEMPOROMANDIBULAR DISORDERS

Disorders of the temporomandibular joints are treated by dentists, but their symptoms are primarily medical—facial pain and limitation of jaw movement, in particular. Moreover, an understanding of these disorders is still evolving, and treatment procedures have not yet become standardized. As a result of these ambiguities and uncertainties, many insurance plans are reluctant to provide coverage.

In recent years, the situation has been clarified to some extent. Many insurers now define *phase-one* TMD treatment (see page 209) as *medical* treatment, and extend coverage under medical insurance. *Phase-two* procedures (see page 214) are defined as *dental*, and can be covered by dental insurance. But this distinction doesn't end all controversy. Some plans still specifically exclude these disorders from coverage.

Therefore, if you need treatment for a TMD, and are a member of a dental or medical plan, you would be well advised to consult the benefits manager of your employer or union, or a representative of the insurance company or service organization that administers the plan, to determine whether you are covered, and if so, to what extent.

ORTHODONTICS

Most conditions that require orthodontic treatment are congenital or arise in early childhood—they are almost certain to be regarded as pre-existing conditions for insurance purposes. Moreover, orthodontic treatment is usually *elective*—it can greatly improve tooth function and appearance, but is not absolutely essential to health. Hence, orthodontics, when not completely excluded from coverage, is likely to be subject to several special limitations.

- Coverage may extend only up to a certain age—19 years, for example. As orthodontics for adults becomes more common, this limitation may eventually be liberalized.
- You may have to choose the orthodontist from a closed panel of practitioners who have agreed to accept assignment.
- Reimbursement for orthodontic treatment may be at a lower percent of total charges than for other dental treatment, and your co-payment may be higher.
- There may be an annual maximum or a lifetime maximum (or both) on benefits paid for orthodontic treatment.
- The course of treatment may have to receive *preauthorization* (see below). In particular, your dentist may have to demonstrate that the proposed treatment is needed to improve function, and not just to improve appearance.

All these considerations make it advisable for you to consult with your benefits manager or an insurance company representative before proceeding with orthodontic treatment.

Orthodontic treatment is likely to extend over more than one year, and to be paid for in installments. Thus, if your membership in a group plan ends while a family member is still in treatment, you may not be covered for the remaining charges. If you enter another plan, however, it may extend coverage for a case in progress.

PREAUTHORIZATION

Many plans require that advanced dental treatment be *preauthorized*. That is, your dentist must submit a treatment proposal, including estimated costs, for approval in advance. Sometimes the dentist must simply fill out an insurance form, or provide a *narrative report*—a written description of the diagnosis and plan for treatment. Some plans require that the dentist submit photographs, x-rays, and models as well. A few insist on having proposed patients examined by their own professional consultants, at least if the treatment will be extensive and costly.

DISPUTED CLAIMS

In rare instances, insurers may *dispute* a claim for payment of dental costs—they may seek to deny the claim or to reduce it, or they may ask for further corroboration. Your dentist may have to provide an additional narrative report with details of your history, diagnosis, and course of treatment. In addition, you may have to undergo an examination by the insurer's professional consultants.

If your claim is not resolved to your satisfaction, you can appeal the decision to the claims supervisor of your plan. In many states, you may also have the right to file a complaint with the state insurance department, and to have the dispute settled by arbitration. Otherwise, if the claim is substantial, you may seek legal counsel and sue the insurer.

However, the best way to avoid disputes and possible disappointment is to discuss the costs of treatment *in advance* with your dentist, and with either the benefits manager of your plan, or a representative of the insurance company that administers the plan.

WORKERS' COMPENSATION AND LIABILITY INSURANCE

The cost of dental treatment may occasionally be covered by other kinds of insurance, rather than a dental plan. For instance, if you require dental treatment as a result of injury from an accident, you may be covered by *workers' compensation* or *liability insurance.*

In virtually every state, workers' compensation insurance covers on-the-job injuries of most employees. It is financed by compulsory contributions from employers, and is administered by the state. Most programs make scheduled payments for various kinds of injuries. Benefits vary widely from state to state, along with limitations and other special conditions.

If you are injured as a result of someone else's negligence, you may be able to recover the costs of treatment from liability insurance. Most injuries result from vehicular accidents, and almost all states require vehicle owners to carry liability insurance. In addition, an increasing number of states have *no-fault* laws, under which specific responsibility for an accident doesn't have to be established.

If you need dental treatment as the result of a vehicular accident, you will submit your claim to the insurer of the other vehicle, or, in a no-fault state, to your own insurer. Some of the same limitations may apply as for dental insurance. Some no-fault states make only scheduled rather than non-scheduled pay-

ments. If you are seeking reimbursement for treatment, the insurer may require a detailed report from your dentist, and sometimes an examination by its own consultants as well. In particular, the insurer will insist on proof that the injury resulted directly from the accident, and not from a pre-existing condition.

If your claim is substantial, you may nonetheless need to consult a lawyer to protect your interests, and you may even have to bring suit. This is especially likely if you are seeking to recover not only treatment costs but also damages for pain or disability resulting from the accident.

MEDICAL INSURANCE

The cost of a few kinds of dental treatment may be covered by a *major medical* insurance policy. For example, phase-one treatment of temporomandibular disorders may be categorized as basically medical in nature. But the procedures most likely to be covered are those of *major* oral surgery upon the jaws—extraction of impacted teeth, for example, or the removal of a cyst or tumor.

MEDICARE AND MEDICAID

Medicare rarely covers the costs of dental treatment. The only exceptions are procedures to correct *dental* conditions that make *medical* conditions worse.

For those who qualify, Medicaid does cover dental treatment. However, care is subject to tight limitations, such as preauthorization for any but routine procedures. Even more important, Medicaid reimbursements are scheduled, and the payments are so low that some practitioners will not accept them.

INSURANCE FRAUD

A few dentists are guilty of submitting false or inflated claims for insurance reimbursement. This is a criminal offense, and you shouldn't acquiesce in it. If you are aware that a claim contains visits you didn't make or procedures you didn't receive, you should report the matter first of all to the dentist, in case the overbilling is accidental. But if the claim is not corrected, or if such "mistakes" occur repeatedly, you have a duty to report the problem to the administrators of your plan. Insurance fraud doesn't just hurt the insurance company or your employer, it hurts *you*.

REDUCING TREATMENT COSTS: TEACHING CLINICS

If the cost of dental treatment—particularly advanced procedures such as orthodontics—will cause you financial hardship, you may be able to obtain treatment through a *teaching clinic*, affiliated with a university dental school or a medical center.

Treatment is provided by dental residents, or by dentists engaged in postgraduate training, under the supervision of experienced professionals. Many such clinics provide a wide range of services, from endodontics to oral surgery. Quality of treatment is likely to be high, and the cost is usually well under the prevailing rates in the area.

Clinic patients may have to sacrifice any one-to-one relationship with a particular practitioner. They must fit their own schedule to that of the clinic, which may be open only at certain hours on certain days. And they must allow time for waiting—waiting for an appointment, waiting to be treated, even waiting to make payments to the clinic cashier.

Also, clinics are mainly concerned with teaching. They select those cases that will best serve that function. So you may apply for clinic treatment and not be accepted.

OTHER ALTERNATIVES FOR LOW-COST TREATMENT

Some people qualify for free or low-cost dental treatment. Members of the armed forces and some federal workers can be treated in federal hospitals. Veterans can obtain dental as well as medical treatment through the VA health system. Employees of universities or medical centers may enjoy reduced rates if their institutions have dental schools or departments. Students at such universities may qualify as well.

DENTAL FRAUD

Dental fraud is fortunately uncommon. If you follow the procedures for choosing a dentist outlined in Chapter 2, you are not likely to encounter it. You should, however, be cautious of any dentist who proposes unorthodox treatment—techniques that are not generally accepted as safe and effective.

Perhaps the easiest and best way to protect yourself is to seek second opinions from other professionals before you undertake any extensive or costly course of treatment. But you should also be wary of practitioners who make the following kinds of claims:

- Their techniques are "special" or "secret," and not available from others.
- Their treatment will provide a much quicker, easier, or less painful cure than established methods.
- The reason that their methods have not been generally accepted is that the "den-

tal establishment" is prejudiced against them, or "out to get them."

- The success of their treatment is "proved" by enthusiastic testimonials from grateful patients.

At present, there are two particular types of therapy that are considered so questionable as to border on fraud: the replacement of amalgam fillings that contain mercury, and special nutritional programs.

REPLACEMENT OF AMALGAM FILLINGS

Mercury is a poison, and in large enough concentrations can do serious harm to the body. In recent years, there have been claims that the mercury in the silver amalgam used for fillings vaporizes and leaks into the system. Some dentists advocate removing all amalgam fillings, and replacing them with composites, gold, or porcelain.

No evidence exists, however, that any significant intake of mercury from fillings takes place, or that any harm to human beings results. A very few patients have a demonstrable allergy to mercury, but the allergic reaction should appear right after the insertion of amalgam, and not after the material has fully hardened. The American Dental Association takes the position that the removal of functional amalgam fillings is ordinarily unnecessary and unwarranted. Moreover, the replacement of fillings has several disadvantages, in addition to the expense of the procedure:

- Removal of a filling inevitably requires enlarging the cavity. The tooth may then require root canal therapy or an artificial crown.
- At present, composites are far less durable and long-lasting than amalgam.
- Gold or porcelain inlays require extensive reshaping of cavities, and are extremely expensive.

SPECIAL NUTRITION THERAPIES

Except in relatively rare instances of allergy to specific substances and of specific deficiency diseases, there is little or no evidence that anything but a normal, balanced diet is needed for oral health. Special diets and massive vitamin supplements have no known value. At best, they are a waste of your money. At worst, they can do you harm. Beware of any dentist who prescribes them.

PART IV

ORAL PATHOLOGY

T W E N T Y - O N E

Disorders of the Teeth, Mouth, and Jaws

Dentistry largely concentrates upon four types of disorder: tooth decay, periodontal disease, traumatic injury, and malfunction of the bite. All these have been discussed extensively in earlier chapters. In addition, however, many other disorders of the mouth are diagnosed or treated by dentists. The study and treatment of these is called *oral pathology*, and the most common of them are described here. For ease of reference, the chapter is divided into three sections: disorders of the teeth, disorders of the soft tissues of the mouth, and disorders of the bones of the jaws.

Many of these conditions will be described as hereditary or congenital. The two terms are often used interchangeably, but they have different meanings. A *hereditary* condition is one that is inherited, genetically, from parents. A *congenital* condition is one that is present at birth. It may be hereditary, but it may, instead, have come about during prenatal development, or during the process of birth.

DISORDERS OF THE TEETH

IRREGULARITIES OF TOOTH SHAPE

Dilaceration. A sharp bend or kink sometimes occurs along the length of the crown or root. The condition is believed to result from pressure, injury, or other trauma that occurred during development, which caused the partly formed crown to be displaced relative to the less developed root. The twisted root of a dilacerated tooth may make root canal therapy or extraction more difficult. Otherwise, the condition is ordinarily harmless.

Fusion. During development, two adjacent teeth may become fused to form a single unit. The condition occurs in both primary and permanent teeth, and the cause is unknown. The fused single unit tends to be narrower than the separate teeth would have been. The irregularity may be unsightly; it may also lead to orthodontic problems. There is also a greater than usual risk of decay along the line of fusion. Otherwise, the condition is harmless.

Gemination. The term comes from a word meaning "twin." During development, the crown of a single tooth may divide partly or completely into twins, over a single root. The condition occurs in both primary and permanent teeth. The cause is unknown. The geminated tooth tends to be wider than normal, and thus may be unsightly or may cause orthodontic problems. Otherwise, the condition is harmless.

Microdontia. The term comes from words meaning "small teeth," and describes a condition in which some or all the teeth are smaller than normal.

Generalized microdontia, involving all or most of the teeth, is rare. It may accompany certain hereditary conditions such as *Down syndrome.* (see pages 269 and 275).

Abnormally small individual teeth occur frequently. Especially common are narrow, pointed lateral incisors, often called "peg laterals" (see page 192). Small individual teeth

may be unsightly, or may cause orthodontic problems. Otherwise, they are harmless.

Anhidrotic ectodermal dysplasia. In this hereditary condition the number of developing teeth is reduced (see page 248), and the teeth that do erupt are malformed. The crowns are small, cone-shaped, and ineffectual for chewing.

Congenital syphilis. A woman infected with syphilis may pass on the disease to her developing fetus. The results may be miscarriage, stillbirth, or birth defects—including defects of the teeth.

Only the permanent incisors and first molars are affected. Some or all of the incisors may be shaped like the blades of screwdrivers—thin from front to back, and tapered on the sides from neck to biting edge. In addition, the biting edges may be notched at the center.

The affected first molars do not have normal cusps. Instead, their biting surfaces are covered with numerous small bumps—a condition called *mulberry molars.*

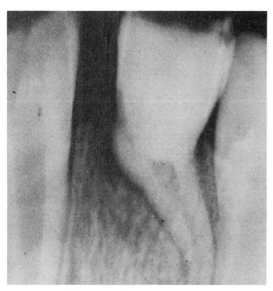

Dilacerated tooth
Radiograph by Jeffrey Leeds

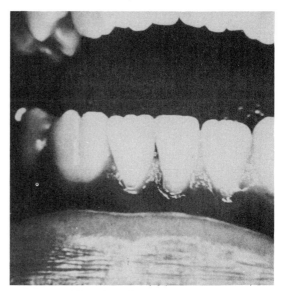

Fused teeth
Photograph by Jeffrey Leeds

These defects are unsightly, and may cause orthodontic problems. Otherwise, the teeth are functional.

Congenital syphilis can be prevented with penicillin or other antibiotics, administered to the mother at any time up to the fourth month of pregnancy.

Syphilis can also cause a variety of mouth sores (see page 254).

IRREGULARITIES IN THE NUMBER OF TEETH

Supernumerary teeth. Extra teeth, beyond the normal number, occur more often among permanent teeth than among primary teeth. The most common of all is a small supernumerary incisor called a *mesiodens* ("middle tooth") that occurs between the upper central incisors.

In some cases, the tendency to produce supernumerary teeth appears to be inherited. Supernumerary teeth are also associated with two hereditary conditions: *cleidocranial dysostosis* and *Gardner's syndrome* (see page 279).

Supernumerary teeth may be unsightly and may cause orthodontic problems. It is often advisable to extract them.

Missing teeth. Missing permanent teeth are more prevalent than missing primary teeth. The tendency is believed to be hereditary.

It is very common for individual teeth to be missing. Those most likely to be missing are lateral incisors, second premolars, and third molars. When teeth are missing within a dental arch, unsightly gaps may occur. Orthodontic problems may also develop. The lack of individual third molars is usually harmless, unless the opposing molars overerupt.

Generalized lack of teeth is rare, and usually occurs only as part of *anhidrotic ectodermal dysplasia*. This hereditary disorder is chiefly characterized by the congenital absence of sweat glands (*anhidrosis*), which makes it impossible for the body to protect itself against high temperatures. In addition, there may be no teeth (*anodontia*), or only a few (*oligodontia*); those teeth that do erupt are small and cone-shaped. For functional chewing, complete dentures are usually necessary.

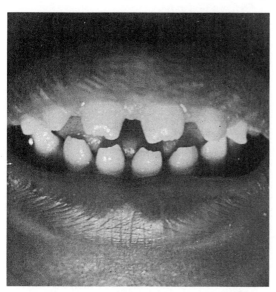

Incisors deformed by congenital syphilis
Photograph by Marie Ramer

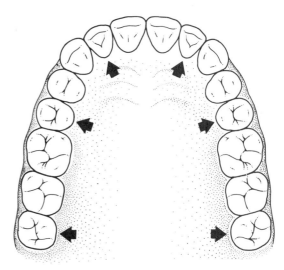

Teeth most likely to be congenitally missing from the jaws

TOOH DISCOLORATION

Tetracycline stain. The antibiotic tetracycline, in any of its several forms, can stain the body's hard tissues, including the developing teeth. Taken by a mother during late pregnancy, tetracycline can stain a baby's primary teeth. Taken by a child, up until the age of about eight, it can stain the permanent teeth (see pages 185 and 193).

The dentin becomes brown or gray, and the stain is difficult to remove. Sometimes it can only be covered up, by such procedures as bonding or veneering, or by the insertion of artificial crowns.

Stain from damaged pulp. When the pulp of a tooth is damaged, usually through inflammation or injury, blood may leak into the tubules in the dentin. Iron in the blood discolors the tooth. The gray stain can sometimes be removed by bleaching, but sometimes it must be covered up (see page 188).

Fluorosis. In some areas, the water supply has very high natural concentrations of fluorides, which can cause a mottled gray or brown discoloration of tooth enamel. This discoloration can often be removed by bleaching (see page 188).

Fluoride toothpaste, fluoride mouthwash, fluoride drops and tablets, and artificially fluoridated water have far lower concentrations of the chemical and will not cause fluorosis when properly used.

Silver amalgam stain. Over time, some of the components of the silver amalgam used for fillings may dissolve and diffuse into the surrounding enamel. The result is a dark gray stain. It can sometimes be alleviated by replacing the amalgam with gold or composite, or by covering it with bonding or a veneer (see page 193).

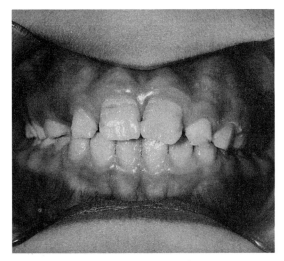

Amelogenesis imperfecta
Photograph by Barry Dale

Discolorations also occur when the tooth structure is defective, as described below.

IRREGULARITIES OF TOOTH STRUCTURE

Defects of Enamel

Amelogenesis imperfecta. The term means "imperfect enamel development." It describes a group of several hereditary conditions, of two basic types. The first, less common type causes *hypoplastic* enamel—a partial or complete lack of enamel. The second, far more prevalent type causes *hypocalcified* enamel—enamel that is deficient in the vital mineral calcium.

The effects of hypoplastic enamel vary widely in severity. They may be no worse than small pits in the enamel surface, which are somewhat susceptible to staining and decay. When severe, the enamel layer may be so thin and imperfect as to give the teeth little or no protection against wear, decay, or fracture.

When teeth with hypocalcified enamel first erupt, they may appear slightly dark in color and dull in surface luster but otherwise normal. The soft, undermineralized enamel, however, becomes darkly stained as it is exposed to food. It is also extremely susceptible to damage from wear and other trauma. The biting edges of the front teeth may become so worn down that they do not meet in chewing (*open bite*).

To protect such weakened teeth, and to improve their appearance, it is often advisable to cover them with artificial crowns soon after they erupt.

Secondary enamel hypoplasia. Diseases and injuries that occur while the teeth are developing may interfere with normal enamel development. These disorders may occur during the pregnancy of the mother, or during early childhood, especially the first year.

The following are among the more common known causes of enamel hypoplasia. In most instances, though, the exact cause is unknown.

• Diseases accompanied by high or prolonged *fever*, especially *exanthematous* (skin rash) viral diseases such as measles, chicken pox, and rubella (German measles). The damage sometimes manifests itself as a horizontal zone of reduced enamel, corresponding to the period of development when the fever occurred.

  Rubella during the first three months of pregnancy is likely to cause several birth defects in addition to defective tooth enamel. Among these may be *cleft palate* (see page 275).

• *Vitamin deficiencies*, especially deficiencies of vitamins A, C, and D. A general improvement in nutrition has made these conditions increasingly uncommon, at least among children in developed countries.

• *Congenital syphilis.* The enamel defects caused by this disorder lead to deformed teeth that look like screwdriver blades (see page 248).

• *Congenital heart disease.* Many inherited birth defects, such as *Down's syndrome* (see pages 269 and 275), include congenital heart defects among their signs. These conditions are associated with a higher than usual occurrence of faulty development of the primary teeth, and delayed eruption of the permanent teeth.

Defects of Dentin and Pulp

Dentinogenesis imperfecta. The term means "imperfect dentin development." In this hereditary condition, the dentin of both the primary and permanent teeth is much softer than normal. The tubules running through it are fewer in number and irregular in shape. Excessive secondary dentin partially or completely fills the pulp chambers and root canals.

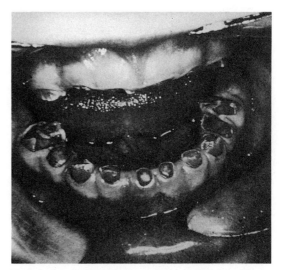

Dentinogenesis imperfecta, also called hereditary opalescent dentin *Photograph by Jeffrey Leeds*

The defective dentin causes the enamel to have a dark bluish or brownish color. The enamel is also noticeably translucent, so the condition is sometimes called *hereditary opalescent dentin*. Because of the soft dentin, the poorly supported enamel is susceptible to chipping. Unless protected, the teeth quickly wear down.

Treatment usually consists of covering the primary and then the permanent teeth with artificial crowns. If the teeth are severely worn down, they may have to be replaced with dentures.

Pulp stones (*pulp calcification*). Small calcified nodules of calcium often form, over time, in the tooth pulp. Ordinarily they are harmless, unless they become large enough to obstruct a root canal, making root canal therapy more difficult.

DISORDERS OF TOOTH ERUPTION

Natal teeth. One or more primary teeth may be present at birth. The cause is unknown. Such teeth are likely to be malformed and immature, and should usually be removed to keep them from falling out and being swallowed.

Impacted teeth. Sometimes a developing tooth, either primary or permanent, cannot erupt properly because it is *impacted* against an adjacent tooth. One cause may be a lack of space on the dental ridge for the tooth to erupt into. Sometimes, however, no cause can be identified (see page 152).

Left untreated, the unerupted tooth may contribute to drifting and malpositioning of the other teeth. Its pressure may also cause resorption of the root of the tooth it is leaning against. Orthodontic treatment may help to provide more space for eruption, and to release the impacted tooth. Occasionally, however, the tooth may have to be surgically extracted.

Ankylosed primary teeth ("submerged" teeth). Normally, as permanent teeth develop and prepare to erupt, the roots of the primary teeth over them dissolve, or *resorb*. The primary teeth then fall out, or *exfoliate*. Sometimes, however, new bone forms around a partly resorbed root, and it becomes *ankylosed*—or locked in place. The primary tooth cannot exfoliate, and the permanent tooth beneath it cannot erupt.

The adjacent permanent teeth are larger, and tend to erupt further than the ankylosed primary tooth, which then looks as if it is "submerged." It is usually extracted surgically to make way for its successor.

PHYSICAL INJURIES TO TEETH

Tooth wear. Over time, teeth are naturally subject to wear. There are three principal forms:

- *Attrition.* Chewing gradually wears down the biting surfaces. The process may be accelerated by imperfections in tooth structure or by bruxism (see below).
- *Erosion.* Acid in food may react chemically with the minerals of the teeth, partly dissolving them.
- *Abrasion.* Tooth surfaces may be ground away by external forces. The toothbrush may be too stiff or applied too vigorously. Toothpaste may be too gritty. Abrasion of individual teeth may be caused by habitually chewing on hard objects such as pipestems, pencils, toothpicks, paperclips, or hairpins.

Bruxism. Habitually clenching or grinding the teeth, which is usually provoked by stress, can both damage the teeth and lead to temporomandibular disorders. Behavioral therapy is often used to alter this response to stress.

Tooth fractures. Teeth become broken for a variety of reasons. They may be injured in accidents or by violence, or they may be broken because the chewing pressures that accompany malocclusion are unbalanced. Teeth are brittle after root canal therapy. Also, aging teeth with narrow pulps tend to be more brittle, and susceptible to fracture.

Fractured teeth can often be restored with inlays, onlays, or artificial crowns. Severely fractured teeth must sometimes be extracted and replaced with bridges or dentures.

Root resorption. The succession of primary teeth by permanent teeth is made possible by the natural resorption of the roots of the primary teeth, which causes them to exfoliate from lack of support.

The roots of permanent teeth may also resorb, a process that endangers their stability and even their survival. The cause is usually some form of external injury, such as infection in the adjacent bone, trauma, the pressure of adjacent impacted teeth (see page 252), or the growth of bone cysts or tumors (see pages 277 and 278).

Less common than external resorption is *internal* resorption. For unknown reasons, a tooth pulp may become inflamed and enlarged, which erodes the dentin around it. The erosion may be revealed as a pink-colored area on the surface (*pink tooth of Mummery*). Eventually it may reach and perforate the surface, and the tooth is often lost.

Ankylosis of permanent teeth. This condition is less common than ankylosis of primary teeth (see page 252).

Avulsed teeth. Trauma may cause one or more teeth to be completely *avulsed*—that is, knocked out of their sockets. If the teeth are immediately reimplanted, the periodontium of the sockets may recover.

DISORDERS AND IRREGULARITIES OF SOFT TISSUES

BACTERIAL INFECTIONS

The mouth contains large numbers of microorganisms—bacteria, viruses, and funguses—at all times. They can be kept in check by good home care, and the body's natural defenses ordinarily keep them from doing harm. But they cannot be completely eliminated, and under certain circumstances they may invade the tissues and cause infection.

The basic regimen of treatment is much the same for all bacterial infections, and for many other inflammatory disorders of the mouth.

- *Antibiotics.* These are the mainstay of treatment for bacterial infection. You can take them in solution—first rinsing the mouth with the solution and then swallowing it—or in tablet form. For serious or far-advanced infections, antibiotics may have to be be injected.
- *Scrupulous home care.* Daily brushing of the teeth, gums, and (especially in later life) the tongue, and flossing between the teeth are absolutely necessary. Any dentures or other restorations should be thoroughly cleaned as well to reduce the levels of bacteria and to prevent tooth decay and periodontal disease.
- *Antiseptic rinses.* These rinses also reduce the levels of bacteria, at least temporarily. If an infection is present, the dentist may prescribe a stronger rinse than any available over the counter.
- *Palliative rinses.* Mouth infections are often accompanied by inflammation and

pain. A simple rinse of warm water (one teaspoon of salt in eight ounces of water) often provides soothing relief. Your dentist may also prescribe a rinse containing an *antihistamine*, such as Benadryl, which tends to reduce inflammation.

- *Topical anesthetics*. These, applied either as rinses or ointments, relieve the pain that often accompanies infection.
- *Corticosteroids*. These relieve inflammation, and hence the pain, that accompanies infection. They must be used sparingly, however, for they actually lower the body's natural resistance to infection.

Canker sores (aphthous ulcers). These small ulcers are covered with a white or gray membrane, and ringed with a red halo. They tend to be quite painful. They may occur singly or in groups on just about any soft tissue of the mouth.

Canker sores are extremely common, and often recur, especially in certain susceptible individuals. Experts do not agree on the basic cause, but most now think it is streptococcal bacteria. However, other circumstances, such as fatigue, psychological stress, physical injury, and allergies, often trigger attacks. Canker sores are also more likely to appear in the mouths of patients with certain diseases of the intestines, such as ulcerative colitis and Crohn's disease. They affect more women than men, and often occur in the days preceding menstruation.

The sores will usually heal spontaneously after a week or two. Antibiotics can sometimes hasten the process. Palliative rinses, topical anesthetics, and corticosteroids often give at least temporary relief from pain. There is, however, no known way of preventing repeated outbreaks.

Syphilis. This sexually transmitted disease is caused by spiral-shaped bacteria called *spirochetes*, of the species *Treponema pallidum*. The lesions of syphilis often appear inside and around the mouth. There are three distinct stages: *primary*, *secondary*, and *tertiary*, and each stage produces distinctive changes in the mouth.

The signs of *primary* syphilis appear after an incubation period ranging from about one week to two months following an initial infection. The main sign is the eruption of a raised, solid, usually painless lesion called a *chancre* (pronounced "shanker"). A chancre may erupt on or near the lips, or on the tongue, palate, gums, or tonsils. In a few weeks, it spontaneously heals and disappears, but the bacteria continue to spread through the body.

Dental signs of *secondary* syphilis begin to appear about six weeks after the primary chancre has healed. Inside the mouth, the most characteristic sign is the eruption of multiple *mucous patches*, painless, grayish-white, irregularly shaped plaques on the mucous membrane. Like chancres, these plaques will spontaneously heal after a few weeks. The disease then enters a *latent* period, with no apparent symptoms.

Both primary and secondary syphilis are extremely infectious. The bacteria are heavily concentrated in the chancre and mucous patches, and can easily be transmitted through breaks in the skin. A dentist treating patients with this disease must take special precautions to avoid being infected.

Tertiary syphilis can appear years later. Soft, rubbery tumors called *gummas* are likely to appear in and around the mouth—especially on the palate. Within these gummas, the tissue dies and sloughs off, leaving hollow, "punched out" ulcers.

In addition, tertiary syphilis often causes the upper surface of the tongue to atrophy, leaving it "bald" and sore—a condition called *glossitis* (see page 267).

Syphilis can be easily treated with an antibiotic such as penicillin but only in its primary and secondary stages. Early diagnosis and treatment are crucial.

Congenital syphilis may be transmitted by an infected mother to the fetus during pregnancy. Its effects include malformations of the teeth (see page 248).

Tuberculosis. Among the symptoms of this chronic disease may be painful, ulcerated lesions inside the mouth, especially on the tongue. Tuberculosis is treated with a variety of antibacterial medications such as isoniazid and rifampin.

Cellulitis. A painful swelling of the soft tissues of the face, often accompanied by fever, cellulitis results from the spread of infection

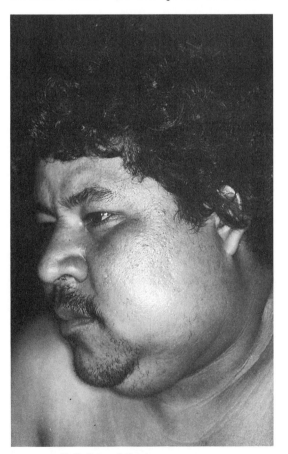

Cellulitis of the jaw
Photograph by Daniel Buchbinder

by staphylococcal and streptococcal bacteria. The bacteria produce enzymes that break down cells and stimulate the formation of pus. The buildup of pus makes the tissues swell, which in turn causes pain.

The infection often occurs when severe decay produces an abscess at the root of a tooth, and bacteria enter the the soft tissues from the bone. It can also result from severe periodontal disease, pericoronitis around a partly erupted third molar, extraction of a tooth, or a jaw fracture.

An especially severe form of cellulitis, *Ludwig's angina*, occurs when the floor of the mouth becomes infected. The swelling pushes the tongue upward and makes swallowing difficult. It may then advance to the throat, and even threaten death by suffocation.

Cellulitis, like other bacterial infections, is usually treated with antibiotics. Local pus pockets may be surgically drained (see page 159).

Actinomycosis. This is a chronic infection caused by common mouth bacteria (*Actinomyces*). Like cellulitis, it often enters the jaw bones and soft tissues through severely decayed or damaged teeth.

The most common symptom is known informally as "lumpy jaw," in which there are one or more knots of swollen tissue under the lower jawbone. Pus-containing abscesses form in these inflamed areas, and often develop channels, or *fistulas*, to the surface, through which the pus drains. Repeated formation of fistulas may cause extensive scarring of the skin.

Actinomycosis is treated with long-term, high-dose antibiotics, can be difficult to eliminate completely, and often recurs.

Sinusitis and other *intracranial infections.* Bacterial infection in the upper jaw, the maxilla, may spread into the cavities that form the *maxillary sinuses.* These may then become infected and inflamed, a condition known as *sinusitis*. Infection may also penetrate other parts of the skull, or *cranium*, and inflame parts of the brain, such as the *meninges*, to cause meningitis.

These infections are serious and potentially life-threatening. Ordinarily they can be controlled by antibiotics, if they are caught early enough.

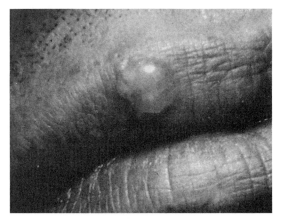

Herpes simplex blister on lip
Photograph by Marie Ramer

VIRAL INFECTIONS

Viral infections differ from bacterial infections in one important respect: they don't respond to antibiotics. If antibiotics are prescribed, it is only to prevent a secondary infection by bacteria.

Some viral infections can be prevented by building up the body's own immune defenses against them, through immunization. Diseases routinely prevented in this way include measles, rubella (German measles), and mumps.

In recent years, *antiviral* medications such as *acyclovir* have shown promise in fighting some viral infections.

Herpes simplex (cold sores: fever blisters). This extremely common infection of the lips and mouth is usually caused by *herpes virus type 1* (herpes virus type 2 causes the sexually transmitted disease *genital herpes*). There are two stages, *primary* and *recurrent*.

Primary herpes simplex results from the first infection by the virus. Because the virus is very contagious, this infection usually takes place before adulthood in a large proportion of the population.

In most people, the primary infection causes no symptoms, or symptoms that are confused with those of some other disorders (such as a cold or flu). Some patients, however, develop *primary herpetic stomatitis*. The gums become inflamed and swollen, and fluid-filled blisters form on the lips and other

soft tissues of the mouth. These blisters often rupture, leaving painful ulcers. In about two weeks, the symptoms spontaneously disappear.

Healing, however, may not be complete. Many infected people will continue to harbor the virus in nearby nerve fibers, and will be susceptible to recurrent attacks.

Recurrent herpes simplex has similar but generally less severe symptoms. The blisters and subsequent ulcers tend to be smaller, and may not be painful. They appear most frequently on the lips, gums, and palate. Healing takes place after about a week.

Recurrent outbreaks are apparently triggered by other conditions. Among the most common are other infections—thus, herpes lesions are commonly called *cold sores* or *fever blisters*. Attacks may also be set off by sunlight, allergies, fatigue, or emotional stress. Among women, they tend to occur more often during menstruation or pregnancy.

There is no cure for either primary or recurrent herpes infection. Antibiotics are not effective, except to prevent secondary infections by bacteria. The antiviral medication acyclovir is sometimes helpful, especially if it is used at the beginning of an attack. Pain may be alleviated by topical anesthetics.

Chickenpox and *shingles*. These two diseases are caused by the same virus: *herpes varicella-zoster (V-z)*.

Chickenpox (*varicella*) is a common, relatively mild *exanthem* (skin-rash disease), which usually occurs in childhood. Sometimes the rash blisters appear inside the mouth, as well as on the skin. Ordinarily, the rash causes no more than moderate discomfort, and heals within two weeks.

The virus, however, may survive in sensory nerve fibers. It is likely to be dormant for many years. It may then cause an outbreak of shingles (*zoster*). Shingles can provoke severe, burning pain, accompanied by a localized rash, and can last two weeks or more. When the virus infects the *trigeminal* nerve of the face, shingles may occur on just one side of the face or inside the mouth.

Shingles is more prevalent and more severe in older people. A single outbreak usually makes the person immune. However, the attack may be followed by *post-herpetic neuralgia*, which causes persistent, disabling pain.

The pain of shingles may be relieved by corticosteroids, and recovery can sometimes be hastened with the antiviral drug acyclovir. There is no cure for the infection itself.

FUNGAL INFECTIONS

Fungi, like bacteria and viruses, occur naturally in the mouth. They are normally kept in check, not only by the body's natural defenses and by regular oral hygiene but also by competition with mouth bacteria. Under certain circumstances, however, fungi may proliferate out of control, overwhelming the natural defenses and causing infections.

Paradoxically, fungal infections often occur following treatment for bacterial infections. When an antibiotic, for instance, sharply reduces the number of bacteria, the fungi, freed from competition, reproduce in great numbers.

Fungal infections are also a common consequence of conditions that weaken the body's immune system. These include other diseases, such as AIDS, and cancer treatment with radiation and chemotherapy (see page 261).

Fungal infections are combated with specific *antifungal* medications, such as *nystatin*, *amphotericin B*, and *miconazole*. Supplements of vitamin B_2 (riboflavin), which build up the body's resistance, can also be helpful.

Candidiasis (moniliasis, oral thrush). This most common of all the fungal infections is caused by the abnormal proliferation of the yeast *Candida albicans*. It is especially prevalent among the very young, the elderly, and patients debilitated by other illnesses.

The main symptom is a creamy, slightly raised plaque, which can appear on any moist surface inside or around the mouth. The plaque is made up of extended yeast colonies; beneath the surface the tissues are red, raw, and painful.

Candidiasis often attacks the tongue, causing burning pain (*glossitis*) and difficulty in

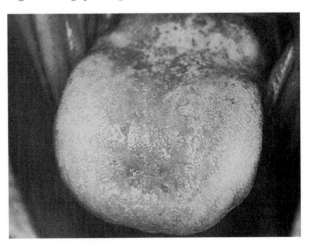

Candidiasis (oral thrush)
Photograph by Marie Ramer

swallowing. The sensation of taste may be diminished or distorted.

Successful treatment must often begin with control of the conditions that have triggered the outbreak. Good hygiene is essential. The infection is combated directly with antifungal medications.

OTHER ERUPTIVE DISORDERS

Fordyce's granules. These small, pale, yellowish granular eruptions may occur individually or in a plaque, usually on the lining of the cheeks. They are believed to be congenital, although they sometimes don't appear until adolescence or adulthood. They are harmless and require no care.

Erythema multiforme. The name of this disease means "many-formed reddening." The main symptoms are skin eruptions, which can take several different forms. Especially common is a red-ringed blister resembling the bullseye of a target. When the disease is especially severe, and inflames the eyes and the genitals, it is called *Stevens–Johnson syndrome.*

The disease often affects the lips and mouth. Blisters form, and then break down into open ulcers that bleed readily. Eating and drinking may be painful. Excessive salivation may cause uncontrollable drooling.

The basic cause is unknown. But the symptoms often appear to be triggered by some other condition. Among younger patients, this is likely to be a disease—especially herpes simplex infection (see page 256). Among adults, the triggering circumstance is more likely to be an allergy, radiation treatment, or a reaction to medication.

The pain of the mouth sores usually can be alleviated with a topical anesthetic. The inflammation can also be treated with a corticosteroid.

Lichen planus. This disorder of the skin is seen especially often inside the mouth. The cause is unknown, but outbreaks often appear to be triggered by emotional stress.

The disease takes two main forms. In the less serious form, small, pale pimples erupt inside the mouth, and become interconnected in a white, lacy network that somewhat resembles a lichen on a rock. These eruptions are usually painless.

The disease also has a more severe, *erosive* form, in which the affected surface is eroded by painful, ragged ulcers. Discomfort may be relieved with a topical anesthetic, and the inflammation reduced with a corticosteroid. There is no permanent cure, and the condition may recur. Furthermore, there is some evidence that in rare instances erosive lichen planus may lead to oral cancer (see page 260).

Leukoplakia. The term means "white plaque." An area on the mucous membranes of the mouth forms a thickened, hardened, whitish patch.

Leukoplakia is believed to result from repeated, chronic irritation. The irritation may be mechanical, such as the pressure of an ill-fitting denture or habitual chewing of the cheek lining. Or it may be chemical; nicotine is the chief offender. A common form of leukoplakia, occurring on the roof of the mouth, is called *smoker's palate* or *nicotine stomatitis.*

Leukoplakia usually isn't painful. The basic treatment is to remove the irritation that causes it. A denture may be refitted to eliminate "high spots," or the patient may stop using tobacco in any form.

Persistent leukoplakia should be checked by *biopsy* (see pages 260–261). About five percent of the plaques eventually become malignant (cancerous).

Erythroplakia. This reddish eruption, which may occur on any of the mucous membranes of the mouth, is no longer believed to be a separate disorder. Instead, it is identified as an early stage of *squamous cell carcinoma*, the most common form of oral cancer (see page 261).

Autoimmune Disorders

Certain eruptive disorders are thought to be caused by an *autoimmune* ("self-immune") reaction. The immune system for reasons that are not well understood, produces antibodies that attack the body's own cells as if they were outside invaders. Autoimmune diseases particularly attack connective tissue, including the subsurface layers of the skin and mouth.

The inflammation seen in these disorders is usually treated with corticosteroids, and often with antibiotics as well, to reduce the risk of secondary infection.

Pemphigus and *bullous pemphigoid*. Although these are classified as skin diseases, they often occur first, or only, in the mouth. They occur mainly among older patients. Both have similar symptoms: the eruption of fluid-filled blisters, or *bullae*, which rupture to produce open, painful, foul-smelling ulcers. Bullous pemphigoid is the less serious of the two—the blisters are less apt to rupture, and they heal faster.

Both disorders are treated with corticosteriods. Foe pemphigus, immunosuppressant drugs are sometimes prescribed as well.

Lupus erythematosus. The most typical symptom of this skin disease is a red, patchy rash that forms a symmetrical, butterfly-shaped pattern across the face. There are two types: one effects only the skin, and the other (*systemic* lupus erythematosus) affects many of the connective tissues of the body.

The skin rash is often accompanied by lesions in the mouth. They usually consist of a hollow area of atrophied tissue, surrounded by a thickened, hardened margin. They may bleed and are often painful.

Scleroderma. The name means "hardened skin," and the main symptom is a stiffening of the subsurface layers of the skin. Other connective tissues may also be involved. Stiffening in the throat may produce a choking sensation. The tongue may become hard and boardlike, making it difficult to speak and swallow. Tissues around the temporomandibular joints of the jaws may become stiff, as may the lips and surrounding skin, so the mouth cannot be opened fully.

The stiffening is caused by excessive concentrations of *collagen* (a protein component of cells) in the tissues. The basic cause is unknown, but an autoimmune reaction may be involved.

The severity of the disorder varies considerably. A mild form affects only limited areas of the skin. A severe form, *systemic sclerosis*, affects many body systems. There is no completely satisfactory treatment. Mild scleroderma often clears up spontaneously. Corticosteroids sometimes give at least partial relief.

BENIGN TUMORS

Tumors are tissue growths, or *neoplasms*. They are classified as *benign*, relatively innocuous, or *malignant*, cancerous. Benign tumors may be difficult to distinguish from malignant ones, and benign tumors may sometimes become malignant. It is therefore advisable to do a *biopsy* on all such growths (see pages 260–261).

Papilloma. This raised, light-colored tumor with a pebbly surface can develop on any of the soft tissues inside the mouth. It is very similar to a wart on the skin, and may sometimes be caused, as warts often are, by a virus.

Papillomas are painless and generally harmless but may be irritatingly intrusive and unattractive. They can be removed surgically but may recur.

Pigmented cellular nevus (pigmented mole). Moles may appear on the soft tissues inside the mouth, just as they do on the skin. They are thought to be hereditary, although they sometimes don't appear until years after birth. Pigmented moles contain a concentration of cells with the dark pigment *melanin*, and may be brown, black, or blue.

Pigmented moles sometimes turn into malignant *melanomas* (see page 262), or they may be merely unattractive. They can be removed surgically.

Fibroma. This common tumor inside the mouth consists of fibrous tissue with a smooth surface. Its cause is unknown. If it is intrusive or unsightly, it can be surgically removed.

Hemangioma. A red or bluish tumor in which blood vessels have proliferated, a hemangi-

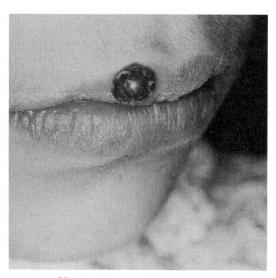

Hemangioma on lip
Photograph by Daniel Buchbinder

oma is usually congenital; it corresponds to a "strawberry" birthmark on the skin. Sometimes, for unknown reasons, it appears later in life. It tends to occur on the lips, tongue, palate, or the lining of the cheeks.

Congenital hemangiomas sometimes disappear spontaneously. If they are intrusive or unsightly, they can usually be removed by a variety of means, including surgery, radiation, medications, or localized freezing.

MALIGNANT TUMORS

Malignant tumors of the mouth (oral cancer) increase with advancing years. More than 90 percent occur after the age of 45. About 30,000 new cases are diagnosed each year, and each year approximately one third of this number prove fatal.

The causes are not completely known. Malignant tumors are especially common among smokers, former smokers, and heavy drinkers.

There are two main kinds of malignant tumor, *carcinoma* and *sarcoma*. Most oral cancers are carcinomas—tumors that arise in the soft tissue closest to body surfaces, such as the outermost layers of the skin, and the epithelial linings of the mouth. Sarcomas arise mainly in bone and muscle tissue (see page 280).

Cancer is most likely to become life-threatening when it *metastasizes*—when cancer cells migrate from the original site and generate tumors in other parts of the body. Oral cancer usually metastasizes by way of the lymph vessels in the head and neck. Conversely, cancer in other parts of the body may metastasize to the mouth, causing tumors there.

All cancers are composed of abnormal cells that reproduce out of control. Often these cells are distinguishable from normal cells only when observed under a microscope. Hence, the diagnosis of cancer is usually based upon a *biopsy*. A small portion of the suspected tissue is collected, from which a number of thin slices are cut, mounted on glass slides, stained, and then examined microscopically.

The success rate of treatment has increased markedly in recent years, especially in patients that have been diagnosed early. There are three main forms of treatment, used alone or in combination: surgery, radiation, and chemotherapy.

Surgery is used to remove tumors at a relatively early stage, before they have metastasized. The object is complete elimination of all cancer cells. If this is accomplished, the chances for recovery are good.

Surgery may require the removal of so much tissue as to be disfiguring. Plastic surgery can sometimes alleviate such disfigurement.

Radiation damages all living cells, but is more harmful to rapidly proliferating cancer cells than to normal cells. It is often used when the cancer is not well enough defined for surgical removal. Early diagnosis greatly increases the chance of success.

Radiation levels that are high enough to kill cancer cells are also likely to damage the surrounding normal tissue. Following treatment of oral cancer, the lining of the mouth, the *oral mucosa*, often becomes inflamed, a condition called *radiation mucositis*. Radiation also reduces resistance to infection, making the mouth more susceptible to attack by bacteria, viruses, and fungi.

When the mouth is irradiated, the salivary glands, which are particularly sensitive to radiation, may also be damaged, and their function may be affected. The reduced production of saliva produces *xerostomia* ("dry mouth"), with several harmful consequences (see page 273).

One of the most severe aftereffects of radiation is an infection of the jawbones, *osteomyelitis* (see page 276).

Chemotherapy is a systemic treatment, used to attack cancer cells that have metastasized from their original site, or to "mop up" cells of a localized tumor that might have been missed by surgery or radiation. It is also used as the sole treatment for certain types of cancer. Chemotherapy employs *cytotoxic* ("cell-poisoning") drugs that act on rapidly reproducing cancer cells. These drugs may be used singly or in combination.

Cytotoxic drugs affect normal cells to some extent, and may produce undesirable side effects, such as nausea, hair loss, and destruction of the blood-forming cells in the bone marrow. Like radiation, they decrease resistance to infections such as herpes simplex and candidiasis.

Because successful treatment depends upon early diagnosis, and because early malignancies are often hard to distinguish from benign tumors and certain mouth sores, your dentist should examine your mouth during your regular dental checkup. If you have a persistent lesion, your dentist may remove a small piece of tissue, under local anesthesia, for biopsy, or may refer you to an oral surgeon or an oral pathologist for diagnosis.

Squamous cell carcinoma. About 90 percent of oral cancer is of this type. The malignant tumor arises in the flattened *squamous* ("scaly")

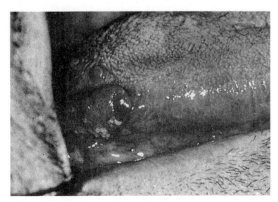

Squamous cell carcinoma on tongue
Photograph by Marie Ramer

cells that form the *epithelium* inside the mouth. The most common site is the tongue, but any of the other soft tissues may be involved, including the lips.

The causes aren't precisely known, but there is a strong association with smoking, heavy drinking, and (on the lips) ultraviolet radiation from sunlight. Squamous cell carcinoma is likely to metastasize, and thus is one of the more dangerous forms of oral cancer.

Malignant melanoma (melanocarcinoma). This is primarily a cancer of the skin, which occasionally occurs in the mouth. Ultraviolet rays from the sun are thought to be a major cause. The cancer arises in cells that contain the dark pigment *melanin,* and may begin as a benign-looking *pigmented mole* (see page 260). The malignant cells reproduce rapidly and often metastasize. Fortunately, malignant melanoma is relatively uncommon inside the mouth. But if you have a dark spot or mole on your skin that persists, becomes larger, or changes color, you should seek professional help.

Basal cell carcinoma. See the discussion of lip disorders, pages 264 and 266.

Kaposi's sarcoma. This used to be a relatively uncommon tumor, occurring mainly in later life among men in certain ethnic groups. However, a severe form of it is now a common symptom of AIDS, which suggests that one of its causes is suppression of the immune system.

The tumors arise in the underlying layers of the skin. They often appear in several places at once, including the soft tissues of the mouth. They are irregularly shaped and contain many small blood vessels, giving them a deep red, brown, or purple color; they also bleed readily.

The tumors are treated with surgery, lasers, and chemotherapy, but since they are often multiple, complete removal is difficult.

BLOOD DISORDERS

Several disorders of the blood cells affect the mouth. The most prevalent symptoms are mouth ulcers, susceptibility to infection, and excessive bleeding, particularly from the gums. These conditions are discussed with disorders that mainly affect the gums (see page 269).

PHYSICAL INJURIES

Physical injuries to the soft tissue of the mouth are caused either by a single episode of trauma, from an accident or by violence, or by repeated irritation. Common sources of such irritation include ill-fitting dentures and other restorations, malposed teeth, harmful habits such as chewing on the lips or cheeks, and new or badly fitting orthodontic appliances.

Traumatic ulcers. These sores may result either from a single injury, such as accidentally biting the tongue, or from repeated irritation. In the mouth, they easily become infected, especially by bacteria, and they are treated much like canker sores (see page 254).

Papillary hyperplasia. An inflammatory overgrowth (*hyperplasia*) of the tissue on the palate, this condition tends to occur under a full upper denture, especially one that does not fit firmly or that is constantly left in the mouth.

Careful, regular cleaning, both of the mouth and the denture, helps prevent this condition, and is also the chief treatment, along with refitting the denture. Sometimes excess tissue must be surgically removed.

Radiation damage. See the discussion of oral cancer, page 261.

Electrical Burns. This type of injury occurs almost exclusively in small children. They have a natural tendency to put things in their mouths and chew them. Unfortunately, it is not uncommon for them to chew through electrical cords until they reach the bare wires, which causes a short circuit and severely burns their mouths.

Electrical injuries are treated like other burns. The damage tends to heal slowly and may be permanently disfiguring.

Cervical–Facial emphysema. During dental treatment—especially oral surgery—air may be injected into the connective tissue, causing swelling in the face or neck. The swelling will usually subside spontaneously in a week. The condition needs to be carefully observed, however. In rare instances, the air may produce a dangerous blood clot in a blood vessel, or the tissues may become infected.

CHEMICAL INJURIES

Aspirin burn. Aspirin is an effective analgesic when taken internally. But sometimes people place it directly on an aching tooth or a mouth sore to relieve pain. Aspirin is a strong acid and can severely burn soft issues, causing a

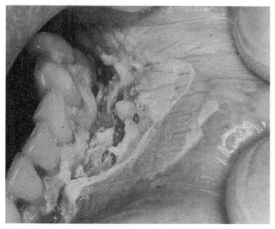

Aspirin burn
Photograph by Marie Ramer

painful, slow-healing wound. It should never be used in this way.

Amalgam tattoo. When teeth that contain silver amalgam fillings are extracted, bits of the fillings often break off, and may remain in the empty socket. When the bone and gums heal, the silver may become visible as dark, gray, or blue spots on the gum surface. The condition is harmless and requires no treatment.

Allergies

Many people are hypersensitive to certain chemicals and other substances. These substances, called *allergens* or *antigens*, provoke the body's immune system to react. Allergic reactions produce such symptoms as headaches, skin eruptions (*eczema* and *hives*), localized swelling (*angioedema*), asthmatic attacks, and hay fever. In some instances, an allergic reaction may produce *anaphylactic shock*, a dangerous condition in which the blood pressure drops too low to maintain body functions.

Allergies are thought to be at least partly hereditary, since they tend to run in families. Allergic reactions within the mouth, however, are relatively uncommon.

Contact Stomatitis. Some individuals are hypersensitive to physical contact with materials used in dental care. Typical allergens include the following:

- Specific metals, such as the nickel in alloys for dental restorations. A few individuals are allergic to the mercury used in silver amalgam restorations, but this is rare.
- Acrylic, a plastic used for dentures, orthodontic retainers, and other restorations. The allergic reaction usually will not occur if the plastic has been properly cured, before it is inserted into the mouth.

- Certain flavoring agents, such as cinnamon oil—used in cleaning agents, mouthwashes, and impression materials—can act as allergens.
- The topical anesthetic procaine, and the local anesthetics injected during treatment, may elicit an allergic response in some people.

Contact stomatitis is best treated by removal and replacement, if possible, of the offending allergen. The inflammatory symptoms are treated much like those of mouth infections (see page 253).

Medication allergies. Much more prevalent than contact stomatitis are allergies to specific drugs. Perhaps the best known of these is the allergy of some individuals to the antibiotic penicillin, but many other types of drugs are known allergens as well.

The reaction to such allergens may include mouth inflammation, or *stomatitis.* In rare instances, the reaction may cause anaphylactic shock (see page 263).

**DISORDERS OF THE FACIAL
NERVES AND MUSCLES**

Trigeminal nerve neuralgia (tic douloureux). The *trigeminal* nerves are the pair of cranial nerves serving most of the face, including the jaws. In trigeminal neuralgia, attacks produce severe, stabbing pain, each lasting seconds or minutes. Usually only one of the pair of nerves is affected, so the pain occurs on just one side of the face. The pain is sometimes accompanied by muscle spasms, from which comes the French name *tic douloureux.* Attacks are often touched off simply by touching some sensitive area, or *trigger zone,* on the skin.

The disorder has no known cause, and is more likely to occur in later years. It is now often treated with *anticonvulsant* drugs such as *carbamezapine (Tegretol),* which are mainly used against epilepsy.

Glossopharyngeal neuralgia. This disorder of the *glossopharyngeal* nerves, which innervate the tongue and throat, produces attacks of severe, sharp pain like those of trigeminal neuralgia, but starting at the base of the tongue and radiating back into the throat. Like trigeminal neuralgia, it usually occurs on only one side, and occurs most often among older people. It, too, is treated with carbamezapine.

Bell's palsy. A disorder of one of the facial nerves, which control the facial muscles. It causes a temporary or permanent paralysis of one side of the face. There is no cure, nor is there any satisfactory treatment for the symptoms, but the condition often goes away spontaneously.

DISORDERS MAINLY AFFECTING THE LIPS

Double lip. This harmless deformity is sometimes congenital, sometimes caused by trauma. A layer of excess tissue, resembling a second lip, forms inside the normal lip. It occurs most often within the upper lip and is usually not visible when the mouth is closed. If the double lip detracts from the person's appearance, it can be surgically removed.

Cleft lip (harelip). This fairly common congenital defect of the upper lip is often accompanied by a separate but closely related defect, *cleft palate* (see page 275).

The cleft arises during prenatal development. It appears along a vertical line from the lip to the nostril, usually on just one side but sometimes on both. It may extend either part or all the way to the nostril. The causes are not known and are probably multiple. The condition tends to run in families, and to occur more frequently in specific ethnic groups, so heredity is probably a factor. But environmental influences during pregnancy may also play a part.

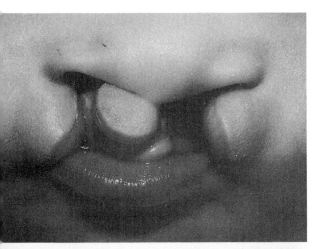

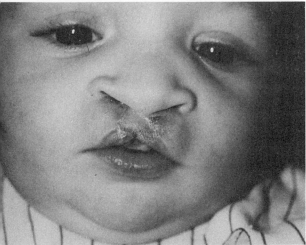

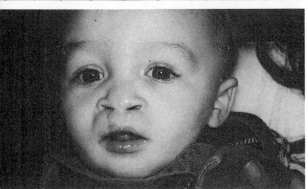

Bilateral cleft lip and cleft palate: before surgery, at four weeks; shortly after surgery, at six months; and at eight months
Photographs by Daniel Buchbinder and Alan Gibbs

By itself, cleft lip is harmless (compared with cleft palate, which can cause difficulties in eating and speaking). It is, however, disfiguring. The cleft is usually closed by plastic surgery a few weeks after birth; further cosmetic surgery may also be needed.

Peutz–Jeghers syndrome (intestinal polyposis syndrome). This main symptom of this hereditary disorder is the growth of small tumors, or *polyps*, inside the intestines. It is also characterized by small dark spots on the skin, especially on and around the lips. The pigmented spots are harmless but may be unsightly.

This condition is closely related to another hereditary disorder, *Gardner's syndrome*, but the oral symptoms are quite different (see page 279).

Angular cheilitis. This inflammation of the corners of the mouth is especially common in later life. It is associated with several underlying conditions, but experts disagree over which of these might be the primary cause:

- *Mechanical irritation.* In later years, loss or wear of the teeth often causes reduction of *vertical dimension* in the bite. The lips overlap more at the corners, and tend to leak saliva. Continuous chafing, plus repeated wetting and drying, irritate the tissues. Attempts to relieve the irritation provoke habitual lip-licking (*perleche*), which, in fact, makes the condition worse.
- *Infection.* The inflamed areas are often found to be infected by the fungus *Candida albicans*. These may be a primary cause of inflammation, or they may more readily invade areas that are already inflamed.
- *Vitamin deficiency.* Vitamin deficiencies, particularly of riboflavin (vitamin B_2), are often associated with angular cheilitis.

The reason may be that the deficiency reduces resistance to infection.

The treatment of angular cheilitis addresses all these conditions. Loss of vertical dimension is corrected with dentures and other restorative dentistry. Infections are combated with antifungal and antibacterial drugs. Nutritional deficiencies are corrected by improved diet and vitamin supplements.

Angioedema (angioneurotic edema). An inflammatory disorder that causes swelling (*edema*) of various body tissues, particularly the lips.

Some forms of the disorder may be hereditary, or the disorder may be provoked by allergies, but in most cases the cause is unknown. The symptoms are successfully treated with antihistamines, sometimes supplemented with corticosteroids, but there is no permanent treatment that will prevent recurrent attacks.

Basal Cell Carcinoma. This form of cancer is very common on the skin of the face, and sometimes appears on the lips. It rarely occurs inside the mouth. It arises in the *basal* cells of the epithelium.

Because this form of cancer occurs so often on the faces of people who spend much time outdoors, ultraviolet radiation from the sun is thought to be a major cause. The tumor grows slowly and seldom metastasizes to other parts of the body, so it is considered far less dangerous than other carcinomas.

DISORDERS MAINLY AFFECTING THE TONGUE

Hairy tongue. This condition tends to occur in later life. The hairlike *filiform papillae* become longer and darker. The causes are unknown and probably multiple. Irritation from tobacco may be a factor.

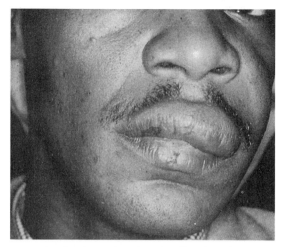

Angioedema (angioneurotic edema)
Photograph by Marie Ramer

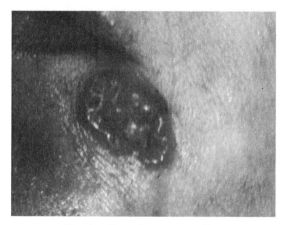

Basal cell carcinoma near lip
Photograph by Marie Ramer

The condition is unsightly but essentially harmless. However, the "hairy" surface is more likely to harbor bacteria and fungi that may cause infection. Brushing the tongue when brushing the teeth is advisable.

Fissured tongue. The tongue surface is normally criss-crossed with a network of shallow furrows, or *fissures*. In later life, some of these fissures may become deeper and more evident. The condition is essentially harmless;

however, irritating food debris may become trapped in the fissures. Brushing the tongue is helpful as a preventive measure.

Sublingual varicosities. On the underside of the tongue, the blood vessels are close to the surface and readily visible. In later life, they may be *varicose*, becoming swollen and prominent. The condition itself is generally harmless.

Ankyloglossia (tongue-tie). A thin, elastic *frenum* (from a word meaning "sail") of muscle tissue connects the underside of the tongue with the floor of the mouth. The frenum may be congenitally short and connected close to the front of the tongue. As a result, the tongue is at least partly "tied" to the floor. Since a freely moving tongue is essential for speech, the frenum may have to be surgically clipped.

Conditions Causing Glossitis

The term *glossitis* means "tongue inflammation." Glossitis is a symptom caused by a wide variety of conditions, including such serious diseases as syphilis. A few of these conditions are painless and harmless, but others cause great discomfort.

The upper surface of the tongue normally contains many cells with thin, hairlike protrusions, called *filiform papillae*. Collectively they give the surface a soft, velvety texture and a pale color. But if the tongue becomes inflamed, some or all of the papillae may atrophy and disappear. The surface looks slick and "bald," and may be more highly colored—bright or purplish red. In addition, the whole tongue may be painful—sore or burning—and swallowing may be difficult.

Median rhomboid glossitis. This is a condition in which an oval or diamond-shaped (*rhomboid*)

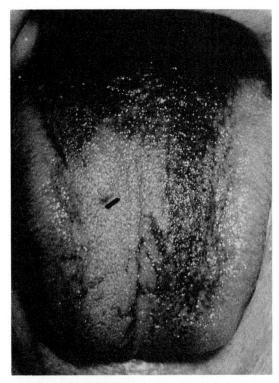

Hairy tongue
Photograph by Marie Ramer

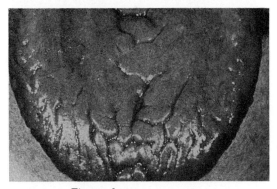

Fissured tongue
Photograph by Marie Ramer

area in the middle of the upper surface lacks filiform papillae. The area is noticeably redder and shinier, but it only appears to be inflamed. The condition is in fact harmless and requires no treatment.

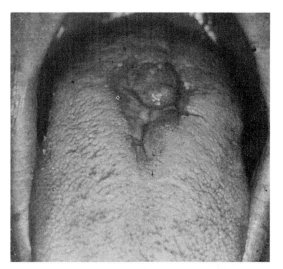

Median rhomboid glossitis
Photograph by Marie Ramer

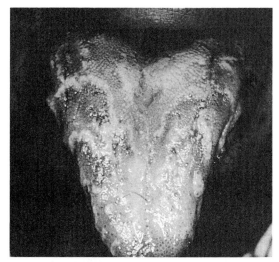

Migratory glossitis (geographic tongue)
Photograph by Marie Ramer

Migratory glossitis (geographic tongue). For no known reason, the filiform papillae in one or more areas of the surface may temporarily break down, revealing irregular red, "bald" patches of the underlying tissue. The edges of these areas are often white or yellowish, and suggest the outlines of a map—hence the name *geographic* tongue. The patches rapidly heal and are succeeded by others in different locations, creating the illusion that they are "migrating" over the surface. Though the condition looks like an inflammation, it is generally harmless.

Candidiasis. This fungal disease often causes inflammation of the tongue (see page 257).

Nutritional deficiency disorders. The lack of sufficient vitamins and minerals in the diet may produce symptoms in the mouth—glossitis, in particular.

Nutritional deficiencies may result simply from poor diet, especially in older people. One common cause, however, is alcoholism, which interferes with the digestion of food.

The principal treatment is correction of the deficiency.

Among the most common nutrients involved are the following:

- *B-complex vitamins.* The B-complex vitamins include *riboflavin* (B_2) and *niacin* (nicotinic acid, nicotinamide). A lack of these vitamins is also believed to contribute to *angular cheilitis* (see page 265).
- *Folic acid.* Deficiency of this vitamin is very common. In addition to poor diet or alcoholism, causes may include the use of medications such as *methotrexate* (used against cancer), *phenytoin* (used to prevent epileptic attacks), and oral contraceptives. Patients undergoing dialysis treatment for kidney disease are also likely to be deficient.

  The deficiency produces *folic acid anemia*, of which glossitis is a common symptom.
- *Vitamin B_{12} (cobalamin).* Deficiency of this vitamin, as of other B-complex vitamins, often causes glossitis. But the deficiency itself is usually caused, not by improper

diet but rather by an *autoimmune* reaction (see page 259). This may produce a serious blood disease, *pernicious anemia*, of which tongue inflammation is a symptom.

- *Iron.* Lack of sufficient iron produces *iron-deficiency anemia*, of which glossitis is a symptom. The deficiency may result from insufficient iron in the diet, particularly among children, pregnant women, and older people. It may also be caused by loss of blood. It is relatively common among women with heavy menstrual bleeding, and people suffering ulcerating diseases of the digestive tract such as stomach ulcers, colon cancer, and hemorrhoids.

  Iron-deficiency anemia is often accompanied by angular cheilitis (see page 265). An especially severe form is called *Plummer–Vinson syndrome.* An obstruction in the throat makes swallowing difficult, and the fingernails become smaller and spoon-shaped. Plummer–Vinson syndrome is also associated with a predisposition to the development of oral cancer.

Conditions Causing Tongue Enlargement (*Macroglossia*)

Lymphangioma. This benign tumor contains a concentration of lymph vessels. It occurs most frequently on the tongue, often causing it to become considerably enlarged. The condition is usually considered to be congenital, and becomes evident early in life. It can be treated surgically.

Down syndrome. A common characteristic of this hereditary condition is an enlarged tongue. The enlargement may be so great as to keep the mouth from closing fully, which, in turn, may contribute to the gum inflammation and periodontal disease that are also typical of this syndrome.

Neurofibroma (von Recklinghausen's Disease). In this hereditary disorder, tumors form in nerve tissue. They often appear on the skin, either as multiple lumps or large, irregular masses. They also sometimes occur in the mouth, especially on the tongue, where they produce a generalized enlargement.

There is no satisfactory treatment. Individual tumors can sometimes be removed surgically, but they are usually too numerous or too extensive to be completely eliminated.

Conditions Causing Taste Loss or Distortion

Many disorders may alter the sensation of taste, either temporarily or permanently. The sensation may be lost entirely, or it may be distorted by unpleasant "phantom" tastes. The following are among the most common of these conditions:

- *Infections.* One example is the viral infection hepatitis, which produces a characteristic bitter taste in the mouth. The common fungal infection candidiasis (see page 257) often affects the tongue, causing both taste loss and taste distortion.
- *Xerostomia (dry mouth).* Food that is not wet can't be tasted. Many disorders of the salivary glands (see page 273) reduce or stop the generation of saliva, making the mouth dry.
- *Medications.* Many kinds of drugs cause or contribute to xerostomia (see list, page 231). Drugs that affect the parasympathetic nervous system, such as antihistamines and antidepressants, may cause taste loss as well. In addition, certain drugs leave unpleasant aftertastes.

DISORDERS MAINLY AFFECTING THE GUMS

Conditions Causing Gum Inflammation

Gum inflammation, or *gingivitis*, results mainly from infection by bacteria, viruses, or fungi. Endocrine disorders and hormone changes also appear to play a role. Gingivitis is treated much like other mouth infections (see page 253).

Acute necrotizing ulcerative gingivitis; desquamative gingivitis; juvenile periodontosis. These three inflammatory diseases of the gums are discussed in detail in Chapter 9.

Herpetic gingivostomatitis. Infection with herpes simplex virus 1 can affect any of the soft tissues in the mouth (see page 256), but inflammation of the gums is especially common.

Diabetes mellitus. The general debilitation produced by this disease greatly reduces the body's resistance to infection. Among the tissues likely to be infected are the gums, which may become severely inflamed, oozing pus and bleeding. Diabetes has no cure, but it can be controlled through diet or insulin (taken by mouth, or injected, or both). Stabilizing the patient helps reduce gum inflammation.

Pericoronitis. This inflammatory infection occurs most frequently in the gums around third molars ("wisdom teeth"), when they fail to erupt completely, usually because they are impacted against adjacent teeth. Bacteria easily work their way into the soft tissue around a partly erupted tooth (see illustration, page 152).

The infection can be combated with antibiotics, and the inflammation relieved by standard methods (see page 152). The best long-range remedy, however, is extraction of the tooth.

Female hormonal changes. Most women are likely to suffer gingivitis at certain times of their lives, when sex hormone levels significantly change. These times are puberty, menstruation, pregnancy, and menopause. In addition, gingivitis is more prevalent among women taking oral contraceptives.

Benign Tumors of the Gums

Certain tumors, which appear as localized growths or swellings, occur either exclusively or predominantly on the gums.

Dental lamina cyst of the newborn (Epstein's pearls). Small, pale nodules sometimes appear on the ridges of the jaws of newborn children, where teeth will later erupt. They are enclosed hollows, or *cysts*, that form from tissues that also generate teeth. They are harmless, and soon disappear.

Congenital epulis. This benign tumor may appear on the gums of newborn children. It occurs more often on the upper jaw, and in girls. The cause is unknown. The growth can be removed surgically.

Pyogenic granuloma. A granuloma is a benign (noncancerous) growth that forms as a response to chronic inflammation. Pyogenic granulomas usually occur on the gums, particularly on the raised triangles of gum tissue between the teeth. They may occasionally appear on other soft tissue of the mouth as well. They grow quickly from a narrow, stalklike base, and then stabilize in size. They can be red, brown, or purple. They bleed easily because of the many small blood vessels they contain.

Pyogenic granulomas are believed to result from mechanical trauma, such as a blow or scratch, followed by bacterial infection. They can affect anyone, but they are especially prevalent among pregnant women; thus, they are called *pregnancy tumors*.

Sometimes these growths will shrink and disappear by themselves. Surgical removal, however, is often advisable. They sometimes reappear after surgery, or because of continued inflammation. To avoid recurrence, it is important to keep the adjacent teeth clean and free of calculus.

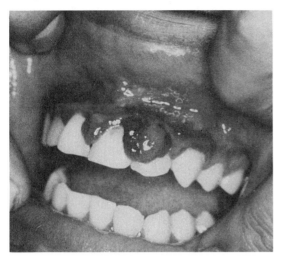

Pyogenic granuloma
Photograph by Marie Ramer

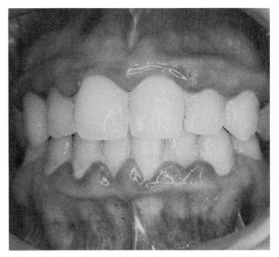

Inflammatory hyperplasia, from severe gingivitis
Photograph by Marie Ramer

Gingival Hyperplasia

Hyperplasia is the generalized overgrowth of tissue through proliferation of its cells. Several conditions cause hyperplasia of the gums. Alleviation of the underlying causes, when possible, is the most effective treatment. The overgrown tissue can sometimes be surgically removed. The inflammatory symptoms that often accompany hyperplasia are treated in much the same way as those of mouth infections (see page 253).

Inflammatory hyperplasia. Inflammation from infections and other disorders may cause the gums to become red, swollen, and tender, and to bleed readily. Periodontal disease is the most common cause. Inflammatory disorders that cause gingivitis may produce hyperplasia as well. Other disorders include the following:

- *Vitamin C deficiency.* The severe lack of vitamin C causes *scurvy*, which was widespread but now, happily, is rare. Even a less severe deficiency, however, can produce inflammation of the gums.
- *Leukemia.* This cancer of white blood cells

(see page 272) may cause the gums to become swollen and tender, and to bleed spontaneously.

Fibrous hyperplasia. Unlike inflammatory hyperplasia, the tissue of *fibrous* hyperplasia is firm and resilient because its cells are rich in the protein *collagen*.

Such overgrown tissues are not tender and do not bleed readily, but they may be unsightly and interfere with normal function. Treatment is correction of the underlying cause, but surgical removal of the hyperplastic tissue is sometimes advisable. These tissues include:

- *Epulis fissuratum.* The most common cause of this fibrous inflammatory hyperplasia is repeated mechanical irritation; the most common irritant is a chafing, ill-fitting denture. Epulis (the term means "upon the gums") tends to occur where the edges of a denture rub against the outer gum.
- *Phenytoin (Dilantin) reaction.* The most widely used drug to prevent seizures in epilepsy is *phenytoin* (trade name *Dilan-*

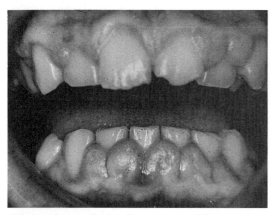

Fibrous hyperplasia of gum, caused by reaction to phenytoin (Dilantin)
Photograph by Marie Ramer

tin). It often produces fibrous hyperplasia as a side effect. Careful oral hygiene sometimes delays or reduces the reaction, and the excess tissue can be removed surgically. Recurrence is likely, however, unless the drug is discontinued or replaced by another.

Bleeding Disorders

Several diseases of the blood cause excessive or prolonged bleeding. In the mouth, such bleeding occurs most often from the gums. Treatment must be directed at the underlying cause.

Aplastic anemia. Many blood cells, including the red blood cells, are produced in the bone marrow. Aplastic anemia results when the marrow fails to form enough of these cells (*aplastic* means "not forming").

About half the cases have no known cause; the other half of the cases appear to result from exposure to radiation or certain chemicals or drugs.

In the mouth, the main symptoms are spontaneous bleeding—especially from the gums—and mouth lesions from infections.

Mouth lesions are treated like other infections (see page 253). The anemia can sometimes be alleviated by blood transfusions.

Hemophilia. In this hereditary condition, the blood lacks a necessary protein, known as a *clotting factor*, that enables it to coagulate. If a blood vessel is damaged, bleeding may be excessive, even life-threatening. The disorder has several forms; the most common is *sex-linked* and affects only males.

Bleeding from the gums and other soft tissues of the mouth may result from even slight trauma. Oral surgery, such as tooth extraction, can be dangerous. In recent years, the risks of hemophiliac bleeding have been considerably reduced, through periodic injections of the missing clotting factor.

Polycythemia. This is also a group of disorders. Here, the proportion of red blood cells is too high, compared with the other components of the blood. There are two main forms:

- Polycythemia *vera* ("true" polycythemia). The bone marrow produces excessive red blood cells for no known reason. Hemoglobin concentration also increases.
- *Secondary* polycythemia. The overproduction of red blood cells here may be due to reduced oxygen intake, from lung disease, heart disease, or high altitude.

The oral symptoms are similar for all forms of the disorder. The high concentration of red blood cells discolor the soft tissues of the mouth, particularly the gums, a dark red or purple, and cause them to bleed readily.

Treatment of polycythemia depends on the form. Secondary polycythemia is treated by correcting the underlying causes. There is no complete cure for polycythemia vera, but it is sometimes relieved by periodically drawing blood from the system and avoiding foods with a high iron content. Radioactive phosphorus is sometimes administered to decrease red blood cell production.

Leukemia. This group of disorders is generally classified as "cancer of the blood." The tissues that produce white blood cells (*leukocytes*), either in the bone marrow or in the lymph system, produce abnormal white blood cells in large numbers, which invade and damage many body organs. Resistance to infection diminishes sharply.

The causes of leukemia are unknown and are probably multiple. Among the factors that may be involved are hereditary predisposition, exposure to radiation, and reaction to certain drugs and chemicals.

Oral symptoms may occur in most forms of leukemia. These include inflamed and swollen gums that bleed easily. Some symptoms are the result not only of the disease itself, but of the radiation and anticancer drugs used to treat it. They are treated in the same ways as mouth infections (see page 253) to make the patient more comfortable and to prevent secondary infection.

The leukemias are very serious diseases, and used to be uniformly fatal. Recent advances in radiation treatment and chemotherapy have greatly improved chances of recovery, or at least temporary remission, especially for the forms that occur in young people.

Thrombocytopenia. Thrombocytes, or *platelets*, are specialized blood cells that aid in the clotting of blood (*thrombos* means "clot"). In thrombocytopenia, the number of platelets is greatly reduced. *Primary* thrombocytopenia is thought to be hereditary. *Secondary* thrombocytopenia appears to be a reaction to radiation or to medications, especially those used in cancer chemotherapy.

Thrombocytopenia is often accompanied by a weakening of the small blood vessels, or capillaries, and a leakage of blood into the surrounding tissue. This is often manifested as *purpura*, or "purpling"—the appearance of red spots, which later darken, on the skin.

Thrombocytopenia tends to produce prolonged bleeding from the gums, due to the low number of platelets. It may also produce spots or patches of purpura on the gums and other soft tissue surfaces of the mouth.

The oral symptoms, though irritating and sometimes alarming, usually require no specific care. The main treatment of the disorder is treatment of the underlying cause, if possible.

DISORDERS OF THE SALIVARY GLANDS

Disorders of the salivary glands can affect the mouth generally, when insufficient saliva is generated.

Xerostomia. "Dry mouth," resulting from insufficient saliva, is a symptom rather than a specific disorder. It has several harmful effects:

- Drying irritates the soft tissues in the mouth, often making them inflamed and painful, and more susceptible to infection.
- Tooth decay and periodontal disease become much more prevalent and severe when the cleansing, antiseptic, and buffering effects of saliva are lost.
- Drying and the lack of antiseptic protection also contribute to bad breath (halitosis).
- Prosthetic dentures, especially *full* dentures, are less stable when there is no thin film of saliva to help them adhere properly.
- The sensation of taste is altered or diminished, and swallowing may become more difficult.

Xerostomia is especially prevalent in later years, and may be part of the natural aging process. Many authorities believe, however, that common disorders of old age, and the methods used to treat them, are more responsible. Among the common causes of xerostomia are the following:

- *Medications.* Many experts consider side effects of drugs to be the most important cause. More than 400 medications have mouth dryness as a potential side effect (see table, pages 231–233).
- *Radiation.* Oral cancer (see page 261) is often treated with X-rays. Radiation penetrates the salivary glands and stops their function, at least temporarily.
- *Dehydration.* Many systemic diseases cause an excessive loss of water from the body. These include diabetes (see page 270) and blood disorders such as leukemia (see page 273) and pernicious anemia (see page 269).
- *Sjögren's Syndrome.* This is now thought to be an *autoimmune* disease (see page 259). It particularly affects the salivary glands and decreases their secretions.

Xerostomia can sometimes be alleviated by increasing the fluid intake or by sucking on sugarless fruit lozenges to stimulate the salivary glands. *Artificial* saliva is especially helpful to denture wearers. Thorough home care is crucial in minimizing decay, periodontal disease, and other oral infection.

Sialolithiasis (Salivary gland stone). Hard, stone-like accumulations of calcium compounds may form in the salivary glands or in the ducts leading to the mouth. Such a stone is especially troublesome if it blocks a duct. When the gland is stimulated by food to produce saliva, the flow is stopped by the obstruction. The fluid builds up pressure in the gland, making it swollen and painful. Salivary stones must usually be removed by surgery.

Mumps. This highly contagious viral infection causes the *parotid* salivary glands to become swollen and painful. Because it is so easily transmitted, it is usually caught in childhood. Immunization is effective, so mumps is becoming increasingly rare.

Tumors. Salivary gland tumors, like tumors elsewhere in the mouth, may be either benign or malignant. Most develop in the parotid glands, causing them to swell. But they may occur in other major glands or in minor glands in the lining of the mouth. Treatment is usually surgical. For malignant tumors, radiation therapy may be used after surgery to make sure no malignant cells survive.

Mucous retention cyst (mucocele). In addition to the three pairs of major salivary glands, there are many small *secondary* or *accessory* glands in the lining of the mouth. Sometimes the duct from such a gland may become severed, usually as the result of minor trauma. The trapped saliva is retained in a hollow pocket, or cyst, which on the surface looks like a blister.

Mucoceles occur most frequently on the lower lip. It is often advisable to remove them surgically.

Sometimes a mucocele forms in one of the major glands under the floor of the mouth, causing it to swell. This type is called a *ranula* (literally "little frog").

DISORDERS OF BONE

DISORDERS OF HEREDITY AND DEVELOPMENT

A number of conditions—some clearly hereditary, others that apparently arise during fetal development—produce malformations of the face, including the jaws. Some are too severe to be corrected, but others can be successfully treated with surgery.

Cleft palate. This fairly common congenital defect of the roof of the mouth often accompanies a separate but closely related defect, *cleft lip* (see page 264).

The cleft originates during prenatal development, along the central line of the palate. Sometimes it involves only the boneless soft palate, but it may divide the bones of the hard palate as well. In more severe instances, the cleft then deviates slightly to one side or the other, and crosses the ridge of the upper jaw. There it may continue as a cleft lip (see illustration, page 265).

The causes of cleft palate are not known and are probably multiple. The condition tends to run in families, and it occurs more frequently in specific ethnic groups, so heredity is probably a factor. But environmental influences during pregnancy may also play a part.

Unlike a cleft lip, which is merely unsightly, a cleft palate can cause significant functional problems, especially if the hard palate and dental ridge are involved. Eating and swallowing may be difficult, and food may spill out of the mouth and into the nose. During infancy, a special nursing bottle and nipple may be needed. Later on, speech is likely to be impaired, since the pronunciation of several sounds depends on the spatial relationship of the tongue with the upper teeth and hard palate. A cleft extending across the upper dental ridge will almost certainly disturb the development and placement of the teeth, so that malocclusion results.

The condition can sometimes be remedied with a special orthodontic device inserted soon after birth, which gently but steadily presses the divided parts of the palate together. A series of such appliances may be required as the jaws grow, until the parts of

the palate meet and form a natural suture.

Otherwise, the basic form of treatment for cleft palate, as for cleft lip, is surgery. Lip surgery is usually performed first, soon after birth, by a plastic surgeon. Palate surgery is performed within a few years, by either a plastic surgeon or an oral surgeon. Malocclusion is treated, starting in later childhood, with orthodontics, restorative dentistry, or both.

Thalassemia (Cooley's anemia). In this serious hereditary disorder of the blood, the bone marrow cannot produce enough normal red blood cells. The disorder occurs mainly in ethnic groups from around the Mediterranean Sea and in the Middle East.

The disorder also may cause the bones of the upper jaw, the maxilla, to grow more than the mandible. The resulting mismatch in jaw sizes may cause a severe *overjet* (see below). Orthodontic treatment is sometimes helpful.

Micrognathia ("small jaw"). The lower jaw, or *mandible*, is much smaller than the upper jaw, (*maxilla*), creating a severe *overjet* (see page 160). This condition is sometimes part of a hereditary syndrome, such as *Pierre–Robin syndrome* or *Treacher–Collins syndrome*.

Prognathism ("forward jaw"). Either the mandible is relatively overdeveloped, or the maxilla is underdeveloped. In either case, the mandible is significantly longer than the maxilla. The lower front teeth close in a *crossbite* in front of the uppers, a *class III malocclusion* (see page 160).

Prognathism, by itself, is a fairly common hereditary variation. It may also be one of the elements of a hereditary syndrome, such as *achondroplastic dwarfism, Down syndrome, cleidocranial dysostosis (Marie–Sainton syndrome),* and *craniofacial dysostosis (Crouzon's disease).*

Facial asymmetry. Slight differences in proportion or form between the sides of the face are normal. Greater differences are likely to be disfiguring, and may cause functional difficulties such as *lateral crossbites* (see page 165).

The asymmetry may result from faulty development of a single bone. The condyle of the mandible, for example, may not be fully developed on one side. Or the defect may be generalized, as in *Goldenhar syndrome* and *hemifacial microsomia*.

DISORDERS OF BONE GROWTH

Fibrous Dysplasia of Bone. Dysplasia means "malformation." This disorder, of unknown cause, makes its appearance in childhood, and usually subsides after puberty. It may occur in a single bone or several bones. A soft form of bone replaces some of the normal bone, which increases in size. The disorder often occurs in the jaws, making them bulge outward.

There is no cure. Surgical "shaving" is sometimes effective in correcting cosmetic deformities.

Paget's Disease (Osteitis Deformans). The Latin name for this disorder means "deforming inflammation of bone." It appears in later life; the cause is unknown, though it may run in families. The principal symptom is abnormal growth of the bones, including the skull. The cranium becomes bigger, and the jawbones grow thicker and wider. The teeth, particularly in the upper jaw, tend to splay outward, and gaps appear between them. The cementum on their roots often becomes abnormally thick (*hypercementosis*).

There is no cure for this disorder. Soreness is treated with analgesics such as aspirin, and with nonsteroidal anti-inflammatory drugs. A synthetic form of the thyroid hormone *calcitonin* may slow the abnormal growth process.

DISORDERS CAUSING BONE LOSS

The primary cause of bone erosion or resorption is inflammation, usually the result of infection or trauma or both. Almost any severe infection of the mouth may affect the bones of the jaw. The most common causes of such infection are tooth decay and periodontal disease.

Osteomyelitis. This serious infection of the bone and bone marrow is usually bacterial in origin. It may follow an injury to the soft tissue, or a tooth extraction or jaw fracture. It is often very painful and persistent, and can seriously erode the bone. The infection may also involve adjacent soft tissue, causing *cellulitis* (see page 255).

The risk of osteomyelitis rises sharply following radiation treatment of the face for cancer. Radiation impairs the circulation and damages the immune system that protects the body against infection. Tooth extraction after radiation of the jaws is especially dangerous. Thus, damaged or decayed teeth are often removed *before* radiation treatment.

Since osteomyelitis is usually a bacterial infection, it is treated with antibiotics. Abscesses in the bone may be surgically opened and drained (see page 158).

CALCIUM DEFICIENCY DISORDERS

Calcium is one of the chief minerals of bone, giving it strength and solidity. Several conditions cause a deficiency of calcium, either in the body as a whole or specifically in the bones. Either way, the mineral structure of the bone tissue is adversely affected. The bones of the jaws are often involved.

Osteoporosis. In the body of the healthy adult, new bone constantly forms, old bone simultaneously dissolves, and the two processes are approximately in balance. With osteoporosis, old bone breaks down faster than new bone forms, apparently because of a lack of calcium. The mineral framework of the tissue becomes thinner and more fragile. The bones are more brittle, and their surfaces are more subject to erosion.

The underlying causes of osteoporosis are not known, and are probably multiple. The following are considered to be either possible causes or contributing factors:

- *Deficiency of calcium in the diet.* The modern adult diet tends to be low in calcium. Calcium supplements can be taken, but they are not always successful in preventing or reversing osteoporosis.
- *Prolonged inactivity and lack of exercise.* Both are at least contributing factors.
- Disorders of the *endocrine glands*, such as *hyperadrenocorticism (Cushing's disease)*.
- *Corticosteroids*, used to treat inflammatory diseases such as rheumatoid arthritis. These medications appear to stimulate, if not cause, osteoporosis.
- *Aging.* Osteoporosis occurs so often among older people, particularly older women, that it is now believed to be one of the natural consequences of aging.
- Osteoporosis often affects the jaws, especially *edentulous* jaws, from which the teeth have been lost. The natural process of *alveolar bone resorption* is accelerated. Dentures become harder to insert firmly and to wear comfortably, and lose their fit more rapidly.

Osteoporosis is treated with calcium supplements, along with vitamin D, or with a synthetic form of *calcitonin*, a hormone produced by the thyroid glands. Among women past menopause, adding the female hormone *estrogen* to this regimen sometimes appears to prevent or minimize the disorder.

Hyperparathyroidism. The four small parathyroid glands produce a hormone that controls the utilization of calcium in the body. Under certain circumstances, such as a tumor on a gland, too much hormone is produced, which causes the bones to lose calcium; this calcium is subsequently excreted from the body.

This disorder often affects the jaws, and a dentist may be the first to diagnose it. In addition to a general demineralization of the bone, similar to osteoporosis, *giant cell granulomas* (see page 278) may form near the roots of the teeth, depriving them of support and allowing them to drift out of position.

Dental splints (see page 130) may help stabilize drifting teeth. The main treatment of the disorder is surgical removal of any tumor or removal of a portion of the glands themselves.

Vitamin D deficiency. Vitamin D affects the ability of the digestive system to absorb calcium. Thus, vitamin D deficiency leads to a deficiency in calcium as well. In infancy and childhood, vitamin D deficiency causes *rickets*, in which the developing bones become fragile and deformed. Modern diet has made this disease rare, at least in developed countries.

In later life, vitamin D deficiency may be caused by disorders such as kidney disease (*chronic renal failure*) or by medications such as the *anticonvulsants* used to treat epilepsy. The result may be *osteomalacia*, or *adult rickets*, which can affect the jaws. The defective, demineralized bone is susceptible to fracture, and may also cause the teeth to loosen.

Dietary vitamin D deficiency is easily treated with an improved diet or a supplement. If the deficiency results from disease or medications, the underlying cause must be treated as well.

CYSTS

Cysts are hollow sacs, usually filled with fluid, that may form in soft tissue or in bone.

They have a wide variety of causes, ranging from heredity to infection. Cysts in the bones of the jaws may make them especially susceptible to fracture, or may cause teeth to be displaced or lost.

The standard treatment is surgical removal (see page 159). Prosthetic dentistry may also be needed to replace missing teeth, and orthodontics to realign teeth that have been displaced. Since cysts may be the precursors of malignant tumors (cancer), they should be *biopsied* (see pages 260–261).

Relatively common forms of cysts include the following:

Primordial cyst. This type of cyst, the result of faulty tooth development, occurs fairly early in life. The tooth—either primary or permanent—fails to develop, and forms a cyst instead.

Dentigerous cyst. A dentigerous, or "tooth-making," cyst occurs late in the development of a permanent tooth, when the crown has fully formed but has not yet erupted. For unknown reasons, a cyst may form in the adjacent bone, usually between the tooth and the surface of the dental ridge.

A dentigerous cyst may cause a more serious disorder if it arises near an impacted tooth, such as a third molar, that cannot erupt properly (see page 252). The cyst may become very large, seriously weakening the bone. Or it may develop into a tumor called an *ameloblastoma* (see page 279).

Apical periodontal cyst. Severe tooth decay and pulp inflammation often produce a pus-filled *abscess* at the apex of the root (see page 63), or they may produce an *apical cyst* in the adjoining bone. Such a cyst may remain following extraction of the tooth; it is then called a *residual cyst.*

Basal cell nevus syndrome. This hereditary condition has a wide variety of symptoms, among which are multiple *basal cell carcinomas* on the skin (see page 266). Recurring cysts in either or both jaws, are also common.

Developmental cysts at fissural boundaries. During the prenatal development of the jaws, the bones on each side join and fuse to form a single maxilla and a single mandible. Sometimes this fusion is not complete, and a cyst forms along the central *fissure.* Such cysts occur most frequently in the roof of the mouth. If they are small and benign, they sometimes do not require surgery.

BENIGN TUMORS

Tumors occur in bone, just as they do in soft tissue (see page 259), and may be either benign or malignant. Even benign tumors can displace or loosen the teeth or deform the jaws. They may also eventually become malignant. It is therefore usually advisable to have them surgically removed (see page 159), which also encourages the regrowth of normal bone tissue. In any event, they should be biopsied to determine if they are malignant.

Central giant cell granuloma. This benign tumor mainly affects children and young adults, and twice as many girls as boys. The fibrous tumor contains a high proportion of *giant cells,* with multiple nucleuses.

Aneurysmal bone cyst. Despite the name, this is thought to be a tumor rather than a cyst. Like giant cell granuloma, it affects mainly young people. The basic cause is believed to be a reaction to trauma. The tumor is mostly fibrous cells in a loose framework, and has many blood vessels so that it bleeds readily if cut during surgery.

Osteoma. This benign tumor consists of proliferating, tightly concentrated *bone* cells. It may enlarge and deform the jaw bones.

The cause of most osteomas, as of other tumors, is unknown. They are a characteristic symptom, however, of a hereditary condition called *Gardner's syndrome* which mainly affects the intestines, but which can also cause multiple tooth impactions of the teeth (see page 252).

Torus palatinus, torus mandibularis, and multiple Exostoses. These are all bony outgrowths (*exostoses*) from the surfaces of the jaws or palate. Torus palatinus is a "bulge" of bone that grows from the center of the palate. Torus mandibularis arises inside one or both sides of the lower jaw. Multiple exostoses are small knobs of bone that grow in rows on the surface of the upper jaw, just above the gumline.

These growths are fairly common. Torus palatinus, in particular, is very common, occurring in about one in four Americans. All forms are generally thought to be hereditary. They are ordinarily harmless, and usually are left untreated. But if the teeth are lost, and a

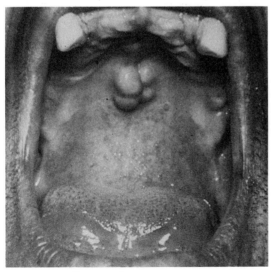

Torus palatinus
Photograph by Barry Dale

complete denture must be fitted, such intrusive growths may have to be removed.

Odontogenic Tumors

A number of tumors of the jaw have their origins from the same kinds of cells that also develop into teeth and periodontal tissues. Thus, they are adjacent to the tooth roots. Known as *odontogenic* ("tooth-generated") tumors, they tend to appear during adulthood. Like other tumors and cysts of the jaws, they can loosen and displace the teeth, and deform the jaws, so they are generally removed surgically. The following are a few of the more common:

Ameloblastoma. This fairly common jaw tumor develops from the cells that produce the enamel layer in a tooth. The tumor itself, however, is soft and fibrous. It often appears under the back molars of the lower jaw—particularly the third molars, or "wisdom teeth." It may become invasive and destructive, or even malignant, and should be carefully and thoroughly removed so as to avoid recurrence.

Periapical cemental dysplasia (cementoma). This benign tumor apparently grows from cells that generate the layer of cementum on the tooth root. Cementomas tend to occur in groups near the roots of the lower incisors, and are more prevalent among women than men.

Cementomas differ from other tumors in at least two important respects. First, they simply replace bone tissue with fibrous tissue so that the jaw usually is not enlarged. Second, their fibrous tissue is nearly as dense and strong as bone itself, so that the teeth do not become loose or displaced. Such tumors, therefore, are usually not treated.

Odontoma. This odontogenic tumor contains fully formed but structurally unorganized tooth tissues. Odontomas usually resemble small, malformed, unerupted teeth. They appear when the permanent teeth are developing and may interfere with the normal pattern of eruption. Odontomas may also grow large enough to deform the jaw.

MALIGNANT (CANCEROUS) TUMORS

Malignant tumors of jaw bones are much less common than those of soft tissues. Individual cancers, such as *round cell sarcoma, chondrosarcoma, osteosarcoma,* and *reticulum cell sarcoma,* take their names from the cells in which they originate. With few exceptions, bone tumors are treated surgically, not with radiation therapy or chemotherapy.

Multiple myeloma. In this common cancer of the bones, certain white blood cells, called *plasma cells,* in the bone marrow become malignant. These cells are ordinarily involved in the immune reaction that protects the body against infection. The malignant cells tend to appear and proliferate in several different bones at the same time, causing hollow, cyst-like erosions, which are often accompanied by swelling and pain. Anemia and increased susceptibility to infection are also important symptoms.

These bone lesions often appear in the jaws, and may be the first sign of the disease. In addition to swelling, pain, and susceptibility to fracture, the lesions may cause the teeth to loosen and drift. The pain and inflammation are treated with analgesics and anti-inflammatory drugs. Radiation therapy and chemotherapy are also used to improve the quality of life, but the disease is invariably fatal.

APPENDIX: DENTAL SCHOOLS AND PROFESSIONAL ORGANIZATIONS

DENTAL SCHOOLS

ALABAMA

School of Dentistry
University of Alabama
1919 Seventh Avenue South
Birmingham, AL 35294

CALIFORNIA

School of Dentistry
University of the Pacific
2155 Webster Street
San Francisco, CA 94115

School of Dentistry
University of California, San Francisco
513 Parnassus Avenue, S630
San Francisco, CA 94143

School of Dentistry
University of California, Los Angeles
53-038 Center for Health Sciences
Los Angeles, CA 90024

School of Dentistry
University of Southern California
University Park-MC 0641
Los Angeles, CA 90089-0641

School of Dentistry
Loma Linda University
Loma Linda, CA 92350

COLORADO

School of Dentistry
University of Colorado Medical Center
4200 East Ninth Avenue, Box C-284
Denver, CO 80262

CONNECTICUT

School of Dentistry
University of Connecticut
263 Farmington Avenue
Farmington, CT 06032

DISTRICT OF COLUMBIA

College of Dentistry
Howard University
600 "W" Street, N.W.
Washington, DC 20059

FLORIDA

College of Dentistry
University of Florida
Box J405, JHMHC
Gainesville, FL 32610

GEORGIA

School of Dentistry
Medical College of Georgia
1459 Laney Walker Boulevard
Augusta, GA 30912-0200

ILLINOIS

School of Dentistry
Loyola University of Chicago
2160 South First Avenue
Maywood, IL 60153

Northwestern University Dental School
240 East Huron Street
Chicago, IL 60611

School of Dental Medicine
Southern Illinois University
2800 College Avenue
Alton, IL 62002

College of Dentistry
University of Illinois
801 South Paulina Street, Room 102–801
Chicago, IL 60612

INDIANA

School of Dentistry
Indiana University
1121 West Michigan Street
Indianapolis, IN 46202

IOWA

College of Dentistry
The University of Iowa
Dental Building
Iowa City, IA 52242

KENTUCKY

College of Dentistry
University of Kentucky
800 Rose Street
Lexington, KY 40536-0084

School of Dentistry
University of Louisville
Health Sciences Center
Louisville, KY 40292

LOUISIANA

School of Dentistry
Louisiana State University
1100 Florida Avenue
New Orleans, LA 70119

MARYLAND

Baltimore College of Dental Surgery
University of Maryland
666 West Baltimore Street
Baltimore, MD 21201

MASSACHUSETTS

School of Dental Medicine
Harvard University
188 Longwood Avenue
Boston, MA 02115

School of Graduate Dentistry
Boston University
100 East Newton Street
Boston, MA 02118

School of Dental Medicine
Tufts University
One Kneeland Street
Boston, MA 02111

MICHIGAN

School of Dentistry
University of Detroit
2985 East Jefferson Avenue
Detroit, MI 48207

School of Dentistry
The University of Michigan
1234 Dental Building
Ann Arbor, MI 48109-1078

MINNESOTA

School of Dentistry
University of Minnesota
515 Delaware Street, S.E.
Minneapolis, MN 55455

MISSISSIPPI

School of Dentistry
University of Mississippi
2500 North Street Street
Jackson, MS 39216-4505

MISSOURI

School of Dentistry
University of Missouri
650 East 25th Street
Kansas City, MO 64108

NEBRASKA

School of Dentistry
Creighton University
2500 California Street
Omaha, NE 68178

College of Dentristy
University of Nebraska Medical Center
40th and Holdrege Streets
Lincoln, NE 68583-0740

NEW JERSEY

New Jersey Dental School
University of Medicine and Dentistry
110 Bergen Street
Newark, NJ 07103-2425

NEW YORK

School of Dental and Oral Surgery
Columbia University
630 West 168th Street
New York, NY 10032

College of Dentistry
New York University
345 East 24th Street
New York, NY 10010

School of Dental Medicine
State University of New York
Rockland Hall–Health Science Center
Stony Brook, NY 11794-8700

School of Dentistry
State University of New York
325 Squire–3435 Main Street
Buffalo, NY 14214

NORTH CAROLINA

School of Dentistry
University of North Carolina
Chapel Hill, NC 27514

OHIO

College of Dentistry
Ohio State University
305 West 12th Avenue
Columbus, OH 43210

School of Dentistry
Case Western Reserve University
2123 Abington Road
Cleveland, OH 44106

OKLAHOMA

School of Dentistry
University of Oklahoma
Health Sciences Center
P.O. Box 26901
Oklahoma City, OK 73190

OREGON

School of Dentistry–Sam Jackson Park
Oregon Health Sciences University
611 Southwest Campus Drive
Portland, OR 97201

PROFESSIONAL ORGANIZATIONS

GENERAL DENTISTRY

American Dental Association
211 East Chicago Avenue
Chicago, Illinois 60611

Academy of General Dentistry
211 East Chicago Avenue
Chicago, Illinois 60611

PERIODONTICS

American Academy of Periodontology
211 East Chicago Avenue
Chicago, Illinois, 60611

PEDIATRIC DENTISTRY

American Academy of Pediatric Dentistry
211 East Chicago Avenue
Chicago, Illinois, 60611

GERIATRIC DENTISTRY

Federation of Special Care Organizations
American Society of Geriatric Dentistry
211 East Chicago Avenue
Chicago, Illinois, 60611

ENDODONTICS

American Association of Endodontists
211 East Chicago Avenue
Chicago, Illinois, 60611

PROSTHODONTICS

Federation of Prosthodontic Organizations
211 East Chicago Avenue
Chicago, Illinois, 60611

ORAL AND MAXILLOFACIAL SURGERY

American Association of Oral and
Maxillofacial Surgery
9700 Bryn Mawr Avenue
Rosemont, Illinois 60018

ORTHODONTICS

American Association of Orthodontists
460 North Lindbergh
St. Louis, Missouri, 63141

TEMPOROMANDIBULAR DISORDERS

American Academy of Craniomandibular
Disorders
10 Joplin Court
Lafayette, California 94549

American Equilibration Society
8726 North Ferris Avenue
Morton Grove, Illinois 60053

DENTISTRY FOR THE MEDICALLY COMPROMISED

American Association of Hospital Dentists
211 East Chicago Avenue
Chicago, Illinois, 60611

Academy of Dentistry for the Handicapped
211 East Chicago Avenue
Chicago, Illinois, 60611

INDEX

Page numbers in *italics* refer to illustrations.